AAOS

Calculations for Medication Administration

Paramedic

Andrew N. Pollak, MD, FAAOS
Series Editor
Medical Director, Baltimore County
Fire Department
Associate Professor
University of Maryland School of Medicine
Baltimore, Maryland

Mithriel Salmon, BS, MT (ASCP),
NREMT-P, LP
LPMH and Associates
University of Texas Medical Branch,
Education Lab Training Specialist
Texas A&M University Galveston
San Antonio, Texas

David S. Pomerantz,
NREMT-B, EMT-P
Deerfield Beach, Florida

JONES AND BARTLETT PUBLISHERS

Sudbury, Massachusetts

BOSTON   TORONTO   LONDON   SINGAPORE

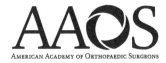

AMERICAN ACADEMY OF ORTHOPAEDIC SURGEONS

World Headquarters

Jones and Bartlett Publishers
40 Tall Pine Drive
Sudbury, MA 01776
978-443-5000
info@jbpub.com
www.jbpub.com

Jones and Bartlett Publishers Canada
6339 Ormindale Way
Mississauga, Ontario L5V 1J2
Canada

Jones and Bartlett Publishers International
Barb House, Barb Mews
London W6 7PA
United Kingdom

Jones and Bartlett's books and products are available through most bookstores and online booksellers. To contact Jones and Bartlett Publishers directly, call 800-832-0034, fax 978-443-8000, or visit our website www.jbpub.com.

Substantial discounts on bulk quantities of Jones and Bartlett's publications are available to corporations, professional associations, and other qualified organizations. For details and specific discount information, contact the special sales department at Jones and Bartlett via the above contact information or send an email to specialsales@jbpub.com.

This textbook is intended solely as a guide to the appropriate procedures to be employed when rendering emergency care to the sick and injured. It is not intended as a statement of the standards of care required in any particular situation, because circumstances and the patient's physical condition can vary widely from one emergency to another. Nor is it intended that this textbook shall in any way advise emergency personnel concerning legal authority to perform the activities or procedures discussed. Such local determination should be made only with the aid of legal counsel.

Production Credits

Chief Executive Officer: Clayton Jones
Chief Operating Officer: Don W. Jones, Jr.
President, Higher Education and Professional Publishing: Robert W. Holland, Jr.
V.P., Sales and Marketing: William J. Kane
V.P., Design and Production: Anne Spencer
V.P., Manufacturing and Inventory Control: Therese Connell
Publisher—Public Safety Group: Kimberly Brophy
Acquisitions Editor—EMS: Christine Emerton
Managing Editor—Public Safety: Carol B. Guerrero
Associate Editor: Amanda Brandt
Senior Production Editor: Karen C. Ferreira

Composition: Shepherd, Inc.
Text Design: Anne Spencer
Cover Design: Kristin E. Ohlin
Photo Research Manager and Photographer: Kimberly Potvin
Cover Image: © Mark C. Ide
Interior Photos: 4–1A, 4–1B, 4–2 Courtesy and © Becton, Dickinson and Company; 4–3 © aaaah/ShutterStock, Inc.
  Unless otherwise indicated, all photographs and illustrations are under copyright of Jones and Bartlett Publishers.
Printing and Binding: Malloy, Inc.
Cover Printing: Courier Stoughton

Library of Congress Cataloging-in-Publication Data
Salmon, Mithriel.
  Paramedic : calculations for medication administration / Mithriel Salmon, David S. Pomerantz.
    p. cm.
  Includes index.
  ISBN 978-0-7637-4683-4
  1. Medicine—Mathematics. 2. Emergency medical technicians. I. Pomerantz, David S. II. Title.
  R853.M3S23 2009
  616.02'5—dc22
                      2008022764
6048

Brief Contents

Contents

Chapter Resources

Paramedic: Calculations for Medication Administration is designed to teach the basic principles of mathematics and apply these principles to cases that paramedics face on the job. Features that reinforce and expand on essential information include:

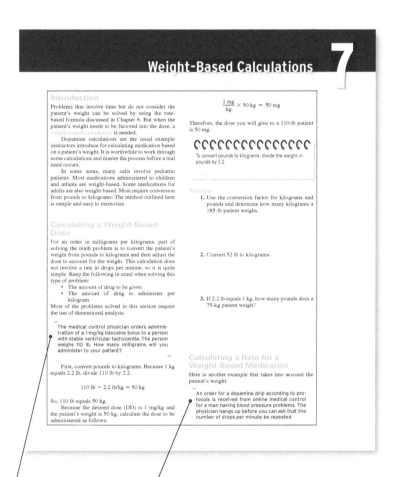

Weight-Based Calculations 7

Introduction

Problems that involve time but do not consider the patient's weight can be solved by using the rate-based formula discussed in Chapter 6. But when the patient's weight needs to be factored into the dose, a weight-based calculation is needed.

Dopamine calculations are the usual example instructors introduce for calculating medication based on a patient's weight. It is worthwhile to work through some calculations and master the process before a real need occurs.

In some areas, many calls involve pediatric patients. Most medications administered to children and infants are weight-based. Some medications for adults are also weight-based. Most require conversion from pounds to kilograms. The method outlined here is simple and easy to memorize.

Calculating a Weight-Based Dose

For an order in milligrams per kilograms, part of solving the math problem is to convert the patient's weight from pounds to kilograms and then adjust the dose to account for the weight. This calculation does not involve a rate in drops per minute, so it is quite simple. Keep the following in mind when solving this type of problem:
- The amount of drug to be given
- The amount of drug to administer per kilogram

Most of the problems solved in this section require the use of dimensional analysis.

The medical control physician orders administration of a 1-mg/kg lidocaine bolus to a person with stable ventricular tachycardia. The person weighs 110 lb. How many milligrams will you administer to your patient?

First, convert pounds to kilograms. Because 1 kg equals 2.2 lb, divide 110 lb by 2.2.

$$110 \text{ lb} \div 2.2 \text{ lb/kg} = 50 \text{ kg}$$

So, 110 lb equals 50 kg.

Because the desired dose (DD) is 1 mg/kg and the patient's weight is 50 kg, calculate the dose to be administered as follows:

$$\frac{1 \text{ mg}}{\text{kg}} \times 50 \text{ kg} = 50 \text{ mg}$$

Therefore, the dose you will give to a 110-lb patient is 50 mg.

To convert pounds to kilograms, divide the weight in pounds by 2.2.

Practice

1. Use the conversion factor for kilograms and pounds and determine how many kilograms a 185-lb patient weighs.

2. Convert 52 lb to kilograms.

3. If 2.2 lb equals 1 kg, how many pounds does a 75-kg patient weigh?

Calculating a Rate for a Weight-Based Medication

Here is another example that takes into account the patient's weight.

An order for a dopamine drip according to protocols is received from online medical control for a man having blood pressure problems. The physician hangs up before you can ask that the number of drops per minute be repeated.

Realistic Paramedic Problems

Math concepts are taught using realistic, relevant examples from the day-to-day job of a paramedic.

End-of-Chapter Problems

Each chapter contains a multitude of practice problems reviewing all of the methods covered in the chapter.

The book concludes with 172 problems representing every type of problem presented in the book.

7. A 51-year-old man is complaining of a severe headache and, after several minutes, becomes unconscious. You attempt intubation, and because of difficulty, the physician gives you an order for rapid-sequence intubation. After a successful intubation and owing to a lengthy transport time, the physician also gives you an order for 0.1 mg/kg of vecuronium to maintain the paralysis of this patient. The patient

10. Your ambulance responds to a patient complaining of chest pain. You find a 47-year-old woman complaining of a heavy feeling in her chest and shortness of breath. Your partner gives the patient oxygen, applies the cardiac monitor, and inserts an IV line. When you look at the monitor, you find that the patient needs cardioversion, and, per protocol, you need to administer etomidate, 0.3 mg/kg, for sedation before the delivery of the shock. Your patient weighs 157 lb. You have 50 mg of etomidate in a 5-mL vial. What is the correct dose, and how much medication will you administer?

11. A patient is having multifocal PVCs at a rate of 10/min. Per protocol, you are directed to administer lidocaine, 1.0 mg/kg, to control the PVCs. The patient weighs 208 lb. You have 100 mg of lidocaine in a 10-mL prefilled syringe. How much medication will you administer?

12. A patient is having cardiac problems. Examination shows uncontrolled atrial fibrillation with an irregular rate of 140 beats/min. The medical control physician orders diltiazem, 0.25 mg/kg. The patient weighs 133 lb. You have ... in a 10-mL vial. What ... how much medica-

Prep Kit

Math Vocabulary

weight-based calculation A medication calculation that takes the patient's weight into consideration; for example, if a dose is ordered per kilogram, the dose must be adjusted to correspond to the patient's weight in kilograms.

Practice Problems

By using the desired dose and the patient's weight, calculate the dose you will administer.

1. A patient is having multifocal premature ventricular contractions (PVCs) at a rate of 20/min. Per protocol, you are directed to administer lidocaine, 1.5 mg/kg, to control the PVCs. The patient weighs 150 lb. You have 100 mg of lidocaine in a 10-mL prefilled syringe. What is the dose (adjusted for weight), and how much medication will you administer?

2. You have a patient who needs cardioversion, and, per protocol, you need to administer etomidate, 0.3 mg/kg, for sedation. The patient weighs 122 lb. You have 50 mg of etomidate in a 5-mL vial. What is the adjusted dose, and how much medication will you administer?

3. A 65-year-old patient is in cardiac arrest. During the resuscitation, you receive orders for 1 mEq/kg of sodium bicarbonate. The patient weighs 128 lb. On hand you have 60 mEq of sodium bicarbonate in 50 mL of solution. What volume will you administer?

4. A female patient takes phenytoin for seizures, and, by protocol, you need to administer 15 mg/kg of the medication to help control seizures. You determine that the patient weighs 130 lb. You have 1 g of phenytoin in a 20-mL vial. What is the adjusted dose, and how much medication will you administer to this patient?

5. A patient is having cardiac problems. An electrocardiogram shows a rapid atrial flutter with a rate of 150 beats/min. The medical control physician orders diltiazem, 0.25 mg/kg. The patient weighs 185 lb. You have 25 mg of diltiazem in a 10-mL vial. What is the adjusted dose, and how much medication will you give?

6. The physician has ordered ketamine, 1 to 2 mg/kg during 1 minute, to help control a patient's pain. The patient weighs 142 lb. You decide to administer 2 mg/kg. You have 150 mg of ketamine in 10 mL of solution. How much medication will you administer to this patient?

... head injury is having difficulty ... but you are unable to intubate ... control physician orders ... 0.8 mg/kg. You determine ... 184 lb. You find 100 mg ... in a 2-mL vial. How much ... you administer?

... multifocal PVCs at a rate ... protocol, you are directed to ... lidocaine, 1.5 mg/kg, to control ... patient weighs 118 lb. You ... lidocaine in a 10-mL prefilled ... much medication will you

... complaining of a "heavy feeling" ... and shortness of breath. The ... uncontrolled atrial fibrillation ... irregular rate of 123 beats/min. ... control physician orders diltiazem, ... The patient weighs 163 lb. You have 20 mg of diltiazem in a 10-mL vial. **What is the adjusted** dose, and how much medication will you give?

16. Your patient is in cardiac arrest. During resuscitation, you receive orders for 1 mEq/kg of sodium bicarbonate. The patient weighs 200 lb. In your drug box you have an ampule of 50 mEq of sodium bicarbonate in 50 mL of solution. What volume will you administer?

20. A patient is having major motor seizures, and, by protocol, you need to administer 15 mg/kg of phenytoin to help control the seizures. You determine that the patient weighs 105 lb. You have 1 g of phenytoin in a 20-mL vial. What is the adjusted dose, and how much medication will you administer?

Answer Key With Explanations

Unlike other math books, this book's Answer Key contains explanations for how the answer was reached. Every step is included; no steps are skipped and no assumptions are made. This allows readers of any comfort level to learn.

Answer Key   179

48. First, recall that 1:1,000 means there is 1 g per 1,000 mL. Because the question asks for milligrams and the concentration is in grams, convert grams to milligrams. (Table 5-1 showed that 1 g equals 1,000 mg.)

$$\frac{1,000 \text{ mg}}{1,000 \text{ mL}} = \frac{?}{1 \text{ mL}}$$

? = 1.0 mg

49. 50% solution = 50 g in 100 mL, or 25 g in 50 mL.

$$\frac{25}{50} = \frac{5}{?}$$

$25 \times ? = 50 \times 5$

$$? = \frac{50 \times 5}{25}$$

$$\frac{250}{25} = 10 \text{ mL}.$$

50. 50% solution = 50 g in 100 mL, or 5 g in 10 mL.

Because there are 5 g in the 10-mL prefilled syringe and the order is to administer 5 g, a calculation is not needed. By administering the whole prefilled syringe, you will administer the required 5 g.

51. First, convert gram to milligrams: 1 g equals 1,000 mg

$$\frac{1,000 \text{ mg}}{50 \text{ mL}} = \frac{400 \text{ mg}}{\text{mL}}$$

Flip the equation:

$$\frac{}{400 \text{ mg}} = \frac{50 \text{ mL}}{1,000 \text{ mg}}$$

$$? = \frac{50 \times 400}{1,000}$$

? = 20 mL.

52. $\frac{500 \text{ mg}}{50 \text{ mL}} = \frac{175 \text{ mg}}{\text{mL}}$

$$\frac{\text{mL}}{175 \text{ mg}} = \frac{50 \text{ mL}}{500 \text{ mg}}$$

$$? = \frac{50 \times 175}{500}$$

? = 17.5 mL.

53. 50% solution = 50 g in 100 mL, or 25 g in 50 mL.

Because you need to administer 25 g and the prefilled syringe contains 25 g/50 mL, you administer the entire prefilled syringe.

54. 10% solution = 10 g in 100 mL, or 5 g in 50 mL.

$$\frac{5 \text{ g}}{50 \text{ mL}} = \frac{4 \text{ g}}{\text{mL}}$$

$$\frac{\text{mL}}{4 \text{ g}} = \frac{50 \text{ mL}}{5 \text{ g}}$$

$$? = \frac{50 \times 4}{5}$$

? = 40 mL.

Because the prefilled syringe contains 20 mL, you will need to administer two prefilled syringes.

55. 25% solution = 25 g in 100 mL, half of which would be 12.5 g in 50 mL.

$$\frac{12.5 \text{ g}}{50 \text{ mL}} = \frac{2.75 \text{ g}}{\text{mL}}$$

$$\frac{\text{mL}}{2.75 \text{ g}} = \frac{50 \text{ mL}}{12.5 \text{ g}}$$

$$? = \frac{50 \times 2.75}{12.5}$$

? = 11 mL.

56. Convert grams to milligrams because this is a lidocaine drip.

$$2 \text{ g} \times \frac{1,000 \text{ mg}}{1 \text{ g}} = 2,000 \text{ mg}$$

$$\frac{2,000 \text{ mg}}{500 \text{ mL}} = 4 \text{ mg/mL}.$$

$$\frac{4 \text{ mg}}{\text{mL}} = \frac{? \text{ mg}}{3 \text{ mL}}$$

$$\frac{? \text{ mg}}{\text{mL}} = \frac{4 \text{ mg}}{3 \text{ mL}}$$

$$? = \frac{4 \text{ mg} \times 3 \text{ mL}}{\text{mL}}$$

? = 12 mg

The concentration is 4 mg/mL. In 3 mL, there would be 3 times that amount, or 12 mg/3 mL.

57. 60% solution = 60 g in 100 mL, or 30 g in 50 mL.

$$\frac{30 \text{ g}}{50 \text{ mL}} = \frac{6 \text{ g}}{\text{mL}}$$

$$\frac{\text{mL}}{6 \text{ g}} = \frac{50 \text{ mL}}{30 \text{ g}}$$

$$? = \frac{50 \times 6}{30}$$

? = 10 mL.

Answer Key   169

Chapter 4
Chapter Problems
Reading and Writing Fractions

1. $\frac{2}{6} \div \frac{2}{2} = \frac{1}{3}$

One third of the ambulances are responding to calls.

2. $\frac{4}{20} \div \frac{4}{4} = \frac{1}{5}$

One fifth of the medics are needed to staff the units this weekend. This also equals 0.20, or 20%:

$$20\overline{)4.00} \quad 0.20$$

3. $\frac{1 \text{ L LR}}{4 \text{ doses LR}}$

Convert L to mL:

$$\frac{1,000 \text{ mL LR}}{4 \text{ doses LR}}$$

Reduce:

$$\frac{1,000}{4} \div \frac{4}{4} = \frac{250}{1} = 250 \text{ mL LR}$$

Each of the four doses of lactated Ringer's should equal 250 mL.

Multiplying Fractions

1. $\frac{4}{1} \times \frac{20}{5} = \frac{80}{5}$

This can be reduced:

$$\frac{80}{5} \div \frac{5}{5} = 16$$

2. $\frac{11}{6} \times \frac{8}{2} = \frac{88}{12}$

This can be reduced:

$$\frac{88}{12} \div \frac{4}{4} = \frac{22}{3}$$

3. $0 \times \frac{6}{8} = 0$

Note that zero times anything is always zero.

Dividing Fractions

1. $\frac{3}{12} \times \frac{2}{1} = \frac{6}{12}$

This can be further reduced to:

$$\frac{6}{12} \div \frac{6}{6} = \frac{1}{2}$$

This also equals 0.5, or 50%.

2. $\frac{7}{8} \times \frac{4}{3} = \frac{28}{24}$

This can be further reduced to:

$$\frac{28}{24} \div \frac{4}{4} = \frac{7}{6}$$

This also equals:

$$6\overline{)7.00} \quad 1.16$$

This can be rounded to 1.2 (recall rounding from Chapter 1).

3. $\frac{76}{128} \times \frac{3}{2} = \frac{228}{256}$

(Recall the manual multiplication method to reach these numbers.)

$$\begin{array}{r} 76 \\ \times\ 3 \\ \hline 228 \end{array}$$

$$\begin{array}{r} 128 \\ \times\ 2 \\ \hline 256 \end{array}$$

This can be further reduced to:

$$\frac{228}{256} \div \frac{4}{4} = \frac{57}{64}$$

Note that if the initial fractions had been reduced to their lowest terms at the outset, the multiplication would have been easier:

$$\frac{76}{128} \div \frac{4}{4} = \frac{19}{32}$$

The equation would then progress as follows:

$$\frac{19}{32} \times \frac{3}{2} = \frac{57}{64}$$

Multiplying and Dividing Complicated Fractions

1. $\frac{12}{3} \div \frac{?}{?} = \frac{12}{3} \div \frac{?}{?} = \frac{96}{21}$

This can be reduced as follows:

$$\frac{96}{21} \div \frac{3}{3} = \frac{32}{7}$$

Hints

Hints boxes give students tips to help them remember methods and solve problems successfully.

Notepad Tips

The notepad contains key concepts in boxes which are easy to locate in the text. They are also compiled in Appendix B for easy reference and review.

---

26   Paramedic: Calculations for Medication Administration

$$\begin{array}{r} 26 \\ \times\,23 \\ \hline 78 \\ +\,52 \\ \hline 598 \end{array}$$

In problems of this type, it is very important to keep your work neat. If the numbers are added into the wrong column, the answer is changed dramatically.

Additional Examples The next two final examples summarize manual mode of multiplication by following the same process. There are comments inserted to make it easy to follow the steps.

Problem:

$$\begin{array}{r} 62 \\ \times\,13 \\ \hline ? \end{array}$$

Foundation number: 62

Multiplier: 13

Estimate: $60 \times 15 = 60 \times 5 \times 3 = 300 \times 3 = 900$

Calculation:

$$\begin{array}{r} 62 \\ \times\,13 \\ \hline 186 \\ +\,62 \\ \hline 806 \end{array}$$

Problem:

$$\begin{array}{r} 36 \\ \times\,12 \\ \hline ? \end{array}$$

Foundation number: 36

Multiplier: 12

Estimate: $35 \times 10 = 350$

Calculation:

$$\begin{array}{r} 36 \\ \times\,12 \\ \hline 72 \\ +\,36 \\ \hline 432 \end{array}$$

Last, but not least, try some problems on your own.

Math **Hints**

Sometimes it is difficult to keep the numbers aligned. Here's a trick. When multiplying the tens number of the multiplier times the foundation number, you can place a zero in the ones place, to "hold" the place. This will remind you not to accidentally place the tens number in the ones place.

$$\begin{array}{r} 36 \\ \times\,12 \\ \hline 72 \\ +\,36 \\ \hline 432 \end{array}$$ A zero holds the "ones" place so you don't accidentally misalign numbers.

Practice

1. $$\begin{array}{r} 54 \\ \times\,83 \\ \hline ? \end{array}$$

    Foundation number: _____
    Multiplier: _____
    Estimate: _____
    Calculation:

    $$\begin{array}{r} 54 \\ \times\,83 \\ \hline \\ + \\ \hline \end{array}$$

    Check against your estimate: Estimate = _____
    Answer = _____

2. $$\begin{array}{r} 26 \\ \times\,77 \\ \hline ? \end{array}$$

    Foundation number: _____
    Multiplier: _____
    Estimate: _____
    Calculation:

    $$\begin{array}{r} 26 \\ \times\,77 \\ \hline \\ + \\ \hline \end{array}$$

    Check against your estimate: Estimate = _____
    Answer = _____

Multiplying Decimals

Multiplying decimals is simple. All you have to do is remember the methods:

Here is a basic decimal point math problem.

...the four doses of lactated Ringer's ...L.

...ce, write the shorthand (fractions) ...blems at the end of this chapter.

g Complicated ...ultiplying, Dividing, ...d Subtracting

...ve spent a lot of time, energy, and ...ering and proving the many rules ...formulas. We should be grateful ...ause that means that we don't have ...ork to take advantage of the rules! ...n the math rules and apply them to ...s, focusing on our patients' needs ...ives. That's good enough most of

...g with fractions, there are many ...culations easier. Writing problems ...s it easier to find the meat of the ...inate the distractions. Simple is ...a medical math, where making a ...e serious consequences.

...math shorthand focuses on rear- ...ns to make them simple to use. As ...the rules, you can move the parts ...until you find the best, easiest-to-

...ply when working with the frac- ...edical math:

...y fractions: First multiply the ...(top numbers) to find the new ...and then multiply the denomi- ...tom numerators) to find the new ...r; then simplify.

...fractions: First invert the second ...p it over), and then multiply the ...as; then simplify.

...an be added or subtracted only ...have the same denominator (a ...minator). Once the denominators are the same, then:

- To add fractions: Add the numerators and keep the common denominator.
- To subtract fractions: Subtract the numerators and keep the common denominator.

How to apply the rules for adding, subtracting, multiplying, and dividing fractions is discussed in the next sections.

Multiplying Fractions

When multiplying fractions, first multiply the numerators to find the new numerator, and then multiply

---

...ons for Medication Administration

Fractions
Multiply: Multiply the numerators, and then multiply the denominators.
Divide: Invert the second fraction, and then multiply.
Add or subtract: Find a common denominator, and then add or subtract the numerators.

the denominators to find the new denominator; then simplify. Here are a few examples.

$$\frac{3}{8} \times \frac{6}{7} = ?$$

Multiply the numerators, and multiply the denominators.

$$\frac{3}{8} \times \frac{6}{7} = \frac{18}{56}$$

This can be further reduced as follows:

$$\frac{18}{56} \div \frac{2}{2} = \frac{9}{28}$$

Here's another example.

$$\frac{2}{8} \times \frac{5}{9} = ?$$

Multiply the numerators, and multiply the denominators.

$$\frac{2}{8} \times \frac{5}{9} = \frac{10}{72}$$

This can be further reduced as follows:

$$\frac{10}{72} \div \frac{2}{2} = \frac{5}{36}$$

Here is a final example.

$$\frac{1}{2} \times \frac{15}{16} = ?$$

Multiply the numerators, and multiply the denominators.

Vocabulary

Vocabulary terms are highlighted within the text and defined at the end of the chapter.

The Language of Math

Prep Kit

Math Vocabulary

decimals   Numbers based on the number 10 and that contain a dot (point) between whole numbers (written to the left of the dot) and numbers that are smaller than whole numbers (written to the right of the dot). The numbers to the right of the dot constitute decimal fractions.

denominator   The bottom part of a fraction, for example, the 10 in $\frac{1}{10}$.

estimate   To make an approximation of a number, rather than an actual calculation.

fraction   A number expressed using a numerator and a denominator, for example $\frac{1}{10}$.

improper fraction   A fraction in which the numerator is larger than the denominator.

mixed number   A number written as a whole number and a fraction.

multiple   A number that can be divided by the original number(s) without a remainder. For example: 5, 10, 15, 20, 25, 30, are multiples of 5, and 24 is a multiple of 6 and 4.

numerator   The top part of a fraction, for example, the 1 in $\frac{1}{10}$.

percentage   A portion of 100, noted with the "%" sign.

proper fraction   A fraction in which the numerator is smaller than the denominator.

round   To express a number as a convenient whole number. A rounded number can be used in a mathematical calculation when estimating.

trick of 5s   A method used to make it easier to multiply by 5, in which a number is multiplied by 10 and the answer is then cut in half.

Table 1-2   Comparing Fractions, Percentages, and Decimals

Fraction	Percentage	Decimal
$\frac{1}{10}$	10%	0.10
$\frac{1}{4}$	25%	0.25
$\frac{1}{2}$	50%	0.50
$\frac{3}{4}$	75%	0.75
1	100%	1.00

32 is 50% (or $\frac{50}{100}$) of 64 oz

32 oz is 50% of 64 oz

Table 1-2 shows a few of the more common numbers that we are comfortable using in all three math languages.

There is a pattern in Table 1-2 that you might recognize. These numbers are familiar when we think of them as money. Remember, as a math rookie, you need only realize that there are three math languages and be comfortable with this concept.

Using decimals provides an easy way to read numbers. Understanding how decimals compare with fractions helps us have a better understanding of numbers, regardless of how they are written.

When a decimal point is used, whole numbers are written to the left of the decimal point; fractions of numbers are written to the right of the decimal point (Figure 1-1).

When we use decimals, we understand that each "place" occupied by a number actually has a value based on a multiple of 10. We can write numbers infinitely on either side of the decimal point as needed. The decimal point indicates which parts are whole numbers (on the left) and which parts are fractions of a number (on the right). To see how this works, look at the construction of the following number written with a decimal:

WWWWW.FFFFF

Starting at the decimal place and working to the left, the W represents whole numbers. The first place to the left of the decimal is the "ones place." The number occupying that place is multiplied by 1 to determine

Whole number ——▶ 7.5 ◀—— Fraction of the number

Decimal point

Figure 1-1 The decimal point is placed between the whole number and the fractions of the number.

its value. The next number to the left of the ones place occupies the "tens place." The number in that place is multiplied by 10 to determine its value. Every number to the left, thereafter, is occupying a place that is the next higher multiple of 10 (for example, 100; 1,000; 10,000).

Math Hints

A multiple of 10 is a number that can be reached when you multiply 10 × 10 enough times. For example:

$$10 \times 10 = 100$$
$$10 \times 10 \times 10 = 1,000$$
$$10 \times 10 \times 10 \times 10 = 10,000$$

These numbers—100, 1,000, and 10,000—are multiples of 10.

That may sound complicated, but you already know this from reading numbers. For example, look at the following number:

1 2 3 4 . 5 6 7

The left side of this number reads "one thousand, two hundred, thirty-four." This isn't anything new. If the number was written as 1,234, it would read the same.

The right side of the decimal point is the fraction side. The numbers occupying this space will always be less than 1. In the preceding example, ".567" appears to the right of the decimal point. Each place represents the number divided by a multiple of 10 (for example, $\frac{1}{10}, \frac{1}{100}, \frac{1}{1,000}$). Follow the breakdown of the right side of the decimal fraction below:

6 is in the tenths place and represents "six tenths" (or $\frac{6}{10}$)

7 is in the hundredths place and represents "seven hundredths" (or $\frac{7}{100}$)

8 is in the thousandths place and represents "eight thousandths" (or $\frac{8}{1,000}$)

Text Format	Fraction Format	Decimal Format
Twenty-five and three hundredths	$25\frac{3}{100}$	25.03
Three and sixty-seven hundredths		
		0.3
	$126\frac{5}{10}$	
Nine hundred eighty-seven thousandths		
	$327\frac{98}{100}$	

2. Fill in the blanks in the chart below. The percentages are filled in for you. You have learned that percentage is one of the three math languages.

Decimal	Fraction	Percentage
1.2		1 and 20 = 120%
3.68		3 and 68 = 368%
	$\frac{25}{100}$	25%
0.10	$\frac{1}{10}$	10%
0.5		50%
	$\frac{75}{1,000}$	7.5%

Instructor Resources

Instructor's ToolKit CD-ROM

ISBN 13: 978-0-7637-5210-1
ISBN 10: 0-7637-5210-X

Preparing for class is easy with the resources found on this CD-ROM, including:

- **PowerPoint Presentations**—Providing you with educational and engaging presentations. Presentations can be modified and edited to meet your needs.
- **Lecture Outlines**—Providing you with complete, ready-to-use lesson plans that outline all of the methods and concepts covered in the text. The lesson plans can be modified and edited to fit your course.
- **TestBank**—Providing you with the additional problems that you can use to create your own exams. Tailor your tests and quizzes easily by selecting, editing, organizing, and printing an exam along with an answer key that includes page references to the text.

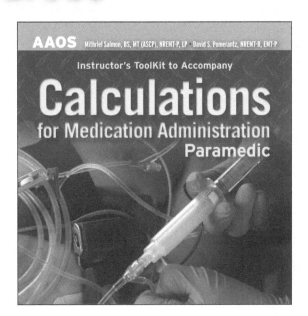

AAOS   Mithriel Salmon, BS, MT (ASCP), NREMT-P, LP · David S. Pomerantz, NREMT-B, EMT-P

Instructor's ToolKit to Accompany
Calculations
for Medication Administration
Paramedic

Technology Resources

Paramedic.EMSzone.com

- **Online Practice Problems**—Students practice with instant results and feedback on incorrect answers.

- **Vocabulary Explorer**—Interactive online glossary to expand student's medical vocabulary.
- **Animated Flash Cards**—Review vital vocabulary and key concepts.

Acknowledgments

The authors wish to thank Leslie Hernandez and Steve Rahm for their support in bringing this project to fruition.

Series Editor

Andrew N. Pollak, MD, FAAOS
Medical Director, Baltimore County Fire Department
Associate Professor, University of Maryland School
  of Medicine
Baltimore, Maryland

Contributors

David S. Becker, MA, EMT-P, EFO
EMS Program Director
Sanford-Brown College
Fenton, Missouri

Reviewers

Gerria Berryman, EMT-P
Educational Coordinator
Emergency Medical Training Professionals
Nicholasville, Kentucky

John Bray, BS, NREMT-P, CCEMT-P
Saint Vincent's Hospital
Manhattan Institute of Emergency Care
New York, New York

Bradley E. Dean, BBA, NREMT-P
Triad Regional Advisory Committee
Wake Forest University Baptist Medical Center/Trauma
  Services
Davidson County Emergency Services
Thomasville, North Carolina

M. John Dudte, MPA, MICT I/C
District of Columbia Fire/EMS Department, Training
  Academy
Washington, District of Columbia

Tim Duncan, RN, CCRN, CEN, CFRN, EMT-P
St. Vincent Mercy Medical Center Life Flight
Toledo, Ohio

Todd Jaynes
Shoshone, Idaho

Louis B. Mallory, MBA, REMT-P
Santa Fe Community College
Gainesville, Florida

Andrew Margolies, EMT-P/CIC
State University of New York at Stony Brook
Stony Brook, New York

Greg Mullen, MS, NREMT-P
National EMS Academy
Lafayette, Louisiana

Laurie Oelslager, EdD, NREMT-P
South Central College
North Mankato, Minnesota

David S. Pomerantz, NREMT-B, EMT-P
Deerfield Beach, Florida

Jennifer Russell, BS EM, EMT-P
Bellingham, Washington

**Scott A. Smith, RN, BSN, BA, CEN, CFRN,
  NREMT-P, I/C**
Sidney, Maine

Karyl White, MS, MICT, IC
Barton County Community College
Great Bend, Kansas

**Matthew Zavarella, RN, NREMT-P, MS, CFRN,
  CEN, CCRN**
Youngstown State University
North Huntingdon, Pennsylvania

Suzan A. Zehner
University of Alaska, Fairbanks
Fairbanks, Alaska

"Math." Saying the word "math" opens up a dialogue in any group.

"I love math!"

"I hate math!"

"I had a math teacher who was absolutely evil."

"Coach was our math teacher. He threw erasers and chalk at us when we fell asleep in class."

"I'm pretty good at math. That's why I do the checkbook in our house."

"I'm lousy at math. I gave up trying to balance my checkbook."

The reality is that we do math every day. If you have a headache, you read the label of the pain reliever to figure out how much to take. If you buy groceries, you comparison shop to get the most for your money. Need bricks to lay down a patio? *Math.* Need paint for a house project? *Math.* Didn't think your last raise was enough to keep up with your bills? *Math again.* You can do math. You are already a very accomplished mathematician.

This text is designed to help you transform the math skills you have already acquired through the course of your daily life. The goal here is to take just a few of the concepts to which you have already been exposed (in the formal, sit-down, classroom style most of us experienced while growing up) and to transform those experiences into tools you can access quickly in the prehospital setting. In this text, you can take your time while solving the same types of math challenges that you will see in the field. Here, math problems are taken apart, the pieces are explained, and the components are then rearranged into something that can be solved quickly and yields an answer that is useful to patients.

Our Approach

The approach contained in these pages is different from that taken in other math texts. Most textbooks use a fairly traditional format for teaching math:

demonstrate how to use different math skills, give examples, and then have a few chapters of "putting it all together." This system, though it works for some math-savvy individuals, is intimidating to most people. By the time you get to the chapters where you are supposed to *put it all together,* you may feel overwhelmed by having to remember the entire scope of skills taught in the previous few hundred pages.

This book approaches the challenges of learning math in terms of levels. Each level of the text gives you the tools needed to immediately solve the math challenges you will find in both the field and day-to-day life. Each chapter builds on the previous one; you master one level before moving to the next. The challenges start off quick and easy. Hints to help understand and process the problem-solving techniques are interjected along the road to resolution.

The first chapters in this book are dedicated to getting you comfortable with using numbers you are already experienced at manipulating (thanks to the U.S. monetary system!), including "1," "2," "5," and "10." Early chapters cover the concept of estimating. Many times in the prehospital setting, obtaining an estimate helps you double-check that your exact answer is correct.

The levels of play (and *play* is precisely what it should be!) will progress by introducing new challenges along with tried-and-true methods for finding their solutions. Your perspective and approach to using math will be altered so that you are ready to accept this challenge while keeping the math organized and simple.

A final suggestion: *Relax.* The calculations presented here are meant to be approached much in the same way that you would pick up a puzzle book to keep you busy on a coast-to-coast flight. There are no tones dropping, no sirens blaring, and no one waiting for you to arrive on scene. You have time to lay out the scratch paper and kick back. Enjoy the challenges and the confidence that comes with mastering the game!

—Mithriel Salmon

Learning the Languages of Mathematics

Numbers are like most things in that the more you use them, the more familiar you become with the way to use them. There are different ways of looking at numbers, and the best, most appropriate way often depends on what you are trying to figure out.

It is easy to get used to math calculations that you perform frequently. For example, when you buy food at the grocery store, you might use addition and subtraction to compare the prices of items. Addition and subtraction become easier as you apply these operations more often.

Learning to look at numbers in different ways helps you to manipulate the numbers and makes calculations and concepts easier to work with. This ease of use comes from reading the numbers and being familiar with the different languages of mathematics.

Introduction to Fractions, Percentages, and Decimals

The three languages we use in prehospital care most often are fractions, percentages, and decimals. The languages of math are actually simple—in fact, you use them every time you pay cash to make small purchases. Percentages are mentioned only briefly in this chapter; they will be covered in more depth with ratios in Chapter 5. In this chapter, your challenge is to understand the relationship between fractions and decimals. It is a snap to move between these two math languages, and calculations are simpler when you take advantage of this concept.

Here is a look at the three languages of math just mentioned.

You drive your unit into the local gas station to purchase fuel while your partner purchases a drink for each of you. The ambulance has a 60-gallon gas tank that is now half full.

Because the 60-gallon tank is half full, you know that you need 30 gallons to fill it. In the languages of math (fractions, percentages, and decimals), "half" can be written as follows:

$$\frac{1}{2} = 50\% = 0.5$$

Simple enough! By recalling lessons learned from your last math class, you can dust off a few skills and rewrite this information a little bit differently without changing the values:

$$\frac{1}{2}\,(\text{fraction})$$

$$50\%\,(\text{percentage}) = \frac{50}{100}$$

$$0.5\,(\text{decimal}) = \text{five tenths} = \frac{5}{10}$$

Fractions and Mixed Numbers

A first step in becoming reacquainted with math languages might be to refresh a few concepts you learned in school. Here is a brief look at how these math languages all say the same thing. As you move through the skills and add tools to your calculation jump bag, you will discover how easy it will be to work with all three languages.

The previous three numbers show three ways to write the same value. To explain further, 50% (or $\frac{50}{100}$) is interpreted as *50 parts of a total 100 parts* or *half* of the total parts.

A fraction is a portion of a whole. Do you remember Grandma's hot apple pie? Cut the pie into sixths and you have six pieces, which make up the whole pie. If you eat one of the pieces, a sixth or $\frac{1}{6}$ of the pie is missing. The sixth or $\frac{1}{6}$ is considered a fraction.

You can relate to fractions by considering money. Take, for example, a one-dollar bill ($1.00). The one-dollar bill represents the whole number or 100% of the object. Each of the four quarters (25 cents each) that make up the dollar is a fourth or $\frac{1}{4}$ of the whole number, or the whole dollar.

Each fraction has a numerator (top number) and a denominator (bottom number). With fractions, there are proper and improper fractions. A proper fraction is one in which the numerator is less than the denominator. For example, the following three fractions:

$$\frac{2}{5} \quad \frac{3}{5} \quad \frac{7}{8}$$

are all proper fractions.

An improper fraction has a numerator that is larger than the denominator.

For example:

$$\frac{14}{5} \text{ (which means } 14 \div 5)$$

An improper fraction can be reduced to a mixed number, which is a number written as a whole number and a fraction.

- In the preceding fraction, divide the numerator (14) by the denominator (5). This gives 2, with a remainder of 4.
- The mixed number can be created by using the 2 as the whole number, the 4 as the numerator, and the 5 as the denominator.
- $\frac{14}{5}$ is an improper fraction and can be reduced to $2\frac{4}{5}$, which is a mixed number.

Percentages

A percentage is a portion of 100, noted with the "%" sign. In other words, $\frac{1}{100}$ equals 1%, $\frac{2}{100}$ equals 2%, $\frac{100}{100}$ equals 100%, and so forth. You are probably already familiar with percentages from exam grades you received throughout school.

Decimals

Decimals may be less familiar to you. Decimals are numbers based on the number 10 and that contain a point between whole numbers and numbers that are smaller than whole numbers. For example:

0.2   2.5   5.6   2.8   1.5   33.33
100.5   200.1   3.2   5.7   10.1

The number to the left of the decimal point is known as the whole number. The number one place to the right of the decimal point is the "tenths" digit. The value of the digit two places to the right of the decimal point is based on a value of hundreds, three places is based on a value of thousands, and so on.

The number in the tenths position can also be expressed as a fraction with a ten in the denominator. For example, 0.1 is equal to $\frac{1}{10}$. The number in the hundredths position can be expressed as a fraction with 100 in the denominator. Therefore 0.01 equals $\frac{1}{100}$, and so on. Table 1-1 ▶ shows these and other examples.

Table 1-1	Comparing Decimals and Fractions
Decimal	Fraction
0.1	$\frac{1}{10}$
0.01	$\frac{1}{100}$
0.001	$\frac{1}{1,000}$
0.0001	$\frac{1}{10,000}$

The first place to the right of the decimal point is the *tenths* place. This means that 0.5 equals five tenths, which can be written as $\frac{5}{10}$. The fraction is interpreted as 5 parts of a total of 10 parts, or half the total number of parts.

The understanding that all these numbers are saying the same thing is a tool that you need for medication dose calculations.

It is well worth spending a few minutes to practice these languages. Math is, after all, a game. In fact, it is a lot like chess. When you play chess, you can move the pieces any way you like, as long as you follow the rules that apply to each individual piece. Similarly, in math problems, you can move the numbers around any way you like, as long as you follow the rules. In chess, the pieces can move in different patterns over the board. In math, the numbers can be moved around (by rewriting them in one of the other math languages without changing the values) as long as the basic rules are followed. To help you practice using these languages, there are practice problems at the end of this chapter, to be completed after mastering this skill level.

Here is another example.

You arrive at a convenience store. Inside the store, your partner gets the 32-ounce soda you requested and buys himself a 64-ounce soda.

Your partner's purchase includes a 32-ounce soda for you and a 64-ounce soda for himself. Here are these numbers written in the different math languages:

32 oz = 64 oz ÷ 2 (You are half as thirsty as your partner.)

32 oz is $\frac{1}{2}$ of 64 oz

Table 1-2 Comparing Fractions, Percentages, and Decimals		
Fraction	Percentage	Decimal
$\dfrac{1}{10}$	10%	0.10
$\dfrac{1}{4}$	25%	0.25
$\dfrac{1}{2}$	50%	0.50
$\dfrac{3}{4}$	75%	0.75
1	100%	1.00

32 is 50% (or $\dfrac{50}{100}$) of 64 oz

32 oz is 0.5 of 64 oz

Table 1-2 ⏴ shows a few of the more common numbers that we are comfortable using in all three math languages.

There is a pattern in Table 1-2 that you might recognize. These numbers are familiar when we think of them as money. Remember, as a math rookie, you need only realize that there are three math languages and be comfortable with this concept.

Using decimals provides an easy way to read numbers. Understanding how decimals compare with fractions helps us have a better understanding of numbers, regardless of how they are written.

When a decimal point is used, whole numbers are written to the left of the decimal point; fractions of numbers are written to the right of the decimal point (Figure 1-1 ▶).

When we use decimals, we understand that each "place" occupied by a number actually has a value based on a multiple of 10. We can write numbers infinitely on either side of the decimal point as needed. The decimal point indicates which parts are whole numbers (on the left) and which parts are fractions of a number (on the right). To see how this works, look at the construction of the following number written with a decimal:

W W W W W . F F F F F

Starting at the decimal place and working to the left, the W represents whole numbers. The first place to the left of the decimal is the "ones place." The number occupying that place is multiplied by 1 to determine

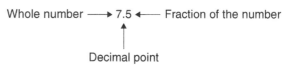

Figure 1-1 The decimal point is placed between the whole number and the fractions of the number.

its value. The next number to the left of the ones place occupies the "tens place." The number in that place is multiplied by 10 to determine its value. Every number to the left, thereafter, is occupying a place that is the next higher multiple of 10 (for example, 100; 1,000; 10,000).

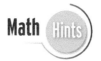

A multiple of 10 is a number that can be reached when you multiply 10 × 10 enough times. For example:

$$10 \times 10 = 100$$
$$10 \times 10 \times 10 = 1,000$$
$$10 \times 10 \times 10 \times 10 = 10,000$$

These numbers—100, 1,000, and 10,000—are multiples of 10.

That may sound complicated, but you already know this from reading numbers. For example, look at the following number:

1 2 3 4 . 6 7 8

The left side of this number reads "one thousand, two hundred, thirty-four." This isn't anything new. If the number was written as 1,234, it would read the same.

The right side of the decimal point is the fraction side. The numbers occupying this space will always be less than 1. In the preceding example, "6 7 8" appears to the right of the decimal point. Each place represents the number divided by a multiple of 10 (for example, $\dfrac{1}{10}, \dfrac{1}{100}, \dfrac{1}{1,000}$). Follow the breakdown of the right side of the decimal fraction below:

6 is in the tenths place and represents "six tenths" (or $\dfrac{6}{10}$)

7 is in the hundredths place and represents "seven hundredths" (or $\dfrac{7}{100}$)

8 is in the thousandths place and represents "eight thousandths" (or $\dfrac{8}{1,000}$)

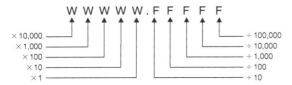

Figure 1-2 Positions before and after the decimal point, shown with their corresponding values.

In other words, 0.678 can be written in a fraction as $\frac{678}{1,000}$.

Figure 1-2 ▲ shows the positions to the right and left of the decimal point and their corresponding values.

Converting Decimals to Fractions and Back

Converting numbers to fractions from decimals is done by writing the whole number (both systems are the same for whole numbers) and then placing the numbers to the right of the decimal over the appropriate fraction. In other words, the place held by the number farthest to the right will be the denominator. For example,

$$1.1 \text{ becomes } 1\frac{1}{10}$$

How is a 0.3 decimal number converted to a fraction? This problem is quite simple. No math needs to be done to figure out how to write 0.3 as a fraction. Just remember that one place to the right of the decimal is the tenths decimal place. Two places is the hundredths place; three places is the thousandths place, and so forth. The decimal number 0.3 is the same as the fraction $\frac{3}{10}$. The final answer can be written as the fraction $\frac{3}{10}$.

Table 1-3 ▶ shows more examples.

The multiple of 10 used in the denominator will have the same number of zeros as the number of places to the right of the decimal point. If the number with decimals is 1.345, the number written with a fraction will be $1\frac{345}{1,000}$, with 1,000 having three zeros.

Table 1-3 Examples of Conversions Between Decimal Numbers and Fractions	
Decimals	Fractions
1.25 ⟵ Two places to the right of the decimal	$1\frac{25}{100}$ ⟵ Two zeros in the denominator
3.75	$3\frac{75}{100}$
75.183	$75\frac{183}{1,000}$
2.7	$2\frac{7}{10}$
3,468.17899	$3,468\frac{17,899}{100,000}$
0.26	$\frac{26}{100}$
0.5	$\frac{5}{10}$

When a number is less than one, a "0" is often placed to the left of the decimal point. Having a zero "hold the place" in front of the decimal point helps to eliminate errors caused by differences in handwriting by clarifying precisely where the decimal is located. In other words, ".5" is often written as "0.5" for clarity.

Moving Numbers in Your Head

Making Estimates

Your mission for this level is to move numbers around in your head quickly by using the tools that you have gathered (and that might have been collecting dust) over the years. These tools include the ability to add, subtract, multiply, and divide. By the completion of this chapter, you will be able to estimate the solutions to math problems. You will also be accomplished at working with multiples of 2, 5, and 10 to facilitate quick and easy problem solving.

Note that although we will be practicing how to estimate, there are cases when estimating may be appropriate and others when exact calculations are critical. Familiarity with administering medications is a critical skill for paramedics. For example, dopamine is an example of a medication that requires exact administration of the correct dose. A dose of dextrose, however, does not need to be as accurate when administered. Estimating is practiced to help you become comfortable using numbers and because estimating is sometimes useful for determining if your calculations are correct. It is imperative that you be familiar with all medications that may be administered and follow your protocols when calculating drug doses.

You have not acquired a calculator in your jump bag in this level. Your tasks will include moving around the EMS station and emergency department setting of your trauma center and quickly finding solutions to the challenges of day-to-day care. The solutions to the challenges you encounter along your path will allow you to make it through your shift with less stress and aggravation than your "not so math savvy" colleagues.

Using the Numbers 2, 5, and 10

You walk into the EMS station at 6:00 AM, sharp and eager to begin your shift. Your station is attached to the emergency department of the level 1 trauma center where you order your medical supplies for the ambulances and work under the supervision of the emergency department physicians who provide medical control.

The crew coming off duty greets you in the bay. The shift captain passes the task of restocking the trucks to your on-coming crew. A quick glance around the four ambulances in the bay reveals that two of the units are stocked and ready to go. That leaves two units that need attention before they can go out on calls.

The crew surveys the two ambulances that need to be restocked and passes a list of needed supplies to you. The chief has been pressured to keep costs at a minimum and stay within her EMS budget and now requires any supply order totaling more than $200 per ambulance per shift to be accompanied by a letter of justification.

In everyday life, you solve math problems all the time. In this setting, you need to solve a variety of math calculations just to get the shift started.

The crew hands you a list of supplies needed for each ambulance. Your task will be to write the requisition in a way that keeps the supply costs for each ambulance to less than $200. With a quick glance you can estimate which way you want to fill out your requisitions. If the total by ambulance keeps your requests under $200, that is the way to go. If ordering supplies from different vendors will keep the cost for supplies on the requisition at less than $200, then that is the way you will write them up.

Rounding To estimate, you will need to know how to round numbers up or down. In most cases, round-

ing simply means that if a number contains a decimal point or fraction, you will change it to a whole number. For example, if one prefilled syringe of lidocaine costs $2.73, it would be easier for you to add it to your calculations if it were a whole number. The number 2.73 is between 2.00 and 3.00. In rounding, 0.50 is the middle point. To round the number, do the following:

- If the number after the decimal is less than 0.50, the number is rounded down. For example, for a number of 2.49 or lower, round down to 2.00.
- If the number after the decimal is 0.50 or more, the number is rounded up. For example, for a number of 2.50, round up to 3.00. Also, for a larger number, for example 2.51 or higher, round up to 3.00.

In this case, because the number is 2.73, round up to 3.00, resulting in an estimation of $3.00 for the prefilled syringe of lidocaine.

In the previous examples, the numbers were rounded up or down to the nearest whole number (2 or 3). You can also round up or down to the nearest multiple of 5, multiple of 10, and so forth. Rounding to multiples of 5 or 10 can make it easier to add numbers in your head because these numbers are familiar—we use multiples of 5 and 10 all the time when we use money.

When rounding to the nearest multiple of 5 or 10, first figure out the halfway point between the two nearest multiples of 5 or 10. To round $2.73 to the nearest multiple of 5, the two nearest numbers are 0 and 5. The halfway point between 0 and 5 is 2.50. Because 2.73 is greater than 2.50, it would be rounded up to 5.

To round $2.73 to the nearest multiple of 10, round down to 0 or up to 10. In this case, the halfway point between 0 and 10 is 5. Because 2.73 is less than 5, it would be rounded down to 0.

Table 1-4 ▸ contains a list of supplies needed for the two ambulances and the price for each supply. Before spending time writing the requisitions, you can quickly estimate the costs by rounding the cost of the items to the nearest multiple of 5. Jot down your estimates, and add up the total in the column at right. (Note that boxes and cases cannot be split for a single order.)

Table 1-5 ▸ shows the correct cost estimates; use this to check your work.

Estimating the total cost of the supplies *per ambulance* results in each requisition totaling more than $200.00. Therefore, you would need to write two letters justifying your orders of more than $200.00.

A side note: if a box of supplies could be split between more than one ambulance, we wouldn't have

6 IV setups

Table 1-4 Sample Table of Supplies Needed for Two Ambulances

Unit 1 Supply List	Price	Estimated Cost
6 IV setups	$150.00/box of 50	
8 500-mL bags of saline	$28.23/case of 10	
4 rolls of roller gauze	$5.00/12 rolls	
2 trauma dressings	$3.00 each	
1 prefilled syringe of promethazine	$3.00 each	
2 prefilled syringes of fentanyl	$3.00 each	
1 large vacuum splint	$15.00 each	
4 nonrebreathing face masks	$25.00/case of 10	
2 nasal cannulas	$23.00/case of 10	
1 package of ECG electrodes	$6.00/pouch	
4 fitted sheets	$40.00/case of 10	
1 bag-mask device	$12.00 each	
1 7.5 ET tube	$4.00 each	
1 end cap CO_2 detector	$15.00 each	
1 tube holder	$8.00 each	
Total		
Unit 2 Supply List	Price	Estimated Cost
4 IV setups	$150.00/box of 50	
4 500-mL bags of saline	$28.23/case of 10	
2 rolls of roller gauze	$5.00/12 rolls	
1 bottle of aspirin	$4.00 each	
1 prefilled syringe of morphine sulfate	$4.00 each	
1 prefilled syringe of lidocaine	$2.73 each	
2 prefilled syringes of epinephrine, 1:10,000	$2.00 each	
1 set of Combipads	$38.00 each	
3 fitted sheets	$40.00/case of 10	
1 bag-mask device	$12.00 each	
1 7.0 ET tube	$4.00 each	
1 end cap CO_2 detector	$15.00 each	
1 tube holder	$8.00 each	
Total		

Table 1-5   Sample of Estimated Costs for Supplies Needed for Two Ambulances

Unit 1 Supply List	Price	Estimated Cost
6 IV setups	$150.00/box of 50	150
8 500-mL bags of saline	$28.23/case of 10	30
4 rolls of roller gauze	$5.00/12 rolls	5
2 trauma dressings	$3.00 each	5
1 prefilled syringe of promethazine	$3.00 each	5
2 prefilled syringes of fentanyl	$3.00 each	5
1 large vacuum splint	$15.00 each	15
4 nonrebreathing face masks	$25.00/case of 10	25
2 nasal cannulas	$23.00/case of 10	25
1 package of ECG electrodes	$6.00/pouch	5
4 fitted sheets	$40.00/case of 10	40
1 bag-mask device	$12.00 each	10
1 7.5 ET tube	$4.00 each	5
1 end cap CO_2 detector	$15.00 each	15
1 tube holder	$8.00 each	10
Total		**$350**
Unit 2 Supply List	Price	Estimated Cost
4 IV setups	$150.00/box of 50	150
4 500-mL bags of saline	$28.23/case of 10	30
2 rolls of roller gauze	$5.00/12 rolls	5
1 bottle of aspirin	$4.00 each	5
1 prefilled syringe of morphine sulfate	$4.00 each	5
1 prefilled syringe of lidocaine	$2.73 each	5
2 prefilled syringes of epinephrine, 1:10,000	$2.00 each	5
1 set of Combipads	$38.00 each	40
3 fitted sheets	$40.00/case of 10	40
1 bag-mask device	$12.00 each	10
1 7.0 ET tube	$4.00 each	5
1 end cap CO_2 detector	$15.00 each	15
1 tube holder	$8.00 each	10
Total		**$325**

to spend as much (for example, above, we've ordered IV setups, roller gauze, and fitted sheets twice—one for each ambulance). But for the purposes of this example, we are assuming that supplies cannot be split between ambulances.

Once you have estimated the cost per ambulance, you can estimate the cost for ordering the supplies from two different vendors. For example, you could order respiratory and cardiac supplies from one vendor and all other supplies from another. Supplies are listed by vendor in Table 1-6 ▼. As before, estimate the cost to the nearest multiple of 5 and write it in the column at right.

Once you have completed your work, check it against the estimates shown in Table 1-7 ▶.

Ordering by vendor means that only one of your orders exceeds the $200.00 limit, and, therefore, you have to write only one letter to justify the order that is more than $200.00. Note that the total numbers of IV setups, roller gauze, and fitted sheets needed for the two ambulances is less than the number in a box or case, so the price is listed only once, rather than twice as in the example estimating for each ambulance.

Therefore, you opt to order by vendor.

Estimating With the Numbers 5 and 10   Estimates are one of the most valuable skills when performing your calculations. *The purpose of estimating the answer to a math calculation is to save time or to ensure that the result from your exact calculation is reason-*

Table 1-6 Sample of Supplies Organized by Vendor

Vendor 1 Order List	Price	Estimated Cost
4 nonrebreathing face masks	$25.00/case of 10	
2 nasal cannulas	$23.00/case of 10	
1 package of ECG electrodes	$6.00/pouch	
2 bag-mask devices	$12.00 each	
1 7.0 ET tube	$4.00 each	
1 7.5 ET tube	$4.00 each	
2 end cap CO_2 detectors	$15.00 each	
2 tube holders	$8.00 each	
1 set of Combipads	$38.00/set	
Total		
Vendor 2 Order List	Price	Estimated Cost
10 IV setups	$150.00/box of 50	
12 500-mL bags of saline	$28.23/case of 10	
2 trauma dressings	$3.00 each	
1 prefilled syringe of promethazine	$3.00 each	
2 prefilled syringes of fentanyl	$3.00 each	
1 large vacuum splint	$15.00 each	
6 rolls of roller gauze	$5.00/12 rolls	
1 bottle of aspirin	$4.00 each	
1 prefilled syringe of morphine sulfate	$4.00 each	
1 prefilled syringe of lidocaine	$2.73 each	
2 prefilled syringes of epinephrine, 1:10,000	$2.00 each	
7 fitted sheets	$40.00/case of 10	
Total		

Table 1-7 Sample of Estimated Costs Organized by Vendor

Vendor 1 Order List	Price	Estimated Cost
4 nonrebreathing face masks	$25.00/case of 10	25
2 nasal cannulas	$23.00/case of 10	25
1 package of ECG electrodes	$6.00/pouch	5
2 bag-mask devices	$12.00 each	25
1 7.0 ET tube	$4.00 each	5
1 7.5 ET tube	$4.00 each	5
2 end cap CO_2 detectors	$15.00 each	30
2 tube holders	$8.00 each	20
1 set of Combipads	$38.00/set	40
Total		**$180**
Vendor 2 Order List	Price	Estimated Cost
10 IV setups	$150.00/box of 50	150
12 500-mL bags saline	$28.23/case of 10	60
2 trauma dressings	$3.00 each	5
1 prefilled syringe of promethazine	$3.00 each	5
2 prefilled syringes of fentanyl	$3.00 each	5
1 large vacuum splint	$15.00 each	15
6 rolls of roller gauze	$5.00/12 rolls	5
1 bottle of aspirin	$4.00 each	5
1 prefilled syringe of morphine sulfate	$4.00 each	5
1 prefilled syringe of lidocaine	$2.73 each	5
2 prefilled syringes of epinephrine, 1:10,000	$2.00 each	5
7 fitted sheets	$40.00/case of 10	40
Total		**$305**

able. If the estimate is in the ballpark of what seems to be a reasonable approach, then spending more time to calculate an exact figure is the next step. Sometimes the estimate is all that is needed.

Here is a recap of how to approach an estimated answer.

When you go out to breakfast with the crew and it is your turn to pick up the check, it is important to know if you have enough money in your wallet to cover the bill. The usual breakfast spot costs about $8 per person for the breakfast buffet, including coffee.

With a total of five people at breakfast, you quickly estimate what you need in your wallet. Estimating $10 apiece for five people adds up to about $50, which provides a bit of room in case one of the crew orders something extra.

Without putting a lot of thought or effort into this calculation, you estimated the amount of money you need to cover the check at breakfast. A closer look at what your brain processed will throw a few solid tools into your paramedic math toolkit.

The number 10 is used in our lives every day, thanks to money calculations. Young children learn to count by tens easily and on their fingers, and from there we grow up practicing using multiples of 10 on a daily basis. You took advantage of this skill when it came to rounding the numbers to estimate the check.

The other number that made estimating the check easy is 5. The total number of people eating equaled 5, and you multiplied that number by 10. We are adept at using nickels and dimes as units of measure every day. Multiplying 5×10 did not cause you to drag out scratch paper to calculate an answer.

If the number of people had totaled eight, you could have just as readily used your estimating skills and rounded the numbers to something easy to use for calculating. This estimate can be done in your head by saying to yourself, "8 people at $10 apiece is $80." If you have $100 in your wallet, you know you have the check covered.

In both cases, you overestimated the check to be safe. In other words, you rounded the numbers *up* to the nearest numbers that were easy to work with.

Now, go back to the problem of deciding how to requisition the supplies for the two units. As part of your job as captain, you have become familiar with the cost of supplies for the station. Although you have not memorized the precise costs, the ballpark figures are not hard to remember. Rounding the cost of each item to a number that is easy to add—say, 5 or 10—makes it possible to figure the total costs for each unit quite easily. In this case, you know you are in the ballpark and the chances for mistakes are slim because the numbers are easy to work with and you have lots of practice using 5 and 10.

Estimating With the Number 2

The tones drop for a one-car motor vehicle crash (MVC). Dispatch confirms that there is only one patient, the driver. You make a quick calculation before sending out a crew on Unit 3 to respond to the call.

You are responsible for the narcotics inventory, and you know that there are two prefilled syringes with fentanyl on board instead of the usual four syringes after the last shift. Other than that, the ambulance is fully stocked. If only one patient is involved in the crash, the transport time is 20 minutes to the trauma center from the scene. Fentanyl can be dosed, per protocol, as 1 to 3 micrograms per kilogram of body weight (µg/kg) twice during the transport. Will there be enough fentanyl for the average patient without restocking?

You quickly *estimate* the solution:
- An average man weighs 200 lb.
- There are 0.45 kilograms per pound. Therefore, kilograms are a bit less than half the weight in pounds: 200 lb divided by 2 is a bit more than 100 kg.
- If the crew can give 1 to 3 µg/kg, then using 2 µg (because it is in the midrange) means the crew needs about 100 × 2 µg of fentanyl on board, or *200 µg of fentanyl* for just one dose.
- Each prefilled syringe contains 100 µg. The crew has 200 µg on board (100 µg × 2 syringes).

The crew has only enough fentanyl on board to administer one dose of fentanyl, not nearly enough to send the unit out.

"Hang on a minute!" you yell to the crew. "You need more fentanyl to roll Unit 3. Go ahead and roll Unit 4; it's fully stocked. If there's a second patient, call for backup."

Estimating whether there was enough fentanyl on board for the call took just a minute. In this case, you used the number 2 to quickly solve the problem and make a decision.

Multiplying and dividing by 2 is a math calculation that most of us can do without a calculator. We usually think of the function as "cutting it in half" or "doubling the amount." Using the numbers 2, 5, and 10 wisely can get you in the ballpark when you need a quick estimate. Now you have a few tools in your jump bag to estimate medication calculations.

Try estimating the groups of numbers at the end of this chapter. Remember to use your estimating tools (the numbers 2, 5, and 10) from your jump bag.

Multiplying and Dividing by 10

Multiplying and dividing by 10 is as simple as moving the decimal point to the left or to the right. The answer is divided by 10 when the decimal point is moved one place to the left and multiplied by 10 when the decimal point is moved one place to the right.

For example:

$$162 \div 10 = 16.2$$

There are two questions to ask at the end of every calculation:
1. Is the answer reasonable? That is, does it make sense?
2. How precise does the math need to be?

Is the answer reasonable?
How precise does the math need to be?

Dividing by 10 moves the decimal point one place to the left. This answer makes sense because 16.2 is smaller than the original number, 162.

The preceding example highlights the importance of transcribing calculations neatly and clearly. If the decimal point is not easily seen in the correct place, the dose can be mistaken for a dose signifi-

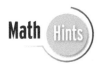

The decimal point in whole numbers is presumed to be positioned after the whole number. Such a number may or may not be written with a zero to make the decimal place obvious. In other words, if the number is "12," the decimal point is assumed to follow the "2," as in 12.0.

cantly smaller or larger than the patient needs and a catastrophic medication error could occur.

Table 1-8 ✦ shows a few examples. In these examples, notice how a zero is used to mark a place before the decimal point when the number is less than 1. As mentioned, this makes it easier to see the decimal point.

In all of these examples, the *answers make sense*. The solutions when the numbers are divided are smaller than the original numbers, and the solutions when the numbers are multiplied are larger than the original numbers. In some cases, such as when multiplying whole numbers, as in the first two multiplication examples in Table 1-8, the decimal point is not shown, but is understood. It is easy to make an error when you move the decimal point, so checking that your answer makes sense is critical.

Administering $\frac{1}{10}$ the prescribed dose or administering 10 times the prescribed dose of a medication can have a dramatic—and sometimes deadly—effect on your patients.

Taking this function to the next step is straightforward. Multiplying by 100 is the same as multiplying by 10 and then multiplying by 10 again. Dividing by 100 is the same as dividing by 10 and then dividing by 10 again.

Follow the examples in Table 1-9 ✦ to see the next step.

Table 1-8 Moving the Decimal Point to Multiply and Divide by Ten	
Multiplying × 10 (decimal point moves right)	Dividing × 10 (decimal point moves left)
12 × 10 = 120	12 ÷ 10 = 1.2
158 × 10 = 1,580	158 ÷ 10 = 15.8
1.5 × 10 = 15	1.5 ÷ 10 = 0.15
0.32 × 10 = 3.2	0.32 ÷ 10 = 0.032

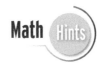

Notice the pattern: When multiplying or dividing by multiples of 10, the decimal point moves one place for 10 (which has one zero), two places for 100 (which has two zeros), and three places for 1,000 (which has three zeros). You can predict correctly that the decimal point will move four places when multiplying or dividing by 10,000, and so forth.

Table 1-9 Moving the Decimal Point to Multiply and Divide by 10, 100, or 1,000		
Multiply × 10 (one decimal place to the right)	Multiply × 100 (two decimal places to the right)	Multiply × 1,000 (three decimal places to the right)
12 × 10 = 120	12 × 100 = 1,200	12 × 1,000 = 12,000
158 × 10 = 1,580	158 × 100 = 15,800	158 × 1,000 = 158,000
1.5 × 10 = 15	1.5 × 100 = 150	1.5 × 1,000 = 1,500
0.32 × 10 = 3.2	0.32 × 100 = 32	0.32 × 1,000 = 320
Divide by 10 (one decimal place to the left)	Divide by 100 (two decimal places to the left)	Divide by 1,000 (three decimal places to the left)
12 ÷ 10 = 1.2	12 ÷ 100 = 0.12	12 ÷ 1,000 = 0.012
158 ÷ 10 = 15.8	158 ÷ 100 = 1.58	158 ÷ 1,000 = 0.158
1.5 ÷ 10 = 0.15	1.5 ÷ 100 = 0.015	1.5 ÷ 1,000 = 0.0015
0.32 ÷ 10 = 0.032	0.32 ÷ 100 = 0.0032	0.32 ÷ 1,000 = 0.00032

The decimal point moves to the left for division.
The decimal point moves to the right for multiplication.

Fill in Table 1-10 ▼ to practice multiplying and dividing by 10.

Here is one more tip for using the number 10 to make life easier when you are doing calculations: The relationship between 5 and 10 can be seen readily. Because 5 is half of 10, when we need to multiply a number by 5, it may be easier to multiply by 10 and then cut the answer in half. We call this the trick of 5s. For example:

12 × 5 is not an obvious answer.

12 × 10 simply enough gives 120.

It may be easier to multiply 12 × 10, get 120 for an answer, and then cut the answer in half to arrive at 60 a little more quickly. This technique is just one more tool for your jump bag.

Try this problem both ways and see how it works for you:

$$14 \times 5 = ?$$

If you multiply this number by 10 and cut the answer in half, the problem becomes

$$14 \times 10 = 140$$
$$140 \div 2 = 70$$

Finally, if you need to multiply by numbers that end in zero, you may be able to rearrange the way that number looks to make the multiplication easier.

Here is an example:

$$18 \times 20 = ?$$

This calculation can be done quickly *in your head* if you think in tens.

Work the answer this way.

First, think 18 × 20 is the same as 18 × 2 × 10.

Take the pieces that are the easiest:

18 × 2 = 36

Then finish the calculation with the last piece.

36 × 10 = 360

More practice problems with this technique appear at the end of this chapter.

Coupling estimating with quick calculations using the numbers 2, 5, and 10 can often give you enough information to make a quick decision. Determining how useful an exact answer will be versus an estimated answer is an important part of providing care. Sometimes estimates are good enough by themselves, for example, when ordering supplies and ensuring that your calculations are reasonable. Sometimes they are used to determine whether a more precise answer makes sense, as in many medication dosing calculations.

Conclusion

Congratulations! You have just finished estimating math calculations in your head and mastered the basics of using decimals. It is quite simple once you see the pattern. Estimating calculations and moving the decimal point are great tools to get you in the ballpark.

Try the problems at the end of the chapter that require you to move the decimal points while you estimate the solutions. Remember to ask yourself whether the answers are reasonable; that determination will help you be sure the decimal point is being moved in the correct direction.

Table 1-10 Practicing Multiplying and Dividing by 10, 100, and 1,000		
Multiply × 10	Multiply × 100	Multiply × 1,000
4 × 10 =	4 × 100 =	4 × 1,000 =
1,893 × 10 =	1,893 × 100 =	1,893 × 1,000 =
2.6 × 10 =	2.6 × 100 =	2.6 × 1,000 =
0.07 × 10 =	0.07 × 100 =	0.07 × 1,000 =
Divide by 10	Divide by 100	Divide by 1,000
4 ÷ 10 =	4 ÷ 100 =	4 ÷ 1,000 =
1,893 ÷ 10 =	1,893 ÷ 100 =	1,893 ÷ 1,000 =
2.6 ÷ 10 =	2.6 ÷ 100 =	2.6 ÷ 1,000 =
0.07 ÷ 10 =	0.07 ÷ 100 =	0.07 ÷ 1,000 =

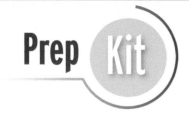

Math Vocabulary

decimals   Numbers based on the number 10 and that contain a dot (point) between whole numbers (written to the left of the dot) and numbers that are smaller than whole numbers (written to the right of the dot). The numbers to the right of the dot constitute decimal fractions.

denominator   The bottom part of a fraction, for example, the 10 in $\frac{1}{10}$.

estimate   To make an approximation of a number, rather than an actual calculation.

fraction   A number expressed using a numerator and a denominator, for example $\frac{1}{10}$.

improper fraction   A fraction in which the numerator is larger than the denominator.

mixed number   A number written as a whole number and a fraction.

multiple   A number that can be divided by the original number(s) without a remainder. For example; 5, 10, 15, 20, 25, 30, are multiples of 5, and 24 is a multiple of 6 and 4.

numerator   The top part of a fraction, for example, the 1 in $\frac{1}{10}$.

percentage   A portion of 100, noted with the "%" sign.

proper fraction   A fraction in which the numerator is smaller than the denominator.

round   To express a number as a convenient whole number. A rounded number can be used in a mathematical calculation when estimating.

trick of 5s   A method used to make it easier to multiply by 5, in which a number is multiplied by 10 and the answer is then cut in half.

Practice Problems

Answer the problems to the best of your ability. If you get stuck, refer back to the chapter to review the concept.

1. Fill in the chart below. Follow the example in the first row.

Text Format	Fraction Format	Decimal Format
Twenty-five and three hundredths	$25\frac{3}{100}$	25.03
Three and sixty-seven hundredths		
		0.3
	$126\frac{9}{10}$	
Nine hundred eighty-seven thousandths		
	$327\frac{98}{100}$	

2. Fill in the blanks in the chart below. The percentages are filled in for you. You have learned that percentage is one of the three math languages.

Decimal	Fraction	Percentage
1.2		1 and 20 = 120%
3.68		3 and 68 = 368%
	$\frac{25}{100}$	25%
0.10	$\frac{1}{10}$	10%
0.5		50%
	$\frac{75}{1,000}$	7.5%

3. Fill in the blanks below.

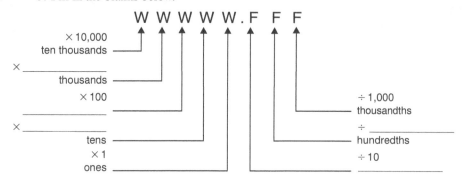

Calculate the following fraction conversions.

4. Convert $\frac{4}{10}$ to a decimal fraction.

5. Convert $\frac{88}{100}$ to a decimal fraction.

6. Convert $\frac{10}{100}$ to a decimal fraction.

7. Convert $\frac{384}{1,000}$ to a decimal fraction.

8. Convert $\frac{5}{1,000}$ to a decimal fraction.

Estimate the answers. Practice rounding the numbers in the following columns into multiples of 2, 5, and 10 for quick calculations. Complete the function indicated. Check your estimated answers with the actual calculated answer in the back of the book.

9. 3 + 7 + 23 + 12

10. 11 + 22 + 33 + 42

11. 76 − 5 + 12

12. 356 − 28

13. 200 ÷ 2

14. 90×11

15. 26×2

16. 3×0.8

17. $76 - 26 - 13 - 6$

Solve the following calculations by moving the decimal point.

18. 1.8×10

19. $1.8 \div 10$

20. 23.8748×100

21. $23.8748 \div 100$

22. 0.6×100

23. $0.6 \div 100$

24. 232.67×10

25. $232.67 \div 10$

26. 232.67×100

27. $232.67 \div 100$

28. $232.67 \times 1,000$

29. $232.67 \div 1,000$

30. 136.278×10

31. 136.278×100

32. $136.278 \times 1,000$

33. $136.278 \div 10$

34. $136.278 \div 100$

35. $136.278 \div 1,000$

36. 186×10

37. 186×100

38. $186 \times 1,000$

39. $186 \div 10$

40. $186 \div 100$

41. $186 \div 1,000$

42. 26.78×10

43. 26.78×100

44. $26.78 \times 1,000$

45. $26.78 \div 10$

46. $26.78 \div 100$

47. $26.78 \div 1,000$

48. 0.3×10

49. 0.3×100

50. $0.3 \times 1,000$

51. $0.3 \div 10$

52. $0.3 \div 100$

53. $0.3 \div 1,000$

Fill in the following table according to the instructions.

54. Use the trick of 5s to solve the following calculations. The column at left shows the problem to be solved. Use the remaining columns to use the trick of 5s (first, multiply by 10, then divide by 2.)

Problem	Foundation Number	$\times$ 10	$\div$ 2
32×5	32		
6.5×5	6.5		
7.36×5	7.36		
0.14×5	0.14		
1.02×5	1.02		

Answer the following word problems.

55. You are ordered to give a patient a medication. When you draw up the medication in your syringe, you only have $\frac{15}{16}$ of the amount you need to give. Even though you do not have the full amount, the physician gives the order to administer the medication. What percentage and decimal fraction of the medication did you administer?

56. A patient is being given a medication in $\frac{1}{6}$ amounts of the supplied dose in one vial. In 1 day, the patient receives the medication 15 times. What is the total percentage and decimal number of vials will you need to have on hand each day to give the proper amount of medication?

57. You are in the field without a calculator or writing materials. You need to give 4.5 times the normal dose of a medication to a patient. The usual amount to be given each time is 3.03 mg. By using an estimate, which of the following should you give?

   A. 1.4 mg

   B. 12.5 mg

   C. 14 mg

   D. 123 mg

58. When responding to a multicasualty incident, you have two groups of patients. In the green group are 57 patients, and in the yellow group are 58. To quickly determine the number of patients in both groups, calculate the total by rounding.

59. You need to give 9 mg of a medication 50 times. Determine the total number of milligrams needed by multiplying or dividing by 10.

Back to Basics: Adding, Subtracting, Multiplying, and Dividing

Introduction

Calculating math problems—even the simplest problems—can be a challenge when there are distractions. Sick patients, anxious family members, traffic, and our own adrenaline are all distractions. Using the skills learned in Chapter 1 and bringing them to the next level in this chapter adds a few methods of getting the correct answer quickly and being assured that the answers are reasonable. It is all about getting back to basics.

Manipulating numbers is the easiest way to use them. You have already taken advantage of this tool when you estimated with groups of numbers. In addition, regrouping numbers so their values do not change (for example, writing 132 as 100 + 30 + 2) can make math simpler.

Addition

Take a look at the following calculation:

$$126 + 362 = ?$$

At first glance, it looks like you will need a piece of paper and pencil to solve this problem and will have to remember how to "carry over" numbers and perform other, more complicated tasks. But watch what happens when you regroup the numbers—it turns this equation into an easy addition problem:

126 is the same as 100 + 20 + 6

362 is the same as 300 + 60 + 2

Here the numbers are rearranged into forms that are easy to add in your head. Solving the new problem is a matter of adding 10s again, as when estimating the answer. Speaking of estimating, did you try it first?

126 is about 125

362 is about 360

Your ballpark answer is about 485.

Now, find the exact answer:

126 is the same as   100 + 20 + 6
362 is the same as   <u>300 + 60 + 2</u>
                      400 + 80 + 8 = 488
(That number is definitely in the same ballpark as the estimate.)

To work this problem in your head, you can look at the "places." Add the hundreds, add the tens, and then add the ones.

Here is another problem:

$$368 + 527 = ?$$

Estimate the answer to the nearest multiple of 10 for a ballpark figure:

$$370 + 530 = 900$$

Now, rearrange the numbers to make them easy to add up:

368 is the same as   300 + 60 + 8
527 is the same as   <u>500 + 20 + 7</u>
                      800 + 80 + 15 = 895
(The estimate was 900.)

This technique works for subtraction, multiplication, and division as well.

Practice

1. $159 + 206 = ?$

2. $361 + 457 = ?$

Subtraction

Try the following problem:

$$127 - 23 = ?$$

Estimate the answer to get a ballpark figure:

127 is about 125

23 is about 25

125 − 25 = 100 for an estimate

Now perform the exact calculation:

For subtraction, leave the first number alone and just "take away" numbers that are easy to use.

127 − 23 can be manipulated like this:

127 − 20 = 107

That leaves 3 more to "take away" so that the entire 23 will have been subtracted as called for by the calculation.

107 − 3 = 104

The actual calculation was:

127 − 20 − 3 = 104 (The estimate was 100.)

Practice
1. 263 − 14 = ?

2. 515 − 36 = ?

Adding Decimals

To add decimals, regular addition is used. The main fact to remember is to align the decimal points of the numbers being added. For example:

$$5.80$$
$$+ \quad 30.3$$

$$1,869.2345$$
$$+ \quad 70.0$$

$$0.0004$$
$$+ 100.07$$

Once the decimal points are aligned, there are columns of numbers to add. However, in some places, there are no numbers, so adding zeros helps keep the columns clear. The following are the three previous examples with zeros added:

$$05.80$$
$$+ 30.30$$

$$1,869.2345$$
$$+ \quad 0070.0000$$

$$000.0004$$
$$+ 100.0700$$

Aligning the decimal point makes it easier to add the correct numbers. Solve the same sample problems, and write in the zeros to help keep the columns clear.

Practice
1.   5.80
   + 30.3
      ?

2. 1,869.2345
   + 70.0
      ?

3.   0.0004
   + 100.07
      ?

Subtracting Decimals

When subtracting decimals, regular subtraction is used, but again, the decimal points of the numbers being subtracted must be aligned. For example:

$$280.40$$
$$- \quad 5.0$$

$$32.485$$
$$- 0.010$$

$$218.64$$
$$- 0.001$$

Again, writing zeros in the places without numbers will clarify the columns. The following are the three previous examples with zeros added:

$$280.40$$
$$- 005.00$$

$$32.485$$
$$- 00.010$$

$$218.640$$
$$- 000.001$$

Solve the same sample problems, and write in the zeros to help keep the columns clear.

Practice

1. 280.40
  − 5.0
  ?

2. 32.485
  − 0.010
  ?

3. 218.64
  − 0.001
  ?

Multiplication

The same technique can be used for solving problems that involve multiplication. Work the following problems by rearranging the numbers. Remember to estimate your answers first.

1. $24 \times 3 = ?$
Estimate the answer: $25 \times 3 = 75$
Calculate the exact answer:

  24×3 can be rearranged as follows:

  20×3 and 4×3

  20×3 is solved by multiplying 2×3 and adding the zero (multiplying by 10) = 60, and then adding $4 \times 3 = 12$

  $60 + 12 = 72$ (The estimated answer was 75.)

Note that you need to *add* the pieces together once you break the numbers down and multiply.

2. $25 \times 11 = ?$
Estimate the answer: $25 \times 10 = 250$
Calculate the exact answer:

25×10 added to $25 \times 1 = ?$ (The 11 has been rearranged into 10 and 1.)

Read the problem this way now: "I need ten 25s and then one more 25 to have eleven 25s." It's fairly simple to do the math now.

$25 \times 10 = 250$ plus one more $25 = 275$ (The estimate was 250.)

3. $81 \times 4 = ?$
Estimate the answer: $80 \times 4 = ?$ Hmmm…. 50×4 will be on the low side, and 100×4 will be on the high side. 80 is almost in the middle of 50 and 100, so the answer should be somewhere near the middle. $50 \times 4 = 200$ and $100 \times 4 = 400$, so the estimate is between 200 and 400, or 300.

  Rearrange the numbers:

  81×4 is the same as 80×4, and an additional 1×4 is needed

  $80 \times 4 = 320$ (8×4, then the answer $\times 10$)

  $1 \times 4 = 4$

  $320 + 4 = 324$

The original estimate indicated the answer was somewhere in the middle between 200 and 400, or 300. That rough estimate was enough to indicate that the calculated answer is in the ballpark: 324 is a reasonable answer.

Here is another example in which the numbers can be rearranged:

$$100 \times 10 \times 6 \times 3 = 18,000$$

This problem can be rearranged like any one of the following equations and will have the same result:

$10 \times 10 \times 10 \times 6 \times 3 = 18,000$

  where "100" is rearranged to 10×10

$100 \times 6 \times 3 \times 10 = 18,000$

  where the numbers are multiplied in a different order and

$10 \times 10 \times 5 \times 2 \times 3 \times 2 \times 3 = 18,000$

  where most of the numbers are written differently

This is a great tool to put on the notepad for future use, as you will see in future chapters.

In the following addition and subtraction examples, it does not matter in what order the operation is completed.

$2 + 3 + 5 = 10$ and $5 + 2 + 3 = 10$

$11 - 5 - 1 = 5$ and $11 - 1 - 5 = 5$

A number can be positive or negative. Positive numbers are the numbers we are used to dealing with—numbers above 0, such as 1, 2, 3, and 4. Negative numbers are numbers that are less than zero and have a negative, or minus, sign in front of them, such as -1, -2, -3, and -4. This information is useful when moving numbers in addition and subtraction problems. To rearrange a problem that involves subtraction, the negative sign must be kept with the negative number. By using this principle, the preceding calculation that uses subtraction may also be written as $-5 + 11 - 1 = 5$, but the "$-$" and "$+$" signs must be kept with the correct numbers.

Practice

1. $36 \times 2 = ?$

2. $118 \times 5 = ?$

Here is a refresher of information from Chapter 1. Solve the following problems by moving the decimal point. Remember that in division, the answers should be smaller than the number being divided.

3. $12.6 \div 10 = ?$

4. $12,356 \div 100 = ?$
   (*Hint:* $12,356 = 12,356.0$)

5. $745.85656 \div 10 = ?$

6. $0.32 \div 100 = ?$
   (*Hint:* The decimal point still moves two places to the left.)

7. $468 \times 1,000 = ?$

8. $4.68 \times 1,000 = ?$
   (*Hint:* The decimal point still moves three places to the right, the same as the number of zeros.)

9. $2.6 \times 10 = ?$

10. $32.6 \times 5 = ?$
    (*Hint:* 32.6×10, then $\div 2$. Remember the trick of 5s?)

Order of Operations   The previous section showed that when only multiplying or only adding and subtracting, the order of the numbers does not matter. This is not the case when the equation includes a mix of different kinds of math, such as multiplication and addition, division and subtraction, division and addition, and multiplication and subtraction. In these cases, math problems follow a rule called order of operations. This rule means that when solving an equation, a certain order must be followed. Specifically, the order of operations is as follows:

1. All operations inside parentheses are done first.
2. All multiplication and division functions are completed, working from left to right in the equation.
3. Last, all addition and subtraction functions are completed, working from left to right in the equation.

What does the order of operations mean to paramedics? In prehospital care, rearranging numbers to simplify problem solving is important for speed and minimizing errors. However, not all numbers in equations can be rearranged and still lead to a correct result. The order of operations needs to be followed, and rearranging the numbers must not result in violation of the order: items in parentheses first, multiplication and division second, and addition and subtraction last.

Here are some examples.

$$10 \times 3 + 4 \div 2 = ?$$

This example contains a mix of multiplication and division. According to the order of operations, the multiplication and division must be done first. This means:

$$10 \times 3 = 30$$
$$4 \div 2 = 2$$

This changes the equation to $30 + 2$, which is now easy to solve. The answer is 32. However, if the preceding equation were solved simply in the order in which it appears and not according to the order of operations, the result would be 17 ($10 \times 3 = 30$; $30 + 4 = 34$; $34 \div 2 = 17$). Parentheses in an equation help to clarify and separate the operations to be done.

The next example shows an equation that includes parentheses. Remember that according to the order of operations, anything in parentheses must be done first, even if the numbers in parentheses are being added or subtracted. Here is an example:

$$(5 + 7) \times 20 = ?$$

Because $5 + 7$ is in parentheses, that part of the equation must be solved first, even though only addition is being done. Therefore, because $5 + 7 = 12$, the equation becomes 12×20. By using skills from Chapter 1, you can break down 12×20 as follows:

$$10 \times 20 = 200$$
$$2 \times 20 = 40$$

Finding the answer is now easy: $200 + 40 = 240$. Note that you could also rearrange 12×20 as follows:

$$4 \times 3 \times 20 = ?$$

This rearrangement is also a bit easier: $3 \times 20 = 60$, and $60 \times 4 = 240$ ($6 \times 4 = 24$, and a zero is added to multiply by 10). The same correct answer, 240, was found in two ways.

Here is one more example, which is more complicated. It mixes all of the elements in the order of operations rule.

$$16 \div 2 + (80 - 5 \times 4) = ?$$

Items in parentheses must be solved first. Within the parentheses, subtraction and multiplication are used. According to the order of operations, multiplication is done before subtraction. Therefore, 5×4 is solved first. It equals 20. The equation within the parentheses therefore becomes $80 - 20$, or 60.

Once the equation in the parentheses has been solved, the parentheses can be removed:

$$16 \div 2 + 60 = ?$$

According to the order of operations, division is done before addition. Therefore, $16 \div 2$ is solved first. Remember from Chapter 1 that dividing a number by 2 is the same as taking its half. Half of 16 is 8. The equation is now:

$$8 + 60 = ?$$

The answer is now clear: 68.

Doing the calculations but ignoring the order of operations gives the wrong answer.

Practice

1. $80 \div 2 + (132 - 12 \times 11) = ?$

2. $16 - 8 + 14 \times 5 \div 2 = ?$

Division

Try the following problem using the tools in your jump bag to estimate and then rearrange and solve: Divide 126 mg into two doses.

1. Estimate the answer: 126 ÷ 2 is more than 100 ÷ 2 = 50 and less than 150 ÷ 2 = 75. (Here, the US dollar is used to make these problems easier: $1.50 ÷ 2 = 75 cents.)
2. The calculated answer should be between 50 and 75. Calculate the answer by rearranging the numbers: 126 ÷ 2 can be rearranged to look like 100 ÷ 2; 20 ÷ 2; and 6 ÷ 2.

$$100 ÷ 2 = 50$$
$$20 ÷ 2 = 10$$
$$6 ÷ 2 = 3$$

Add up the pieces (it's now quick and easy), and the answer is 63. The estimated answer was between 50 and 75.

The more practice you have in rearranging numbers to make the math simple, the easier the problems become. All math problems in this text, which represent all you will need to know for calculations for medication administration, can be broken down into simple components.

The problems at the end of this chapter will give you more practice and point out hints for rearranging the problems in an easy format. This is where the games begin—when you pull out the tools in your jump bag to make calculations quick and easy.

Practice

1. Divide 200 mg into 8 doses.

2. Divide 153 mg into 3 doses.

When the Calculator Batteries Die

There comes a time in every calculator's life when the batteries die. In this technology-driven age, we are humbly reminded that the old-fashioned way of doing things is worthy of mastering. Multiplication and division are two math operations that become easier with practice. Calculators are a gift of speed and ease when the batteries work and a handicap when the batteries die or the wrong buttons are pressed.

Mastering division and multiplication in "manual mode" provides you and your patients with a safety net when the batteries die, the power fails, and the backup method is your brain power. They are skills worth investing in, and it is important to become comfortable with the techniques that dictate how you will get your answers in manual mode.

Multiplication and division are performed by following a pattern of steps. No fancy footwork is needed, but keeping the work neat will go a long way in keeping the calculations accurate.

Keep your work neat! This will help you avoid misaligning numbers, resulting in inaccurate calculations.

Multiplying in Manual Mode

Multiplying numbers that have two or more digits each is performed by using one number as the foundation number and then dissecting the other number. The purpose of setting up the calculation this way is to take advantage of the same rules that allow multiplication of numbers in any order, to rearrange the way numbers look, and to break the calculation into simpler pieces. The shorthand for multiplying these numbers in manual mode facilitates keeping things lined up, neat, and easy to work the math.

Follow along with the reasoning behind this example:

$$\begin{array}{r} 26 \\ \times\, 23 \\ \hline \end{array}$$

In multiplication, when problems are set up like this (stacked on top of one another), we call the top number the foundation number and the bottom number the multiplier.

In this problem, "26" is the foundation number. Remember that numbers can be multiplied in any order, so either number, 26 or 23, can be set up as the foundation number.

Next, look at the number 23 from a different perspective. The math rule says that 23 can be rearranged. To multiply in the manual mode, the answers to each piece of the problem need to be placed in columns. What you are actually doing is multiplying the foundation number by the pieces of the multiplier.

In the manual mode for multiplication, the number 23 can be written in the following manner:

23 is equal to 2×10 plus 3×1.

In our system of math, the following statements are true:

2 is in the "tens place" and, therefore, represents "2 tens" or "2×10."

3 is in the "ones place" and, therefore, represents "3 ones" or "3×1."

Likewise, in the number 26, "2" is in the tens place, and "6" is in the ones place. The next step is to work the calculation, step by step, in manual mode.

Here is the pattern for manual mode multiplication:

A. Estimate the answer.

B. Do the calculation. Multiply the foundation number by each piece of the multiplier.

C. Add up the like pieces.

Having broken down the multiplier into understandable pieces, the answer will make sense when the calculation is performed and the pieces placed in the correct columns.

Estimate the Answer Begin by estimating the answer.

$$\begin{array}{r} 26 \\ \times\ 23 \\ \hline ? \end{array}$$

26 is approximately 25

23 is approximately 20

25×20 can be rearranged to be $25 \times 2 \times 10$

$25 \times 2 = 50$, and $50 \times 10 = 500$

The estimated answer is 500. Both of the original numbers were estimated on the low side of the original number (25 is less than 26 and 20 is less than 23), so the estimated answer should be *more* than 500, and the actual answer should be more than 500.

Do the Calculation Now perform the actual calculation. The following shows you step by step how this is done.

Multiply the foundation number by each piece of the multiplier. Start by multiplying the number in the ones place, in this case 3, by each number in the foundation number. In this case, $3 \times 6 = 18$. Because the answer is more than 10, the 8 is noted under the line and one 10 is carried over to the tens place. Follow along here:

$$\begin{array}{r} 26 \\ \times\ 23 \\ \hline 8 \end{array}$$

Here the "8 ones" are noted in the ones place under the line where the final answer will be calculated. A "1" is noted over the "tens place" to represent 1 group of 10. This is often said as, "Put down the 8 and carry the 1 (ten)."

The next step is to multiply the 3 times the 2 (tens) in the foundation number.

$$\begin{array}{r} 26 \\ \times\ 23 \\ \hline 78 \end{array}$$

This would be $3 \times 2 = 6$ (*tens*). There is still one more group of ten to add (remember the 1 that you placed above), therefore 7 (*tens*) need to be noted in this first step.

The foundation number has now been multiplied by 3 ones from the multiplier. We move on to multiplying the foundation number by 2 tens from the multiplier. Follow along here.

$$\begin{array}{r} 26 \\ \times\ 23 \\ \hline 78 \\ 2 \end{array}$$

2 (*tens*) $\times$ 6 = 12 (*tens*). Because the multiplier is in tens, the answer will be in tens. The answer goes in the tens place under the 7 in 78.

The pattern from above is repeated when writing an answer that has 2 digits, so this time it will be, $2 \times 6 = 12$; "Put down the 2 and carry the 1 (hundreds this time)."

The last numbers that need to be multiplied are the 2 tens in the multiplier by the 2 tens in the foundation number.

$$\begin{array}{r} 26 \\ \times\ 23 \\ \hline 78 \\ 52 \end{array}$$

2 (tens) $\times$ 2 (tens) = 4. One more hundred (1) needs to be added from the last step, and then the answer, 5, is noted under the 78 in the hundreds space.

Add Up the Pieces Finally, all the ones, tens, and hundreds are added up for the answer.

$$
\begin{array}{r}
26 \\
\times\ 23 \\
\hline
78 \\
+\ 52 \\
\hline
598
\end{array}
$$

In problems of this type, it is very important to keep your work neat. If the numbers are added into the wrong column, the answer is changed dramatically.

Additional Examples   The next two final examples summarize manual mode of multiplication by following the same process. There are comments inserted to make it easy to follow the steps.

Problem:

$$
\begin{array}{r}
62 \\
\times\ 13 \\
\hline
?
\end{array}
$$

Foundation number: 62

Multiplier: 13

Estimate: $60 \times 15 = 60 \times 5 \times 3 = 300 \times 3 = 900$

Calculation:

$$
\begin{array}{r}
62 \\
\times\ \mathbf{13} \\
\hline
186 \\
+\ 62 \\
\hline
806
\end{array}
$$

$3 \times 2 = 6;\ 3 \times 6 = 18$
$1 \times 2 = 2\ ;\ 1 \times 6 = 6$

Problem:

$$
\begin{array}{r}
36 \\
\times\ 12 \\
\hline
?
\end{array}
$$

Foundation number: 36

Multiplier: 12

Estimate: $35 \times 10 = 350$

Calculation:

$$
\begin{array}{r}
36 \\
\times\ \mathbf{12} \\
\hline
72 \\
+\ 36 \\
\hline
432
\end{array}
$$

$2 \times 6 = 12;$ note the "2" and carry the 1
$2 \times 3 = 6$ plus 1 (carried over) $= 7$
$1 \times 6 = 6;\ 1 \times 3 = 3$

Last, but not least, try some problems on your own.

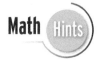

Math Hints

Sometimes it is difficult to keep the numbers aligned. Here's a trick. When multiplying the tens number of the multiplier times the foundation number, you can place a zero in the ones place, to "hold" the place. This will remind you not to accidentally place the tens number in the ones place.

$$
\begin{array}{r}
36 \\
\times\ 12 \\
\hline
72 \\
+\ 360 \\
\hline
432
\end{array}
$$
A zero holds the "ones" place so you don't accidentally misalign numbers.

Practice

1.
$$
\begin{array}{r}
54 \\
\times\ 83 \\
\hline
?
\end{array}
$$

Foundation number: _____
Multiplier: _____
Estimate: _____
Calculation:

$$
\begin{array}{r}
54 \\
\times\quad 83 \\
\hline
 \\
+\_\_\_ \\
\hline

\end{array}
$$

Check against your estimate: Estimate = _____
Answer = _____

2.
$$
\begin{array}{r}
26 \\
\times\ 77 \\
\hline
?
\end{array}
$$

Foundation number: _____
Multiplier: _____
Estimate: _____
Calculation:

$$
\begin{array}{r}
26 \\
\times\quad 77 \\
\hline
 \\
+\_\_\_ \\
\hline

\end{array}
$$

Check against your estimate: Estimate = _____
Answer = _____

Multiplying Decimals

Multiplying decimals is simple. All you have to do is remember the methods:

Here is a basic decimal point math problem.

$$\begin{array}{r} 24.6 \\ \times\ 2 \\ \hline ? \end{array}$$

Note that in this problem, the top number has a number in the tenths position after the decimal point. Here is a panic-free way to solve this problem. The decimal point is between the 4 and the 6, also known as the ones and tenths positions. Take out the decimal point temporarily from the equation, and simply multiply whole numbers.

$$\begin{array}{r} 246 \\ \times\ 2 \\ \hline 492 \end{array}$$

By multiplying the whole numbers (246 × 2), you get an answer of 492. Now place the decimal point in the answer one place to the left because the problem had only one decimal place. For every problem with a decimal point, the decimal value needs to be shown in the answer. In other words, if the original number had a number in the tenths position after the decimal point, the answer needs to have a number in the tenths position after the decimal point.

$$\begin{array}{r} 24.6 \\ \times\ 2 \\ \hline 49.2 \end{array}$$ 1 place to left

Your answer should be 49.2. Here is another problem.

$$\begin{array}{r} 14.2 \\ \times\ 3 \\ \hline ? \end{array}$$

$$\begin{array}{r} 142 \\ \times\ 3 \\ \hline 426 \end{array}$$

There is one decimal point value, so move the decimal point one place to the left.

$$\begin{array}{r} 14.2 \\ \times\ 3 \\ \hline 42.6 \end{array}$$ 1 place to the left

The answer is 42.6.

For every number after the decimal point in the original problem, place the decimal point that many spaces to the left in your answer.

If your problem has one number after the decimal point, your answer will have one number after the decimal point. If your problem has two numbers after the decimal point, your answer will have two numbers after the decimal point, and so forth.

What happens if there is more than one number after the decimal point? For every number after the decimal point in the original numbers in the problem, place the decimal point the same number of spaces to the left in your answer. Here is an example:

$$\begin{array}{r} 10.53 \\ \times\ 5 \\ \hline 52.65 \end{array}$$ 2 places to the left

What happens if both numbers in the problem have a decimal point? Follow the same concept. Count the total numbers after the decimal points in the original problem, and then place the decimal point the same number of places to the left in the answer. Here is an example.

$$\begin{array}{r} 5.6 \\ \times\ 2.5 \\ \hline ? \end{array}$$

In this problem, there are two decimal places (*do not count the decimal points, count the places*). This means that the answer will include two decimal places. Now, solve this problem using manual multiplication skills from earlier in this chapter.

$$\begin{array}{r} ^{3} \\ 5.6 \\ \times\ 2.5 \\ \hline 280 \end{array}$$ ←— Note the first line of work.

$$\begin{array}{r} ^{1} \\ 5.6 \\ \times\ 2.5 \\ \hline 280 \\ \underline{112\ } \\ 14\ 00 \end{array}$$

←— Place a zero to hold the ones position in the second line of work.

←— Insert the decimal point two places to the left.

As with the other problems, the only difference with this one is that the decimal point is being moved two places instead of one.

Now, look at solving a similar problem with a mix of numbers—one with one number after the decimal point, and another with two numbers after the decimal point.

$$
\begin{array}{r}
5.6 \\
\times\ 2.57 \\
\hline
?
\end{array}
$$

Remember what you have learned.

$$
\begin{array}{r}
{\scriptstyle 4} \\
5.6 \\
\times\ 2.57 \\
\hline
392
\end{array}
$$
←—— One line of work

$$
\begin{array}{r}
{\scriptstyle 3} \\
5.6 \\
\times\ 2.57 \\
\hline
392 \\
2800
\end{array}
$$
←—— Place a zero to hold the ones place in the second line of work.

$$
\begin{array}{r}
{\scriptstyle 1} \\
5.6 \\
\times\ 2.57 \\
\hline
392 \\
2800 \\
\underline{11200} \\
14.392
\end{array}
$$
←—— Place two zeros to hold the ones and tens places in the third line of work.
←—— Insert the decimal point three places to the left.

Try another problem.

$$
\begin{array}{r}
{\scriptstyle 2} \\
1.8 \\
\times\ 8.23 \\
\hline
54
\end{array}
$$
←—— One place value

$$
\begin{array}{r}
{\scriptstyle 1} \\
1.8 \\
\times\ 8.23 \\
\hline
54 \\
360
\end{array}
$$
←—— Place a zero to hold the ones place.

$$
\begin{array}{r}
{\scriptstyle 6} \\
1.8 \\
\times\ 8.23 \\
\hline
54 \\
360 \\
\underline{14400} \\
14.814
\end{array}
$$
←—— Place two zeros to hold the ones and tens places.
←—— Insert the decimal point three places to the left.

Note that in this problem the decimal point was inserted three places to the left. When setting up this type of problem on a piece of paper or white board, it is very important to align the lines of work carefully; otherwise, the wrong answer may be the result. Also, be sure to write legibly. Try some more problems to become comfortable with multiplying decimals.

Math Hints

Remember to align your work when multiplying in manual mode.

Practice

1. $\begin{array}{r} 6.3 \\ \times\ 4 \\ \hline ? \end{array}$

2. $\begin{array}{r} 20.28 \\ \times\ \ \ 2 \\ \hline ? \end{array}$

3. $\begin{array}{r} 3.87 \\ \times\ 4.5 \\ \hline ? \end{array}$

4. $\begin{array}{r} 100.5 \\ \times\ 2.5 \\ \hline ? \end{array}$

Dividing in Manual Mode

Dividing in manual mode, much like multiplying in manual mode, is simply breaking a calculation into its pieces. Keeping the work neat helps prevent calculation errors. Estimating the answer helps ensure that calculations are in the ballpark. Once the pattern for setting up a division problem in manual mode is understood, the calculations using larger numbers become simple.

Follow this example for setting up a division calculation in the manual mode.

$$369 \div 3 = ?$$

This is rewritten in manual mode shorthand as $3\overline{)369}$.

369 is the *foundation number*

3 is the *divisor*

The number 3 is divided into each of the pieces of the foundation number, starting with the largest number. The answer to each piece of this calculation, which is the maximum number of times that the divisor can go into the foundation number, is written on top of the line.

Here is the pattern:

$$3\overline{)369}^{?}$$

Calculate the number of times the divisor will go into the largest number (the first number—in this case, the 3, which is in the hundreds place): "3 goes into 3 one time." The number 1 is placed above the 3 in the foundation number on the line.

$$3\overline{)369}^{1}$$

The next step is to divide 3 into the next largest number, 6 (in the tens place), the maximum amount of times possible and note it above the line.

$$3\overline{)369}^{12}$$

"3 goes into 6 two times." The number 2 is placed above the 6 on the line.

Finally, "3 goes into 9 three times." The number 3 is placed on the line above the 9.

$$3\overline{)369}^{123}$$

This is read as, "Three hundred sixty-nine divided by three equals one hundred twenty-three," which is also the same as $369 \div 3 = 123$.

In prehospital medication calculations, rounding off a number to the nearest tenth (1 decimal place to the right) is as specific as necessary (see the note on clinical significance at the end of this chapter).

Math **Hints**

To figure out the number of times a number will go into another, figure out the largest number that you can multiply the divisor by without exceeding the value of the number you are dividing into. See the following example:

$$3\overline{)527}^{?}$$

Here, the maximum number of times 3 can be divided into 5 is just 1 ($3 \times 2 = 6$, which is greater than 5, so 2 cannot be used. The 1 must be used because $3 \times 1 = 3$, which is less than 5).

Another example:

$$2\overline{)862}^{?}$$

This is an easy one: 2 goes into 8 exactly 4 times because $2 \times 4 = 8$. Because the value of 8 was not exceeded, 4 can be used.

In the previous example, the numbers divide evenly, that is, when 2 is divided into 862, the result is a whole number rather than a whole number with a fraction. This is not always the case. The next few examples demonstrate how to calculate dividing in the manual mode when the pieces cannot be divided evenly. The pattern for dividing these problems is a little different. The answers are noted in columns (similar to multiplying in the manual mode). Follow this calculation:

$$3\overline{)127}^{?}$$

The first step is to divide 3 (the divisor) into 1 (from the foundation number). The answer is "0" because 3 cannot be divided into a smaller number. The "0" is noted above the 1 over the line.

$$\frac{0}{3\overline{)127}}$$

Because 3 could not be divided into 1, the next step is to divide 3 into 12 the maximum number of times. The 1 (*hundreds*) is not ignored but is used with the next number (in this case, 2).

"3 goes into 12 four times."

$$\frac{0\,4}{3\overline{)127}}$$

The 4 is written above the line, over the 2. The next step is to divide "3 into 7."

$$\frac{04\,2}{3\overline{)127}}$$

Because 3 does not divide evenly into 7, there is some left over. In this example, "3 goes into 7 two times with 1 (*ones*) left over." The answer to this calculation, 127 ÷ 3, is *42 with a little left over.* If this answer is precise enough, the calculation is finished. If a more precise answer is needed, the pattern can be carried out further.

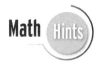

Math (Hints)

In division, the first zero that holds the place can be "dropped" (no longer written) when the calculation is complete. It does not have any numeric value and is only written to keep the numbers properly aligned during the calculation.

Before continuing with the calculation, apply the problem 127 ÷ 3 to a real-world example. Imagine that the entire box below represents 127 parking spaces at a hospital.

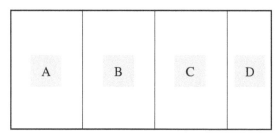

The lot will be divided into three groups of parking spaces that include emergency department parking,

reserved staff parking, and visitor parking. The CEO wants to divide the lot into even sections for aesthetic reasons.

In this example, A, B, and C represent equal areas of 42 parking spaces each, and D represents the "little bit that is left over." A decision needs to be made about what to do with that little bit. Section D needs to be divided by 3 as well. The answer will be a *fraction* of the original sections. Remember from Chapter 1 that another way to express a fraction is in decimal form.

$$\frac{42}{3\overline{)127}}$$

This calculation can be carried out further. Follow along through the rest of the calculation and discover the pattern.

$$\frac{42}{3\overline{)127}}$$

First, draw the line out farther and put a decimal point after the 42, keeping the work neat and organized. The decimal point signals the beginning of the fraction (parking spaces in "D" divided by "3" in the divisor).

Next, place a decimal point in the foundation number and expand the places used to divide by adding zeros after the decimal point.

$$\frac{42.}{3\overline{)127.00}}$$

The "1" that was left over in the first calculation was 1 *ones,* and the leftover 1 needs to be further divided by 3. The leftover 1 is next to the zero in the tenths position; therefore the 3 now needs to be divided into 10. The written form looks like this:

$$\frac{42.}{3\overline{)127.00}}$$

This notation is usually called "carrying over": the number 1 is *carried over* in another form.

Now the division remains easy, and this pattern is continued until an answer that is precise enough for what the problem asked for is found or an answer without a fraction *left over* is found.

Follow along to the completion of this calculation: 3 divided into 10 (*tenths*) the maximum number of times is 3 with *1 left over.*

$$\begin{array}{r} 42.3 \quad \nearrow \\ 3\overline{)127.0\,0} \end{array}$$

Now there is *one left over in the hundredths place.* Again, 3 is divided into 10 the maximum number of times. The result is "3" with 1 left over, and a pattern is developing.

$$\begin{array}{r} 42.33 \quad \nearrow \\ 3\overline{)127.00} \end{array}$$

It is time to decide how far this calculation needs to be carried out, or *"How significant will a more precise calculation be?"* The answer is read across as "42 and 33 hundredths." The CEO and architect agree that this calculation is precise enough.

Recall that earlier most medication calculations will be calculated to the nearest tenth. To do this, use rounding skills from Chapter 1: 42.33 would be rounded down to 42.3. Remember, if the number in the hundredths position were higher than 5, the number would be rounded up to 42.4.

Here is another calculation to illustrate the pattern for division.

You have 4 drawers to store medications in the supply closet. There are 230 boxes of medications to store. If the stock is stored with an equal number of boxes in each drawer, how many boxes will be placed in each?

Set up the problem:

$$\begin{array}{r} ? \\ 4\overline{)230} \end{array}$$

$$\begin{array}{r} 0 \\ 4\overline{)\,30} \end{array}$$

The 4 cannot be divided into 2 because 4 is larger than 2. The place is "held" with a 0.

$$\begin{array}{r} 05 \\ 4\overline{)23\,0} \end{array}$$

The 4 is divided into 23: 4×6 is 24, which is more than 23. Therefore, 5 must be used. The result is 5, with 3 left over. The 5 is noted on top of 23, and the 3 left over is noted below, ready to become part of the next step.

$$\begin{array}{r} 057 \\ 4\overline{)23\,0} \end{array}$$

The 4 is now divided into 30. The result, 7 ($4 \times 7 = 28$), is noted above the 0, and the 2 that is left over is noted below and ready to become part of the next step.

$$\begin{array}{r} 057 \\ 4\overline{)230\,0} \end{array}$$

In this step, a decimal place and a zero are inserted to hold a place for the next step. There is no numeric value to these notations until a number is carried over from the previous step. The decimal must also be placed in the answer.

Now, you can divide 4 into 20.

$$\begin{array}{r} 057.5 \\ 4\overline{)230\,0} \end{array}$$

The 4 divided into 20 is 5 without any left over. The 5 is noted in the answer above the line, and the 0 holding the place at the start of the answer can be removed because it does not have a numeric value.

To decide if the answer to the original problem, $230 \div 4$, is reasonable, the answer, 57.5, can be rounded down to 50 because it is an easy number to work with: $50 \times 4 = 200$, so 57.5 is definitely in the ballpark. Next, the original question needs to be revisited. The challenge was to determine how many boxes could fit in each of the four drawers if the boxes were divided up evenly. The 230 boxes cannot be divided evenly in the 4 drawers, so a decision needs to be made about combining a few boxes or agreeing to have an unequal number of boxes in some drawers. Looking at a problem from this point of view and going back to the original question gives a means of deciding how far to carry out division problems. Try a few problems on your own. Use the space below each problem to do your work.

Practice

1. $7\overline{)6,901}$

2. $4\overline{)51.32}^{\,?}$

3. $12\overline{)4{,}896.7}^{\,?}$

```
           181.176
      51)9,240.000
         51
         414
         408
          60
          51
          90
          51
         390
         357
         330
         306
          24
```

Dividing Decimals

Dividing decimals is simple. When the divisor, or number that is being divided into another number, contains a decimal, move the decimal point the same number of places to the right in the divisor and the foundation number. For example:

$$0.2\overline{)15.144} \qquad 0\,2\overline{)15\,1\,44}$$

The calculation is then completed as usual.

$$\begin{array}{r} 75.72 \\ 2\overline{)15\,1.\,44} \end{array}$$

$$\begin{array}{r} 75\,72 \\ 2\overline{)151\,44} \end{array}$$ ←——— The decimal point goes directly above its place in the foundation.

Here is another example. Note that the decimal point needs to be moved two places to the right, but there is only one number after the decimal point in the foundation number. In this case, a zero is added to hold the place, just as in the second and third lines in manual multiplication.

$$0.51\overline{)92.4} \qquad 0\,51\overline{)92\,40}$$

The calculation is then completed as usual.

Practice

1. $0.1\overline{)12.34}^{\,?}$

2. $0.82\overline{)83.12}^{\,?}$

3. $0.08\overline{)267.8}^{\,?}$

The Clinical Significance of Medication Calculations

In the world of prehospital care, paramedics frequently have to make estimates while performing math calculations. The answer to every calculation does not need to be exact. Many times, the use of an estimate of the patient's weight to calculate a dose rather than a precise weight will not have a significant effect on the calculation of a patient's medication dose.

Consider a patient who is not able to tell you his or her weight. Pain medication is dosed per kilogram of weight. When was the last time you heard this conversation when medications were being prepared?

"Hey! How much you think this guy weighs?"

"He's a pretty big guy, maybe 350 lb. You can probably give him the whole thing without a problem!"

Many medications will have an established range for a proper dose. For example, your protocols may specify that fentanyl is to be dosed at 1 to 3 µg/kg of body weight. Factors to be considered in such cases include the patient's age, the extent of the patient's injuries, the number on the pain scale that the patient assigns to the pain, and the patient's individualized response to fentanyl. These are a lot of factors to consider when calculating a dose for your patient.

When is an exact calculation needed rather than an estimate to determine the dose to administer to a patient? The answer to this question depends on clinical significance. *If the exact number resulting from a calculation will have a clinically significant effect for the patient, an exact calculation is needed. If a reasonable estimate used as the basis for determining a dose will be equally effective as an exact calculation and within standard operating practices, the estimate is appropriate.*

Notes throughout this text will help you realize when exact dosing is—or is not—clinically significant. There is a lot of value in spending extra time in calculations that are precise while sharpening your math skills, but it is important to recognize how much precision is needed in calculations and use as little time as possible in calculations for the maximum benefit of your patient.

Review of Using Estimates

In this chapter, you have learned simple methods of addition, subtraction, multiplication, and division and used the estimating and rounding skills you learned in Chapter 1. Here are some last examples.

Use estimates to complete the problems in this section. Remember to round off to numbers that are easy to use and manipulate. These problems are designed so that you can start off by using the simplest methods of estimating groups of numbers. As you advance through the problems, you will learn how to create simple calculations from what at first glance seem to be complex questions.

Remember, these are *estimated* answers. If you approach these calculations from a different direction (for example, by rounding off a little differently), your answers should still be in the same ballpark. Ask yourself two questions at the end of each problem:

- Is the answer reasonable?
- Do I need to be more precise? (How precise is clinically significant?)

Estimate the total of the following numbers. Use the math tools in your jump bag (not a calculator) to make the math simple. Some notes will be provided to give you additional hints about how to obtain an answer quickly and easily.

1. $3 + 9 + 17 = ?$

2. $7 + 9 + 27 = ?$

3. $3.7 + 15.2 + 22 = ?$

After you have worked out your answers, check the answer key in the back of the book to see if you were right. Note that 15.2 and 22 were rounded *down* in problem 3. The nearest easy number to work with is usually the number of choice. The exception may be when a buffer is needed. For example, when you were calculating the cost of breakfast for the crew in Chapter 1, rounding *up* helped you calculate enough to cover the bill.

4. $47.4 + 143 + 56 = ?$

5. $262 + 298 = ?$

In problem 5, a faster way to estimate the total would be to realize that 262 is about halfway between 200 and 300. Another estimate could be between

200 + 300 and 300 + 300—that is, "somewhere between 500 and 600."

Now that you have estimated answers for all of these problems and you have added estimating as a tool in your jump bag, you may want to grab a calculator and find the exact answers to problems 1 through 5. Compare the answers that you estimated with the exact answers that the calculator gives, and then ask yourself, "When will the estimated answer be close enough?" (How precise is clinically significant?) That is a question that will be revisited often in this text.

Manually find the solutions to the following problems using the tools in your jump bag. Regroup the numbers to first estimate the answers, and then solve each problem to find the exact answer. Remember to use regrouping to make the calculations easy.

6. 160 lb ÷ 2 = ?

7. 36 × 7 = ?

Is your answer reasonable?

Conclusion

Addition, subtraction, multiplication, and division skills are the basis of math. By using these skills and your estimating abilities, you will develop habits that will minimize your errors in the field and help ensure the safety of your patients. Complete the practice section at the end of this chapter to review what you have learned. And remember, most errors can be caught by asking yourself if the answer makes sense!

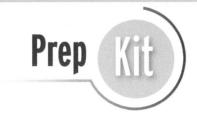

Math Vocabulary

divisor A number that is divided into another number.

foundation number In multiplication, the first number being multiplied; in division, the number being divided into.

multiplier In multiplication, the second number being multiplied.

order of operations The rule in math that indicates that calculations in parentheses must be done first, multiplication and division second, and addition and subtraction last.

Practice Problems

Solve the following addition problems.

1. 36
  + 48

2. 28
  + 49

3. 66
  + 25

4. 45
  + 30

5. 126
  + 96

6.   88
  + 219

7. 165
  + 303

Solve the following subtraction problems.

8. 49
  − 12

9. 33
  − 17

10. 71
   − 44

11.   324
      − 249

12.   101
      − 74

13.   676
      − 564

14.   522
      − 333

Solve the following multiplication problems.

15.   13
      × 7

16.   23
      × 8

17.   45
      × 66

18.   50
      × 17

19.   156
      × 60

20.   357
      × 230

21.   444
      × 321

Solve the following division problems.

22. $42 \div 15$

23. $76 \div 13$

24. 120 ÷ 7

25. 189 ÷ 44

26. 434 ÷ 129

27. 300 ÷ 30

28. 550 ÷ 80

29. 1,000 ÷ 125

Solve the following problems involving the addition of decimal fractions.

30.   5.6
       + 3.8

31.   6.92
       + 14.19

32.   69.48
       + 597.67

33.   157.82
       + 59.46

34.   548.87
       + 234.78

Solve the following problems involving the subtraction of decimal fractions.

35.   6.4
       − 3.7

36.   12.84
       − 9.95

37. 356.7
− 74.56

38. 700.06
− 53.5

39. 1,254.73
−   8.094

Solve the following calculations.
(*Hint*: Remember the order of operations!)

40. $4 \times (23 - 3) + 6 \div 2 =$

41. $(26 \times 2) - 1 + 5 + 8 \div 4 =$

42. $10 \times 2 \times 6 \times 3 \div 2 + 5 - 1 =$

43. Arrive at the answer to the following calculations quickly by following the first example and then completing the table below.

	Estimate	Break it up	Calculate the answer	Check against your estimate
274 + 324	275 + 325 = 600	270 + 4 + 300 + 20 + 4	270 + 20 = 290 4 + 4 = 8 + 300 = 598	Estimate = 600 Answer = 598
278 − 46				
81 × 4				

Solve the following word problems.

44. Your county has five ambulance companies that operate within the county. Each company has a minimum of four ambulances, one has seven, and another has nine. What is the total number of ambulances available to respond within the county in a mass-casualty incident?

45. Your ambulance service has 35 employees, including a chief and an assistant chief. Recently, four people quit, and two were fired. Three new employees have been hired. How many people do you need to hire to have full staffing?

46. Your supervisor ordered 27 cases of IV fluid; 14 are 1,000-mL bags and come with 12 bags in each box. The remaining 13 are 500-mL bags and come with 24 bags in each box. You have been asked for an inventory of the total number of bags received.

47. Your agency responded to 5,000 calls last year. You were on duty 122 days. About how many calls did you respond to?

48. A patient takes 4.75 mg of a medication 6 times per day. What is the total amount of medication taken in 1 day? What is the total amount taken in 1 week?

49. In 1 day, you have to fill up the gas tank in your ambulance four times: the first time, 33.89 gallons; the second time, 24.20 gallons; the third time, 29 gallons; and the fourth time, 16.65 gallons. How much gas did you obtain during your shift?

50. There are a possible 300 points on your paramedic midterm exam. Your instructor forgot to calculate your score, so you need to determine it. In part I, you missed 7.5 points. In part II, you missed 23.75 points. In part III, you missed 19.3. What was the total number of points you earned, and what was your score (percentage of correct answers)?

Solve the following problems multiplying decimals.

51. 12.3
× 2

52. 53.14
× 5

53. 8.2
× 4.1

54. 25.11
× 4.63

Solve the following problems dividing decimals.

55. 0.2)12.78

56. 0.34)89.13

57. 0.04)965.42

58. 0.50)8,756.11

Units of Measurement

Let's take a look at a few systems of measurement.

- **Metric system**: The metric system is based on the decimal system and uses the gram as the basic unit of weight. The metric system is based on units of 10. This system has been widely adopted in the health care field.
- **Apothecary system**: The apothecary system is the oldest system used by pharmacists or chemists today. During the 20th century, the apothecary system was largely replaced by the metric system. In rare cases, medications may still be measured with the apothecary system.
- **Household system**: Household measures, such as teaspoons, fluid ounces, and tablespoons, are commonly used to measure medications at home. You should be familiar with this system in case you are asked to convert values to the metric system.

Table 3-1 ▾ and Table 3-2 ▸ show common units of measure for volume and weight in all three systems. Your work in paramedic calculations will almost exclusively involve the metric system.

The Metric System

The metric system was originally proposed in 1670 by Frenchman Gabriel Mouton and came into use in the 1790s when Louis XVI ordered a group of scientists to create a standard unit of measure. In that period, weights and measures consisted of various types of measurements for length, weight, area, volume, and

Table 3-1   Common Units of Measure: Volume

System	Unit	Abbreviation
Metric	Liter	L
	Milliliter	mL
	Cubic centimeter	cc
Apothecary	Minim	min
Household	Teaspoon	tsp
	Tablespoon	tbsp
	Fluid ounce	fl oz
	Cup	c
	Pint	pt
	Quart	qt
	Gallon	gal

Table 3-2   Common Units of Measure: Weight

System	Unit	Abbreviation
Metric	Kilogram	kg
	Gram	g
	Milligram	mg
	Microgram	μg or mcg
Apothecary	Grain	gr
Household	Ounce	oz
	Pound	lb

time. In France before the metric system was created, there may have been more than 800 different types of measurements! An idea to create a shorter, abridged metric system with one measure per physically measurable quantity was born.

Early developers of the system wanted to create a single system of units, and prefixes were born. Some of the prefixes you might recognize are macro-, milli-, kilo-, and micro-. By using the new system of units and prefixes, there came into existence one way to quantify weights and measures, which was much simpler to use. These prefixes helped simplify measurement units.

Today the metric system is the most commonly used system of measurement. The system is devised around the number 10. This metric system is used worldwide in science and medicine.

As a student, you will have to have a thorough understanding of the metric system because you will be dealing with medication administration and drug doses in milligrams (mg), micrograms (μg), grams (g), and other units of measurement.

Introduction to Using the Number 1

The number 1 can be represented by an endless number of formats. When the numerator (top) and denominator (bottom) of a fraction are the same, the value is always equal to 1. In other words, all of the following fractions are equal to one:

$$\frac{1}{1} \qquad \frac{25}{25} \qquad \frac{0.879}{0.879}$$

and so on. This is true because any number divided by itself equals one, and a fraction is essentially a division problem. For example, let's say you divide an apple pie into eight slices. If you are served 8 of the 8 slices $\left(\dfrac{8}{8}\right)$, you have the entire pie $\left(\dfrac{8}{8} = 1 \text{ pie}\right)$. If you decide that you would prefer only 1 of the 8 slices $\left(\dfrac{1}{8}\right)$, you have a fraction of the pie.

The many ways that 1 can be expressed provide flexibility in solving problems. A convenient expression for the number 1 can be used to rearrange formulas and make them simpler to work with.

Multiplying and Dividing by the Number 1

Multiplying any number by 1 does not change the value; this idea is called the identity property. For example, if a dose of 25 g of glucose is multiplied by 1, the result is still 25 g of glucose. The same holds true for dividing by the number 1. A dose of 2 mg of morphine divided by 1 still results in 2 mg of morphine.

How can we take advantage of this principle? It is useful in the old "compare apples with apples" rule that you have undoubtedly heard before. To be able to work out some math problems, the numbers have to be in the same units (apples and apples; grams and grams; milligrams and milligrams). Life is not always that convenient, of course. Sometimes a few milligrams of a medication are needed, but the medication is prepared in grams. That is when the "don't compare apples with oranges" issue comes up.

But what if you could change the oranges to apples? In other words, what if you could make the units of measure in your problem *all* look like apples? This is one of the places where the number 1 helps out.

The number 1 can also help you stay organized when performing our math calculations. The following problem is an example:

$$25 \times \frac{3}{4} = ?$$

The problem gives a whole number and a fraction (apples and oranges). In this case, rewriting (not "changing") 25 to another form helps keep the numbers straight and reduces errors. Specifically, 25 can be rewritten into a fraction format because any number with a denominator of 1 is equal to itself. Reading this statement as "25 ones" makes this point clearer.

$$\frac{25}{1} \times \frac{3}{4} = ?$$

Now the problem includes only fractions (apples and apples).

The number 1 can often be used to simplify calculations that have large numbers, particularly calculations in which fraction shorthand is used to clarify the problem being solved. The answer will be the same if you simplify (reduce) the fractions, but often the calculations are simpler. Here is an example:

$$\frac{25}{50} = ?$$

This fraction can be reduced by using the number 1 as follows:

$$\frac{25}{50} \div \frac{25}{25} = \frac{1}{2}$$

The fraction was reduced by dividing the numerator and denominator by "1," or $\dfrac{25}{25}$.

Finally, the following example shows how the word "of" can represent a fraction in a word problem:

A hypoglycemic patient needs some glucose. You opt to administer 25 mL of the 50 mL D_{50} in the ampule stored on your unit.

In fraction shorthand, this would be written as follows:

$$\frac{25 \text{ mL } D_{50}}{50 \text{ mL } D_{50}}$$

The line separating the numerator from the denominator represents "of" in the statement. You want to administer a portion (or fraction) of the ampule: 25 is half of 50, or 50% of the ampule. Written in decimal form, this would be 0.5, so half of the ampule would be given. This was an easy example. The next section will show how to work with fractions in which the answer is not so obvious.

Practice

1. $\dfrac{12}{24} \div \dfrac{3}{3} = \dfrac{4}{?}$

2. $\dfrac{4}{8} \div \dfrac{2}{2} = \dfrac{?}{4}$

3. $\dfrac{2}{4} \div \dfrac{2}{2} = \dfrac{1}{?}$

In the preceding problems, the original fraction from problem 1 $\left(\dfrac{12}{24}\right)$ was simplified three times by dividing the new fraction, which has the same value as the original fraction but a new look, by another expression of the number 1. It is perfectly acceptable to simplify any fraction using a few steps if the largest expression of the number 1 is not readily obvious. In this case, if dividing $\dfrac{12}{24}$ by $\dfrac{12}{12}$ had been done first, the simplest form of the fraction would have been achieved in one step.

Changing the preceding answers to the decimal format would be easy:

4. $\dfrac{4}{8} = ?$

5. $\dfrac{2}{4} = ?$

6. $\dfrac{1}{2} = ?$

Reducing Fractions With Ease

Another option for finding the solution to this calculation is to *simplify* or *reduce* the fraction before calculating the answer. When a fraction is reduced, problems that initially seem complicated often are much simpler, and estimating and calculating the so-

lution becomes fairly easy. The purpose of simplifying fractions is to make them easier to use in larger, more complex equations. The easier the numbers are to work with, the less likely you are to make a mistake in solving the problem.

The rule for reducing a fraction is to *find a number that can be divided evenly into the numerator and the denominator of the fraction.* With small numbers, as in the preceding calculation, finding a number that can be divided into the numerator and the denominator is straightforward:

$$\dfrac{25 \text{ mg}}{50 \text{ mg}}$$

25 and 50 can be divided by 25 evenly.

$$\dfrac{25}{50} \div \dfrac{25}{25} = \dfrac{1}{2}$$

This calculation reduces to $\dfrac{1}{2}$.

A closer look at the process reveals how the number 1 made it all happen. The original number was actually divided by the number 1, which was expressed as $\dfrac{25}{25}$ in this case. Dividing any number by 1 does not change its value, and that fact makes life's calculations simpler.

Practice reducing a few fractions, using the number 1.

Practice

1. $\dfrac{10}{100} = ?$

2. $\dfrac{18}{32} = ?$

3. $\dfrac{90}{255} = ?$

Converting to Decimal Format

Much of volume administration is done in decimal format, so here it would be helpful to take the calculation one step further and convert $\frac{1}{2}$ to decimal format. To express this fraction in decimal format, divide the numerator by the denominator:

$$2\overline{)1.0} \quad 0.5$$

The answer is 0.5.

Examples of Reducing Fractions

Here are some more examples.

1. $\frac{125}{1,000} = ?$

   The first number that can be divided evenly into the numerator and the denominator is 25. You can likely handle this problem without a calculator.

   $$\frac{125}{1,000} \div \frac{25}{25} = \frac{5}{40}$$

   The original fraction is now expressed as $\frac{5}{40}$.

   It is not difficult to see that this fraction can be simplified further by dividing the numerator and denominator by 5:

   $$\frac{5}{40} \div \frac{5}{5} = \frac{1}{8}$$

   The original problem of $\frac{125}{1,000}$ is now expressed as $\frac{1}{8}$, after dividing the fraction by various forms of the number 1 a couple of times. It is easier to work with smaller numbers, and errors are less likely during calculations.

   To write this fraction in decimal format, the denominator would be divided into the numerator by using manual division learned in Chapter 2.

   $$8\overline{)1\,0\,0\,0} \quad 0.1\,2\,5$$

   The answer is 0.125.

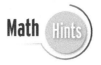

Math **Hints**

Instead of going through the motions of dividing the numerator and denominator by 10, recall how you learned to divide by 10 in Chapter 1: Simply move the decimal point one place to the left. An easier way to see this is to cross out the zeros:

$$\frac{32\,0}{64\,0}$$

Any time you have zeros holding the same place in a number (here, they are both in the tens place), they can be omitted.

2. $\frac{320}{640} = ?$

   Divide the numerator and the denominator by 10:

   $$\frac{320}{640} \div \frac{10}{10} = \frac{32}{64}$$

   Divide the numerator and the denominator by 2:

   $$\frac{32}{64} \div \frac{2}{2} = \frac{16}{32}$$

   Divide the numerator and the denominator by 16:

   $$\frac{16}{32} \div \frac{16}{16} = \frac{1}{2}$$

   In this case, $\frac{320}{640}$ can also be expressed as $\frac{32}{64}$, $\frac{16}{32}$, and $\frac{1}{2}$. All of the simplifying was accomplished by dividing the fraction by the number 1 expressed as another fraction. It also would have been correct to divide this fraction by 1 using $\frac{16}{16}$, $\frac{2}{2}$, or any other expressed form of the number 1 that divides evenly into the numerator and the denominator of the fraction. The answer would have been the same.

3. $\dfrac{250}{400} = ?$

$$\dfrac{250}{400} \div \dfrac{10}{10} = \dfrac{25}{40}$$

$$\dfrac{25}{40} \div \dfrac{5}{5} = \dfrac{5}{8}$$

4. $\dfrac{150}{300} = ?$

$$\dfrac{150}{300} \div \dfrac{10}{10} = \dfrac{15}{30}$$

$$\dfrac{15}{30} \div \dfrac{15}{15} = \dfrac{1}{2}$$

Rule of multiplication: When all numbers are being multiplied, the order in which they are multiplied does not matter; the numbers can be rearranged with no change in the answer.

Practice

1. $\dfrac{6}{168} = ?$

2. $\dfrac{56}{42} = ?$

3. $\dfrac{24}{1,600} = ?$

Reducing Complicated Fractions: Making Complicated Fractions Simple

Pulling out the notepad we can use the rule of multiplication along with what we understand about the number 1 to make life easier in solving these math challenges.

When all of the numbers in an equation involve the same kind of math, for example, only multiplication, the order in which the numbers are multiplied does not matter. The order only matters when there are mixed types of math in one problem (for example, multiplication and subtraction). (Recall the order of operations.)

Here is an example of how to simplify a problem that looks complicated:

$$\dfrac{12.5 \times 18 \times 6}{9 \times 3 \times 12.5} = ?$$

A few math rules are needed from your jump bag. This is a multiplication problem.

- Because there are no other types of math, such as addition or subtraction, the multiplication can be done in any order.
- The numbers can be rearranged in a multiplication problem and not change anything.

The first thing that stands out in this problem is that 12.5 is in the numerator and the denominator of this equation.

$$\dfrac{12.5}{12.5} = 1$$

Two important points follow:

- Multiplying any number by 1 does not change the value of anything.
- If 1 is left in the equation or if 1 is taken out of the equation, the value of the equation remains the same.

Here is the rewritten equation to illustrate the advantage of the number 1 coupled with the multiplication rule about rearranging numbers.

$$\dfrac{12.5 \times 18 \times 6}{12.5 \times 9 \times 3}$$

Now it is easy to see the 1 expressed as $\dfrac{12.5}{12.5}$.

Removing the number 1 does not change the value of anything, so this problem can be rewritten as:

$$\dfrac{18 \times 6}{9 \times 3}$$

This shows why like numbers that appear in the numerator and the denominator of fractions can be crossed out.

$$\frac{12.5 \times 18 \times 6}{12.5 \times 9 \times 3}$$

Prehospital calculations can be made even easier. The original equation looked like this:

$$\frac{12.5 \times 18 \times 6}{9 \times 3 \times 12.5}$$

When it was rearranged, it looked like this:

$$\frac{18 \times 6}{9 \times 3}$$

The rearrangement did not change the value.

The next trick from your math jump bag helps rearrange this problem yet again without changing the value. Some of the numbers can be rewritten into their parts. The equation changes from this:

$$\frac{18 \times 6}{9 \times 3}$$

to this:

$$\frac{9 \times 2 \times 3 \times 2}{9 \times 3}$$

By using the number 1 again, you can eliminate any expression of 1 from the problem without changing anything.

Cross out the number 1:

$$\frac{9 \times 2 \times 3 \times 2}{9 \times 3}$$

You can cross out $\frac{9}{9}$ and $\frac{3}{3}$.

The equation now looks like this: 2×2, which is now easy to solve, and the result is 4.

Here is another example. Simplify the following calculation:

$$\frac{15 \times 16 \times 10.5}{3 \times 8 \times 16}$$

It is easy to pick out the number 1 in at least one form immediately: 16 appears in the numerator and the denominator of this fraction. If the numbers are rearranged by using the rule of multiplication on the note pad, 16 can be placed over 16 in the fraction, and the

number 16 can be crossed out in the numerator and the denominator (which is just removing the number 1).

$$\frac{16 \times 15 \times 10.5}{16 \times 3 \times 8}$$

The result is:

$$\frac{15 \times 10.5}{3 \times 8}$$

Using another trick of rearranging numbers from your math jump bag gives an equation that might look like this:

$$\frac{3 \times 5 \times 10.5}{3 \times 8}$$

in which the number 1 is in the form of $\frac{3}{3}$.

Eliminating this expression of the number 1 (again, not changing any values) leaves this equation:

$$\frac{5 \times 10.5}{8}$$

By using the tricks in your jump bag, you have rearranged the fraction without changing any values or calculating any numbers from the original equation:

$$\frac{15 \times 16 \times 10.5}{3 \times 16 \times 8} \text{ to } \frac{5 \times 10.5}{8}$$

To simplify the numerator, 5×10.5 can be rephrased as:

5×10 and 5×0.5

$5 \times 10 = 50$

$5 \times 0.5 = 2.5$ (remember 0.5 equals half; half of 5 is 2.5)

$50 + 2.5 = 52.5$

This is now a division problem. Solve the division by using the manual mode from Chapter 2:

$$8\overline{)\begin{smallmatrix}0 6.5 6 \\ 52.5 0\end{smallmatrix}}$$

The problem could be carried out further, but because only the tenths place is usually needed in prehospital care, the answer can be rounded to 6.6 and be considered accurate.

These proven math rules will make the math much easier as you advance through more involved medication calculations.

The challenges presented in this section are examples of fractions being simplified (reduced) by using the number 1. Fill in the missing number in each example.

Practice

1. $\dfrac{28 \times 3 \times 88}{15 \times 7 \times 44 \times 3} = \;?$

2. $\dfrac{5 \times 15 \times 100}{15 \times 11 \times 2 \times 25} = \;?$

3. $\dfrac{12 \times 21 \times 10.5}{6 \times 8 \times 21} = \;?$

Conclusion

Fractions allow writing problems in simpler ways. A pediatric patient who needs only a fraction of an adult dose may receive the appropriate amount of medication based on your calculation using fractions. Later, in the discussion of medications based on weight, you will apply the skills you have mastered here and use fractions to determine the appropriate rate of a medication drip, such as dopamine.

The calculations can be written quickly using fractions as "math shorthand." The math can be done swiftly and without error by reducing the fractions into simpler, easier-to-solve calculations. Whether the numbers are given in decimals or in fractions, you can also move easily between the two systems and treat your patients safely and accurately.

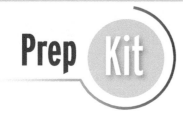

Math Vocabulary

apothecary system   The oldest system used by pharmacists and chemists, which has been replaced by the metric system in most situations.

household system   A system of measurement commonly used to measure medications at home, such as teaspoons, fluid ounces, and tablespoons.

metric system   The system of measurement recognized as the international standard for measurement, which is based on units of 10 and uses decimals.

reduce   To simplify a fraction, accomplished by dividing the same number into the numerator and the denominator.

Practice Problems

Simplify the following problems by using more than one expression of the number 1.

1. $\dfrac{125}{150}$

2. $\dfrac{80}{100}$

3. $\dfrac{126}{144}$

4. $\dfrac{16}{24}$

Convert each of the following to a decimal.

5. $\dfrac{125}{150}$

6. $\dfrac{80}{100}$

7. $\dfrac{126}{144}$

8. $\dfrac{16}{24}$

9. $\dfrac{7}{8}$

10. $\dfrac{4}{9}$

11. $\frac{5}{16}$

12. $\frac{6}{32}$

13. $\frac{25}{32}$

14. $\frac{41}{64}$

15. $\frac{34}{55}$

16. $\frac{76}{32}$

17. $\frac{28}{5}$

18. $\frac{88}{24}$

19. $\frac{40}{60}$

20. $\frac{84}{8}$

21. $\frac{67}{68}$

22. $\frac{63}{62}$

23. $\dfrac{104}{58}$

29. $\dfrac{62}{100}$

24. $\dfrac{70}{32}$

30. $\dfrac{33}{99}$

25. $\dfrac{5}{55}$

31. $\dfrac{25}{100}$

Simplify each of the following by filling in the blanks.

26. $\dfrac{144}{164} \div \dfrac{2}{2} = \dfrac{}{82} \div \dfrac{2}{2} = \dfrac{36}{}$

32. $\dfrac{6}{18}$

27. $\dfrac{80}{100} \div \dfrac{2}{2} = \dfrac{}{50} \div \dfrac{2}{2} = \dfrac{20}{} \div \dfrac{5}{5} = \dfrac{4}{}$

Simplify the following practice problems by reducing the fractions. Each problem can be divided by the number 1 expressed as a fraction. (Do not solve the equations here; solving will be learned in the next chapter.)

33. $\dfrac{4}{6} \times \dfrac{2}{4}$

Simplify the following fractions by using the number 1. Follow this example:

$\dfrac{20}{100} \div \dfrac{20}{20} = \dfrac{1}{5}$

28. $\dfrac{18}{27}$

34. $\dfrac{18}{24} \times \dfrac{6}{9}$

35. $\dfrac{5 \times 4 \times 8}{2 \times 2 \times 5}$

41. $\dfrac{55 \times 22 \times 9}{2 \times 11 \times 3}$

36. $\dfrac{3 \times 7 \times 8}{14 \times 4 \times 3}$

42. $\dfrac{66 \times 4.5 \times 70}{9 \times 6 \times 7}$

37. $\dfrac{6 \times 9 \times 32}{8 \times 3 \times 2}$

43. $\dfrac{14 \times 56 \times 80}{7 \times 7 \times 8}$

38. $\dfrac{15 \times 16 \times 15}{5 \times 2 \times 3}$

44. $\dfrac{23 \times 26 \times 29}{58 \times 13 \times 46}$

39. $\dfrac{12 \times 25 \times 30 \times 7}{5 \times 4 \times 6 \times 7}$

45. $\dfrac{44 \times 56 \times 81}{28 \times 9 \times 11}$

40. $\dfrac{10 \times 20 \times 30}{2 \times 4 \times 5}$

46. $\dfrac{36 \times 72 \times 60 \times 15}{9 \times 12 \times 10 \times 5}$

47. $\dfrac{800 \times 150}{400 \times 50}$

48. $\dfrac{1{,}000 \times 500 \times 100}{100 \times 50 \times 10}$

49. $\dfrac{45 \times 50 \times 55 \times 75}{9 \times 10 \times 11 \times 15}$

50. $\dfrac{47 \times 76 \times 50}{38 \times 23.5 \times 10}$

51. $\dfrac{60 \times 300 \times 42}{30 \times 30 \times 6}$

52. $\dfrac{15 \times 5 \times 15}{75 \times 75 \times 75}$

Find the fractions in the following word problems. Then convert them to decimals (carrying out two decimal places) and/or percentages as requested.

53. Of the 12 members in your EMT class, 10 passed the written exam on the first attempt. Express this as a decimal and a percentage.

54. Your EMS agency has 8 medics; 5 are men and 3 are women. What proportion is men?

55. Your ambulance service has 23 stretchers. The replacement schedule calls for replacement every 5 years. Of the 23, 14 are 5 years old, 5 are 2 years old, and 4 are 3 years old. What percentage needs to be replaced this year?

56. Your service transported 1,240 patients last year; 745 were male and 495 were female. What percentage were male?

57. Your community has 243 residents; 199 are female and 44 are male. What percentage are female?

58. In a customer feedback survey for the month, your service received 74 responses. Of the people who responded, 70 reported your service as excellent, 2 reported satisfactory service, and 2 reported poor service. What percentage reported excellent service?

59. In the previous question, what percentage reported poor service?

60. Your paramedic book has 51 chapters. You have read the first 8 chapters. How much have you read?

61. In paramedic school, in your first 80 attempts to start an IV, you were successful 67 times. What is your success rate?

62. Your favorite baseball team, the St Louis Cardinals, has won 56 of the first 75 games played this season. What is the team's winning percentage?

63. You have 145 red pencils, 56 blue pencils, and 83 yellow pencils. What percentage of the pencils are blue?

64. The ambulance service you work for has 18 ambulances but only 11 are in working order today. To track the number of units available to be put in service on a daily basis, the supervisor requests that you track the percentage of ambulances that are in working order. What would today's rate be?

65. You and a friend go fishing. You catch 15 fish, and he catches 12. What percentage of the total did your friend catch?

66. You are reading a fiction book with a total of 744 pages. You have read 333 pages. How much of the book have you read?

67. Your neighborhood has 35 houses. Of the total, only 25 have school-age children. What percentage is that?

68. Your child's basketball team has won 13 of 31 games. What is its winning percentage?

69. You entered a pie-eating contest. The person with the winning percentage will be declared the winner of the contest. You eat 4 of 6 pies. What percentage is that?

Simplify the following word problems by reducing the fractions. (Do not solve the equations here, just simplify them.)

70. Multiply 34 times 45 times 66 divided by 17 times 9 times 11.

71. Multiply 30 times 40 times 50, and divide by 3 times 4 times 5.

72. Multiply 20 times 80, and divide by 10 times 8.

73. Multiply 40 times 25 times 90 divided by 8 times 5 times 9.

74. Multiply 12 times 36 times 32 divided by 4 times 9 times 8.

75. Multiply 100 times 200 times 300 divided by 50 times 40 times 30.

76. Multiply 44 times 55 times 66 divided by 11 times 11 times 6.

77. Multiply 120 times 40 times 500 divided by 60 times 20 times 100.

78. Multiply 36 times 90 times 14 divided by 12 times 10 times 7.

79. Multiply 16.4 times 6.4 times 8 divided by 4.1 times 3.2 times 4.

80. Multiply 3.5 times 4.5 times 5.5 divided by 7 times 9 times 11.

81. Multiply 21 times 2 times 11 divided by 4 times 84 times 22.

82. Multiply 10 times 5 times 10 divided by 5 times 2 times 5.

83. Multiply 39 times 14 times 16 times 64 divided by 13 times 16.

85. Multiply 51 times 17 times 8 divided by 17 times 4.

84. Multiply 15 times 16 times 7 times 8 divided by 5 times 4 times 7 times 2.

86. Multiply 23 times 13 times 14 divided by 69 times 39 times 5.

Introduction

Medication administration is an important function of an EMS prehospital care provider. It is vital to have knowledge of prehospital medications and their routes of administration, including the use of prefilled syringes and single-dose vials and in intravenous fluids. Sloppy administration of medication can result in adverse outcomes for patients and adverse legal consequences for paramedics and their employers.

This chapter begins with a temporary step away from math to give some context for the problems to come. The discussion starts with routes of administration, principles of medication administration, and the forms in which a medication may be packaged. Then the use of fractions will be discussed.

Parenteral Administration of Drugs

Parenteral administration of drugs is an alternative way to provide medication to patients without going through the gastrointestinal tract (enteral administration). Prehospital care providers are familiar with administering liquid, tablet, and capsule forms of medications enterally. Common parenteral routes include intravenous (IV; into a vein), subcutaneous (SC; under the skin), and intramuscular (IM; into muscle). In some cases, the parenteral route is faster for getting the medication into the body.

Syringes and Needles

Medical syringes were once made of metal or glass and required cleaning and sterilizing before they could be used again (Figure 4-1 ▾). Today, syringes are constructed of plastic and are used once and thrown away. Syringes are clearly marked in cubic centimeters (cc; for example, 3 cc, 5 cc, 10 cc, and 50 cc. Note that cubic centimeters are the same as milliliters [mL],

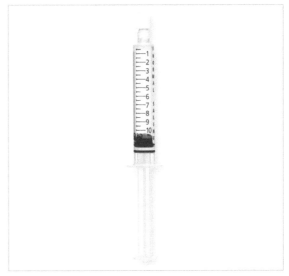

Figure 4-2 A prefilled syringe.

and milliliters is often the term used in physician orders and in textbooks). Some syringes come prepackaged and prefilled with medication (Figure 4-2 ▲) and are usually used for one dose and discarded.

Syringes used in the field may have a hypodermic needle attached or a place to attach a needle. A hypodermic needle is a needle that easily punctures tissues, blood vessels, and IV medication ports. Most SC or IM medication delivery methods use a hypodermic needle. (A hypodermic syringe is a small-caliber syringe that usually is used to inject medication by the SC route.)

Medication Packaging

Most prehospital medications will be packaged in a variety of containers. Here are some examples of the packaging:

- Glass ampules
- Single- and multiple-dose vials
- Prefilled syringes
- Nonconstituted drug vials
- Intravenous medication fluids

Most prepackaged medications will be in single-dose vials or prefilled syringes. Larger glass vials contain multiple doses. These larger vials may come packaged in either plastic or glass containers. Some of the vials have a self-sealing rubber top that prevents leakage after punctures, thus allowing multiple needle punctures for access to the medication. A thin-necked, cone-shaped glass vessel containing medication is called an ampule (Figure 4-3 ▸). Ampules usually

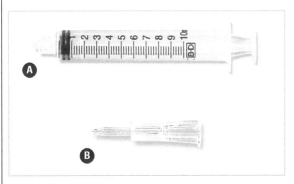

Figure 4-1 **A.** Needleless syringe. **B.** Cannula.

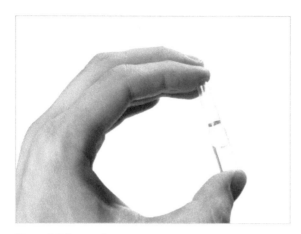

Figure 4-3 An ampule.

come packaged for doses ranging from 1 to 5 mL. Ampules are also single-dose vials.

Understanding Drug Labels

As defined by the US Food and Drug Administration (FDA), a drug is any substance (other than food or a device) intended to diagnose, cure, mitigate, treat, or prevent conditions in a living organism. Many products may appear, at first glance, to not be drugs that fit this description. Did you know that mouthwash, for example, is considered a "drug?" There are two types of drug classifications in the United States:

- *Over-the-counter (OTC) drugs.* Medicines available without a physician's prescription (sometimes called nonprescription drugs). The OTC medicine labels are standardized and follow strict FDA guidelines that offer all of the basic facts about a product. They contain relatively easy-to-understand words and have a consistent style. Everything from mouthwash to cough medicine has labels with detailed information that is arranged in the same format.
- *Prescription drugs.* Medications that require a prescription from a physician or other qualified health professional

Interpreting Drug Orders

Prehospital EMS care providers are responsible for understanding exactly what is asked when a physician gives an order to administer a drug or medication to a patient. A good rule of thumb when receiving a verbal order (for example, by telephone or radio from medical control) is to write the order down and repeat it back to the physician.

Six Rights of Medication Administration

To help ensure that you have some degree of success in medication administration and to reduce errors,

you should be familiar with the six rights of medication administration.

1. Right patient
2. Right medication
3. Right dose
4. Right route
5. Right time
6. Right documentation

Right Patient

The number one priority when administering a medication is that you are administering the right medication to the right person. When more than one person is being treated, there is a chance that a medication will be given to the wrong person. Some form of positive identification is required, for example, asking a patient to tell you his or her name rather than asking "Are you Mr Jones?" and sometimes two forms might be needed.

Right Medication

A common mistake that is made in the prehospital setting is the selection of the wrong medication to be used. Some prehospital EMS care providers may have more than 60 drugs available in the drug box. The typical containers of drugs in the drug box are vials, prefilled syringes, and ampules, which may be stored in boxes designed especially for the containers, for example, a box that holds 12 ampules. Many of the containers and boxes have similar shapes and colors, and different doses might come in similar containers. Therefore, it is essential to read the label on the box and vial or other medication container carefully.

Even have your partner do a quick look to be sure you are administering the right drug.

Right Dose

One of the number one medication mistakes for paramedics and other health care professionals is medication dosing errors. Medication doses that could be mistaken for one another without careful checking are epinephrine 1:1,000 and epinephrine 1:10,000. Common mistakes can easily be remedied by continuing education or studying when you have downtime at the station or at home. Single-dose medications are extremely helpful for reducing dosing errors, but medication doses for children and for IV infusion require calculations, thus leaving more room for error. The study of mathematics and practice both are needed to be proficient.

Right Route

Many prehospital EMS care providers have at their disposal a variety of methods for medication administration such as IV, sublingual (SL), rectal, IM, and nebulizer. It is your responsibility to be familiar with the different medication administration routes that your service uses. Some medications can be administered by more than one route, so be sure to know what route the physician is ordering.

Right Time

Many orders you receive may include the instruction "STAT," requiring immediate intervention on your part. Medication administration in a timely manner is important to increase the chance of patient survival and recovery. Physicians might ask that you administer more than one medication dose before arrival at the emergency department. When it comes to IV drip infusions, time is critical. The physician's orders may require certain amounts of medication to be infused over a lengthy period (for example, lidocaine, dopamine, and nitroglycerin).

Right Documentation

"If it was not documented, you did not do it." This can be a double-edged sword when it comes to accountability for patient care. Always document all interventions during transport, and always document any refusals of, delays in, and reactions to administration of medication. The fact that the patient is being delivered to a higher authority in the hospital does not mean your patient care reporting responsibilities end. The EMS report will follow the patient and become a part of the permanent medical record. It will be maintained in the patient's files at the hospital. Documentation helps provide continuity of care when the nurses and physicians treating the patient refer to your report for interventions while the patient was in your care. In addition, if something were to happen to your patient long after transfer to the hospital staff, you and your report may be required to pay a visit to the court system.

Back to the Math: Introduction to Fractions

Now that we have reviewed some basic information about medication administration, the focus of the rest of the chapter is back to math. In this chapter, fractions are discussed.

Fractions are a form of shorthand that can make math problems much easier. This chapter first addresses how to read the shorthand, next how to write the shorthand, and, finally, how to manipulate fractions to be simpler to take advantage of the shorthand.

Understanding how to simplify fractions is a large part of prehospital medication calculations. Understanding how to use the number 1 to reduce

fractions—a skill introduced in Chapter 3—can make problem solving simple. Learning to read the problem and then write the information in a format that is easy to use in mathematical calculations is your next challenge.

Reading and Writing Fractions

Fractions are a shortcut for writing a sentence when you are talking about a piece, or a few pieces, of one thing. The line separating the two parts of the fraction (the top is the numerator; the bottom is the denominator) can be read as "of" or "divided by." Remembering how to read the fraction makes working with a fraction easier.

Here is an example to see how this works. The following glucose calculation is rewritten as a fraction to demonstrate how all fractions may be used as a form of mathematical shorthand.

> You need to administer only *2 g* **of** *the 25 g* of dextrose in the prefilled syringe in your ambulance.

You can write the same math expression in a fraction:

$$\frac{2\ g}{25\ g} \longleftarrow \text{(The line means "of" or "divided by")}$$

This expression can also be read as "2 g **divided by** 25 g." (It is up to you whether to read the problem using "of" or "divided by.") The fraction may need to be simplified in a more involved calculation, but leaving it as is may also work in some cases.

Once the problem has been written in fraction shorthand, the solution is as easy as punching the numbers into the calculator: 2 ÷ 25. By using the manual math skills you learned earlier, you should get an answer of:

$$25\overline{)2.00}^{\ 0.08}$$

Here are a few more examples. Follow the same pattern for taking the information out of the written problem and rewriting it as a fraction.

1. Your patient needs a promethazine (Phenergan) suppository for nausea. Based on protocols, you decide that a dose of 12.5 mg is appropriate. The medication box contains a suppository with 25 mg of the drug. How much of the 25-mg suppository will you give the patient?

Set up the problem in math shorthand (*fractions*). You need to give your patient 12.5 mg of promethazine. You have 25 mg of promethazine in a suppository. The line in a fraction can mean "of," so your patient will get 12.5 mg *of the 25 mg* in a suppository. In shorthand, you can write this as follows:

$$\frac{12.5 \text{ mg promethazine}}{25 \text{ mg promethazine}}$$

(the part of the suppository you want to administer)
(the *whole dose* in the suppository available)

Note that the units of measure (mg promethazine) have been written beside the numbers in both parts of the fraction. Not labeling the numbers you jot down is the easiest way to lose track of what you are figuring out—and an easy way to make a mistake.

To find the answer, punch the numbers into your calculator: 12.5 ÷ 25, or use your manual math skills:

$$25\overline{)12.5} = 0.5$$

Your patient will receive 0.5 of the whole dose available (or half; see Chapter 1). In other words, in this case you will administer half of the suppository.

2. You are going to administer 5 mg of morphine to your patient by the IV route. The prefilled syringe in your medication box contains 10 mg. What *part of the whole* dose of morphine do you need to administer?

The shorthand for this problem would be written as follows:

$$\frac{5 \text{ mg morphine}}{10 \text{ mg morphine}}$$

Punch "5 ÷ 10" in your calculator (the line in the fraction means "divided by"), or use your manual math skills:

$$10\overline{)5.0} = 0.5$$

The answer is 0.5, or half of the dose available.

Half a dose will usually be too vague an amount to administer to a patient. This calculation gives you an idea of how much to administer. In reality, you would calculate the exact volume to administer, which is covered in Chapter 6.

3. You have a 1,000-mL bag of normal saline (NS) and need to give your patient a 250-mL bolus. How much of the bag do you need to give?

In other words, your patient needs 250 mL *of the 1,000-mL* bag of NS. The shorthand is written as

$$\frac{250 \text{ mL NS}}{1,000 \text{ mL NS}}$$

Punch "250 ÷ 1,000" into your calculator, or use manual math to find the answer:

$$1,000\overline{)250.00} = 0.25$$

The answer is 0.25, or $\frac{1}{4}$ of the bag.

To *divide,* fraction shorthand can also be used because the line separating the numerator and denominator of a fraction represents division. For example, to divide 500 mL of lactated Ringer's solution (LR) into two doses, the shorthand is written as follows:

$$\frac{500 \text{ mL LR}}{2 \text{ doses LR}}$$

To solve the problem, punch the numbers into a calculator to solve the problem "500 mL LR ÷ 2 doses LR," or use manual math:

$$500 \div 2 = 250$$

Reviewing this problem shows that the shorthand was merely rearranged:

$$\frac{500 \text{ mL LR}}{2 \text{ doses LR}} = 500 \text{ mL LR} \div 2 \text{ doses LR}$$

Try writing the shorthand for the next few practice challenges. Remember to label the units and keep your work neat. That way, you give yourself the best opportunity to avoid simple errors and set the stage for rechecking your calculations when the need arises. There is no need to do anything here except to get comfortable writing the shorthand and enjoy playing with the numbers.

1. Two of the six ambulances in the county are currently responding to calls. How much of the workforce is responding to calls? *Write the shorthand.*

2. You need 4 of the 20 medics available to staff the units this weekend. How much of the workforce is needed at the station for the weekend? *Write the shorthand.*

3. Your medical control physician orders you to administer 1 L of lactated Ringer's solution to your patient. He directs you to divide the fluid into four doses over the long transport. How much fluid will each dose contain? *Write the shorthand.*

Working out the shorthand for these three problems means reading the words and jotting down the information as it is presented in the text. Get rid of the extra words that are distracting, and list only what is needed to figure out these problems.

1. This problem shouts to be written in shorthand when it says "two of the six." Because the line in a fraction can be read as "of," it is an easy step to jot down a quick notation for the problem:

$$\frac{2 \text{ ambulances}}{6 \text{ ambulances}}$$

The question asks, "How much of the workforce is responding to calls?" Your shorthand (fraction) makes perfect sense. You would

now reduce the fraction as follows, using your skills from the previous chapter:

$$\frac{2}{6} \div \frac{2}{2} = \frac{1}{3}$$

One third of your ambulances are responding to calls.

2. This problem contains the phrase "4 of the 20 medics," which immediately suggests math shorthand with the line in the fraction representing "of." This can be written as the following fraction:

$$\frac{4 \text{ medics}}{20 \text{ medics}}$$

This reads just like the sentence in the problem. You would then reduce it as follows:

$$\frac{4}{20} \div \frac{4}{4} = \frac{1}{5}$$

This now answers the question. One fifth of the medics are needed to staff the units this weekend. This also equals 0.20, or 20%:

$$20\overline{)4.00}^{0.20}$$

3. This problem contains another key word, "divide." The line in a fraction can also be read as "divided by." In this case, the shorthand is:

$$\frac{1 \text{ L LR}}{4 \text{ doses LR}}$$

Milliliters are the usual unit of measure when using less than 1 L. Because 1 L equals 1,000 mL, the equation can also be written as follows:

$$\frac{1,000 \text{ mL LR}}{4 \text{ doses LR}}$$

This can be further reduced to:

$$\frac{1,000}{4} \div \frac{4}{4} = \frac{250}{1} = 250 \text{ mL LR}$$

Therefore, each of the four doses of lactated Ringer's should equal 250 mL.

For more practice, write the shorthand (fractions) for the practice problems at the end of this chapter.

Rearranging Complicated Fractions: Multiplying, Dividing, Adding, and Subtracting

Mathematicians have spent a lot of time, energy, and brain power discovering and proving the many rules that apply to math formulas. We should be grateful for their effort, because that means that we don't have to duplicate their work to take advantage of the rules! We can simply learn the math rules and apply them to our own challenges, focusing on our patients' needs and our everyday lives. That's good enough most of the time.

When working with fractions, there are many tricks to make calculations easier. Writing problems in shorthand makes it easier to find the meat of the problem and eliminate the distractions. Simple is good, especially in medical math, where making a math error can have serious consequences.

Working with math shorthand focuses on rearranging the fractions to make them simple to use. As long as you follow the rules, you can move the parts of fractions around until you find the best, easiest-to-solve format.

Three rules apply when working with the fractions needed for medical math:

1. To multiply fractions: First multiply the numerators (top numbers) to find the new numerator, and then multiply the denominators (bottom numerators) to find the new denominator; then simplify.
2. To divide fractions: First invert the second fraction (flip it over), and then multiply the two fractions; then simplify.
3. Fractions can be added or subtracted only when they have the same denominator (a common denominator). Once the denominators are the same, then:
   • To add fractions: Add the numerators and keep the common denominator.
   • To subtract fractions: Subtract the numerators and keep the common denominator.

How to apply the rules for adding, subtracting, multiplying, and dividing fractions is discussed in the next sections.

Multiplying Fractions

When multiplying fractions, first multiply the numerators to find the new numerator, and then multiply

---

Fractions
Multiply: Multiply the numerators, and then multiply the denominators.
Divide: Invert the second fraction, and then multiply.
Add or subtract: Find a common denominator, and then add or subtract the numerators.

---

the denominators to find the new denominator; then simplify. Here are a few examples.

$$\frac{3}{8} \times \frac{6}{7} = ?$$

Multiply the numerators, and multiply the denominators.

$$\frac{3 \times 6}{8 \times 7} = \frac{18}{56}$$

This can be further reduced as follows:

$$\frac{18}{56} \div \frac{2}{2} = \frac{9}{28}$$

Here's another example.

$$\frac{2}{8} \times \frac{5}{9} = ?$$

Multiply the numerators, and multiply the denominators.

$$\frac{2 \times 5}{8 \times 9} = \frac{10}{72}$$

This can be further reduced as follows:

$$\frac{10}{72} \div \frac{2}{2} = \frac{5}{36}$$

Here is a final example.

$$\frac{1}{2} \times \frac{15}{16} = ?$$

Multiply the numerators, and multiply the denominators.

$$\frac{1 \times 15}{2 \times 16} = \frac{15}{32}$$

This fraction cannot be further reduced.

You may have noticed something about the equations that can be further reduced. If the fractions in the equation could be further reduced but are not, the answer can also be further reduced. If the fractions in the initial equation cannot be further reduced, the answer is less likely to be able to be further reduced. For example, in the second problem above, the initial equation could have been reduced as follows:

$$\frac{2 \times 5}{8 \times 9} = \frac{1}{4} \times \frac{5}{9} = \frac{5}{36}$$

Note that by initially reducing $\frac{2}{8}$ to $\frac{1}{4}$, the same answer is reached as earlier.

However, note that in the third example, because neither of the initial fractions can be reduced, the answer cannot be reduced either:

$$\frac{1 \times 15}{2 \times 16} = \frac{15}{32}$$

Practice

Try your hand at a few multiplication problems.

1. $\frac{4}{1} \times \frac{20}{5} = ?$

2. $\frac{11}{6} \times \frac{8}{2} = ?$

3. $0 \times \frac{6}{8} = ?$

Dividing Fractions

Division is the opposite of multiplication in the math world. That means that the two operations are related, and that principle can make the math easier.

As stated, *the rule for dividing fractions is to flip (invert) the second fraction and then multiply.* For example, if the problem is:

$$\frac{2}{3} \div \frac{8}{9}$$

the math rules say to flip the second fraction and then multiply the two new fractions:

$$\frac{2}{3} \times \frac{9}{8} = \frac{2 \times 9}{3 \times 8} = \frac{18}{24}$$

Now we can punch the numbers into a calculator: $18 \div 24$ or reduce this as follows:

$$\frac{18}{24} \div \frac{6}{6} = \frac{3}{4}$$

This also equals:

$$4\overline{)3.0\ 0}^{\,0.7\ 5}$$

Here is another example:

$$\frac{3}{4} \div \frac{2}{10} = ?$$

Flip the second fraction, and then multiply the numerators and the denominators.

$$\frac{3}{4} \times \frac{10}{2} = ?$$

The second fraction is flipped, and then the numbers can be multiplied.

$$\frac{3}{4} \times \frac{10}{2} = \frac{30}{8}$$

This can be further reduced as follows:

$$\frac{30}{8} \div \frac{2}{2} = \frac{15}{4}$$

A later section shows how to write this fraction so that the numerator is not larger than the denominator.

This fraction can also be written in decimal format:

$$4\overline{)15.\,0\,0}\quad 3.\,7\,5$$

Practice
Try a few practice division calculations:

1. $\dfrac{3}{12} \div \dfrac{1}{2} = ?$

2. $\dfrac{7}{8} \div \dfrac{3}{4} = ?$

3. $\dfrac{76}{128} \div \dfrac{2}{3} = ?$

The answers are provided in the back of the book.

The rules stay the same even when the shorthand *looks* complicated, and full advantage can be taken of the rules that govern the multiplication and division of fractions to make complicated problems *look* simple. Note that nothing in the calculations is changing except the arrangement of the numbers—that is, the values and results are not changed.

Multiplying and Dividing Complicated Fractions
Look at the following shorthand and follow along as it is rearranged to create a simpler form of the same problem.

$$\dfrac{\frac{3}{4}}{\frac{1}{2}} \times \dfrac{7}{8} \over \frac{4}{8}$$

At first glance, this problem looks incredibly complicated, but watch what happens when it is simplified by using the multiplication and division rules.

$$\dfrac{\frac{3}{4}}{\frac{1}{2}} \longleftarrow \text{Means "divided by"}$$

Or,

$$\dfrac{3}{4} \div \dfrac{1}{2}$$

This can also be written as:

$$\dfrac{3}{4} \times \dfrac{2}{1} = \dfrac{6}{4}$$

By the rule of dividing fractions: "invert and multiply"

Now the calculation is simplified to:

$$\dfrac{\frac{6}{4} \times \frac{7}{8}}{\frac{4}{8}}$$

Next, multiply the top fractions to simplify the way they appear:

$$\dfrac{6}{4} \times \dfrac{7}{8} = \dfrac{42}{32}$$

At this point, punch the numbers into a calculator (42 ÷ 32) or, better yet, keep simplifying the way the calculation looks:

$$\dfrac{\frac{42}{32}}{\frac{4}{8}}$$

This is just another shorthand form for "divided by," so rewrite it. Remember—to divide fractions, the rule is "invert (flip) and multiply."

$$\dfrac{42}{32} \times \dfrac{8}{4} = \dfrac{336}{128}$$

Hint: Recall manual multiplication:

$$42$$
$$\times\ 8$$
$$336$$

$$32$$
$$\times\ 4$$
$$128$$

Now it is a matter of punching the numbers into a calculator for 336 "divided by" 128, or 336 ÷ 128.

$$\frac{336}{128} \div \frac{16}{16} = \frac{21}{8}$$

Or, in decimal format:

$$8\overline{)21.\,0\ 0\ 0}\quad 2.\,6\ 2\ 5$$

Of course, shorthand that looks like the preceding problem will rarely be encountered in our day-to-day lives. The point is that a very complicated-looking calculation was simplified without doing any real math solving until the last step. The biggest part of the challenge was rearranging the numbers until they were in the simplest form possible. The challenge becomes a game: Can you detect all of the places where the numbers can be rearranged to create a simple format?

Reducing Fractions Before Doing the Math Another way to approach the problem is to reduce the fractions before multiplying and dividing. This approach makes the math simpler because you are using smaller numbers that are more familiar. Try this approach with the previous example:

$$\frac{\frac{3}{4}}{\frac{2}{1}} \times \frac{7}{8}$$
$$\frac{4}{8}$$

Begin with this.

$$\frac{3}{4} \times \frac{2}{1} = \frac{6}{4}$$

At this point, the fraction can be reduced as follows:

$$\frac{6}{4} \div \frac{2}{2} = \frac{3}{2}$$

Now this fraction can be inserted into the initial equation:

$$\frac{\frac{3}{2} \times \frac{7}{8}}{\frac{4}{8}}$$

Next, multiply the top fractions:

$$\frac{3}{2} \times \frac{7}{8} = \frac{21}{16}$$

The initial equation will now look like this:

$$\frac{\frac{21}{16}}{\frac{4}{8}}$$

Because when dividing fractions the rule is invert (flip) and multiply, the rewritten initial equation will now look like:

$$\frac{21}{16} \times \frac{8}{4}$$

Note that $\frac{8}{4}$ can also be reduced as follows:

$$\frac{8}{4} \div \frac{4}{4} = \frac{2}{1}$$

The revised initial equation is now:

$$\frac{21}{16} \times \frac{2}{1} = \frac{42}{16}$$

Finally, this can be further reduced as:

$$\frac{42}{16} \div \frac{2}{2} = \frac{21}{8}$$

This results in the same answer, and, as earlier, equals 2.625 in decimal form.

Practice
Here are a few more practice challenges. The objective is to rearrange the fractions (the shorthand for a more complicated challenge) into their simplest form.

Math **Hints**

Remember that whole numbers can be expressed as fractions. (Recall using the number 1 from Chapter 3.)

1. $\dfrac{\dfrac{12}{3}}{\dfrac{7}{8}} = ?$

2. $\dfrac{12 \times \dfrac{5}{6}}{\dfrac{4}{5}} = ?$

3. $\dfrac{\dfrac{9}{18} \times \dfrac{3}{6}}{\dfrac{3}{6}} = ?$

All of the preceding examples may have the answers simplified by using the skills applied in previous chapters. The exercises show how to move the parts of fractions without changing the values or affecting any of the answers. It is clear that seemingly complex fractions can be rearranged to a simpler form *before* calculating the answers. Once again, simplicity works to reduce math errors, and the whole calculation is significantly less intimidating.

Adding and Subtracting Fractions

Addition and subtraction of fractions require talking about "apples and apples." In this case, the numerators tell what part of the whole (denominators) are dealt with. Recall the third rule of fractions mentioned earlier, which means that fractions with dif-ferent denominators cannot be added or subtracted. Therefore, an additional step is needed to ensure that the *denominators are the same number* (to compare apples with apples).

Try thinking about the idea of a common denominator this way: Suppose you have roast beef, tuna fish, and ham in your refrigerator, and you have 25 friends coming over for lunch. It is easier to determine if you have enough food to feed everyone if you think of the food in terms of "sandwiches." "Sandwiches" is the common denominator!

$$\frac{1}{4} + \frac{1}{3} = ?$$

The denominators are different in this example, so the first step is to find a common denominator—that is, a number that is common to both fractions. In this example, 4 and 3 are the denominators. To find a new common denominator, look for a number into which 4 and 3 can be divided evenly.

The simplest way to find a common denominator is to multiply the two current denominators. This approach works well if the numbers are relatively small:

$$4 \times 3 = 12$$

In this case, 12 can be the new common denominator.

The next step is to adjust the fractions in the original example to reflect the new common denominator. Remember, only the way math statements look can be changed—not their value. Because the denominator has increased, the numerators need to increase so that the value of the fraction does not change.

The two parts of the original equation were:

$$\frac{1}{4} \text{ and } \frac{1}{3}$$

With the new common denominator of 12, the following remain to be determined:

$$\frac{1}{4} = \frac{?}{12} \quad \text{and} \quad \frac{1}{3} = \frac{?}{12}$$

or,

$$\frac{1}{4} \times \frac{?}{?} = \frac{?}{12} \quad \text{and} \quad \frac{1}{3} \times \frac{?}{?} = \frac{?}{12}$$

We can use the number 1 to change the way these fractions are expressed without changing the value. Knowing that the goal is to have a new denominator of 12, search for numbers that can be multiplied with the original denominators and have 12 as the answer.

In the first fraction, the denominator is 4; 4 × 3 = 12. If the numerator of the first fraction (that is, 1) is also multiplied by 3, the entire fraction has been multiplied by 1 (that is, $\frac{3}{3}$), and the new expression that results from this operation uses the new common denominator of 12.

$$\frac{1}{4} \times \frac{3}{3} = \frac{\text{(new numerator)}}{12}$$

$\frac{3}{12}$ is the new expression of $\frac{1}{4}$ using the common denominator of 12.

The second fraction also needs to be expressed with the new common denominator, 12:

$$\frac{1}{3} \times \frac{4}{4} = \frac{\text{(new numerator)}}{12}$$

Multiplying by $\frac{4}{4}$ (1) results in $\frac{4}{12}$, which shares the new common denominator. Now the original challenge can be rewritten as follows:

$$\frac{3}{12} + \frac{4}{12} = ?$$

The numerators can be added together (remember the rules of the game), and the denominator remains 12. The solution is $\frac{7}{12}$.

The same rule applies to subtraction. A common denominator is needed to subtract two fractions. Here is an example.

$$\frac{2}{5} - \frac{3}{10} = ?$$

In this example, a common denominator must be found. Both denominators, 5 and 10, can be divided evenly into 10. Conveniently, one of the fractions is already expressed with 10 as the denominator, so only one fraction needs to be expressed differently. Determine what form of the number 1 should be used to change the way $\frac{2}{5}$ is expressed:

$$\frac{2}{5} \times \frac{?}{?} = \frac{\text{(new numerator)}}{10}$$

When the expression is written in this form, it is not difficult to see that 5 × 2 = 10. Therefore, use:

$$\frac{2}{5} \times \frac{2}{2} = \frac{?}{10}$$

to find the new fraction. When the numerator and the denominator of the original fraction are multiplied, the new form of the fraction is $\frac{4}{10}$.

$$\frac{2}{5} \times \frac{2}{2} = \frac{4}{10}$$

The original problem is now written:

$$\frac{4}{10} - \frac{3}{10} = ?$$

Remember, when adding and subtracting fractions, the denominator stays as is. The solution is $\frac{1}{10}$.
Here is another example before you practice:

$$\frac{2}{3} + \frac{1}{2} = ?$$

The common denominator is 6 (using 3 × 2 from the two denominators).

$$\frac{2}{3} = \frac{2 \times 2}{3 \times 2} = \frac{4}{6}$$

By using "1" in the form of $\frac{2}{2}$, determine how $\frac{2}{3}$ will look with "6" in the denominator.

$$\frac{1}{2} = \frac{1 \times 3}{2 \times 3} = \frac{3}{6}$$

By using "1" in the form of $\frac{3}{3}$, determine how $\frac{1}{2}$ will look with 6 in the denominator.
Now the addition is simplified:

$$\frac{4}{6} + \frac{3}{6} = \frac{7}{6}$$

Simplifying Improper Fractions You may have noticed that in some cases, the answers result in a numerator that is larger than the denominator. Such a fraction is called an improper fraction. It can be further reduced so that the numerator is always smaller than the denominator.

Recall from Chapter 3 that the number 1 can be expressed in a fraction as any number over itself. So in the previous example, $\frac{6}{6}$ is equal to one. Because the fraction is $\frac{7}{6}$, it is equal to more than one. The fraction will be equal to 1 plus whatever is remaining. Subtract $\frac{6}{6}$ from $\frac{7}{6}$ to find out what is left:

$$\frac{7}{6} - \frac{6}{6} = \frac{1}{6}$$

Therefore, $\frac{7}{6}$ is equal to $1\frac{1}{6}$.

Practice

1. $\frac{1}{10} + \frac{4}{10} = ?$

2. $\frac{3}{4} - \frac{2}{4} = ?$

Conclusion

Now you have learned some background on medication administration, how fractions apply to medication administration, and how to multiply, divide, add, and subtract simple and complicated fractions. After practicing, you will be ready to take these skills to the next level with ratios in Chapter 5.

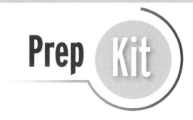
Prep Kit

Math Vocabulary

ampule   A thin-necked, cone-shaped glass vessel; a common way of packaging medications.

common denominator   A denominator (bottom part of a fraction) that is the same number in several fractions. For example, $\frac{3}{10}$, $\frac{4}{10}$, and $\frac{5}{10}$ have the common denominator of 10.

intramuscular   A medication route in which medication is administered into muscle (IM).

intravenous   A medication route in which medication is administered through a vein (IV).

parenteral   An alternative way to provide medication to patients without going through the gastrointestinal tract.

subcutaneous   A medication route in which medication is administered under the skin (SC).

syringe   A device used to inject fluid into or withdraw fluid from the body by way of the vein through an IV catheter. Syringes are also used to administer intramuscular and subcutaneous medications.

unit of measure   The type of measurement used to note a quantity (volume, weight, length, area, and so forth); units can be in the metric system (for example, mg, g, mL), the British imperial system (for example, pint, quart), or other systems.

Practice Problems

Write the shorthand for the following examples.

1. 16 of 20 medics need to renew certification.

2. 20 mg of the 100 mg of IV medication

3. 5 of the 50 vials have arrived by mail.

4. 7 of 10 students aced their tests.

5. 13 of 25 calls this week required CPR.

Multiply the following fractions.

6. $\frac{2}{3} \times \frac{1}{2}$

7. $\frac{7}{6} \times \frac{3}{4}$

8. $\frac{32}{34} \times \frac{4}{5}$

Divide the following fractions.

9. $\dfrac{2}{3} \div \dfrac{1}{2}$

10. $\dfrac{7}{6} \div \dfrac{3}{4}$

11. $\dfrac{32}{34} \div \dfrac{4}{5}$

Simplify the following fractions.

12. $\dfrac{\dfrac{2}{3} \times \dfrac{1}{2}}{\dfrac{4}{5}}$

13. $\dfrac{\dfrac{16}{32} \div 2}{\dfrac{1}{2}}$

14. $\dfrac{\dfrac{3}{4} \times \dfrac{12}{16}}{\dfrac{\dfrac{1}{2}}{\dfrac{1}{4}}}$

15. $\dfrac{\dfrac{12}{24}}{\dfrac{1}{2}} \times \dfrac{\dfrac{18}{9}}{\dfrac{4}{2}}$

Find the common denominators. (*Hint:* There are several possibilities, but the smallest common denominator is usually the easiest to use in solving calculations.)

16. $\dfrac{3}{4} + \dfrac{6}{7}$

17. $\dfrac{4}{6} + \dfrac{2}{3}$

18. $\dfrac{7}{8} + \dfrac{9}{10}$

19. $\frac{2}{3} + \frac{3}{4} + \frac{9}{12}$

Solve the following calculations. Hint: Find a common denominator first.

26. $\frac{3}{4} + \frac{6}{7}$

20. $\frac{2}{3} - \frac{1}{2}$

27. $\frac{4}{6} + \frac{2}{3}$

21. $\frac{9}{10} - \frac{3}{4}$

28. $\frac{7}{8} + \frac{9}{10}$

22. $\frac{3}{6} - \frac{1}{4}$

29. $\frac{2}{3} + \frac{3}{4} + \frac{9}{12}$

23. $\frac{66}{100} - \frac{2}{25} + \frac{1}{5}$

30. $\frac{2}{3} - \frac{1}{2}$

24. $\frac{50}{100} - \frac{1}{4}$

31. $\frac{9}{10} - \frac{3}{4}$

25. $\frac{7}{21} - \frac{2}{7}$

32. $\frac{3}{6} - \frac{1}{4}$

33. $\dfrac{66}{100} - \dfrac{2}{25} + \dfrac{1}{5}$

35. $\dfrac{7}{21} - \dfrac{2}{7}$

34. $\dfrac{50}{100} - \dfrac{1}{4}$

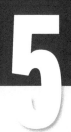

Introduction

In Chapter 4, you learned about fractions. This chapter will explore other ways to use fractions in paramedic calculations: as ratios and proportions. You will learn how setting up proportions can help you solve a multitude of problems.

A ratio is an expression in math that states a relationship between two numbers. It is written as follows:

$$1:6$$

This ratio states that there is 1 of one item for 6 of every other item. For example this ratio could be used if, in a classroom, there was one teacher for every six students.

A proportion is essentially two ratios that equal one another in value. A proportion is set up as follows:

$$1:6 = 2:12$$

This can also be written as:

$$\frac{1}{6} = \frac{2}{12}$$

Proportions are often used when you need to find one piece of a math problem. They are used to compare two things: You have this much, and you need this part of it. Ratios are set up like fractions, which are then solved by using proportions. Like units are set up on top (as the numerators), and like units are set up on the bottom (as the denominators). Labeling units is extremely important in all math problems, and solving proportions is no different. Omitting the labels (units) from the setup of the math puzzle is asking for trouble. The labels keep you on the right path, and then the math gets very easy.

The "Cross Multiply and Divide Method"

To write a proportion, set it up as two fractions that are equal to each other:

$$\frac{A}{B} = \frac{C}{D}$$

When a proportion is set up, it helps to know that you can flip both sides of the equation without changing the value. Therefore, the following proportion is also true:

$$\frac{B}{A} = \frac{D}{C}$$

One of the most useful concepts in solving fraction problems is the cross multiply and divide method. The arrows show the cross multiplication, and $A \times D = C \times B$ is the result, as follows:

$$\frac{A}{B} \times \frac{C}{D}$$
$$A \times D = C \times B$$

By using this principle, the original equation can become:

$$A = \frac{C \times B}{D}$$

Or it can become:

$$\frac{1}{B} = \frac{C}{D} \times A$$

(Because A moves to the other side of the equation, it is replaced by a 1.)

An entire proportion can be flipped without changing its value, so the whole equation could also be flipped to look like this:

$$B = \frac{D \times A}{C}$$

By using the rules of cross multiplying and dividing, you will be able to solve any proportion.

$$(A \times D) \div B = C$$
$$(D \times A) \div C = B$$
$$(B \times C) \div A = D$$
$$(C \times B) \div D = A$$

Numerators and denominators can be moved around by cross multiplying with the opposite side of the equation.

According to the cross multiply and divide method, with the following equation as a basis:

$$\frac{A}{B} = \frac{C}{D}$$

any of the following equations are true:

$$(A \times D) \div B = C$$
$$(D \times A) \div C = B$$
$$(B \times C) \div A = D$$
$$(C \times B) \div D = A$$

Here are some proportions to solve by using the cross multiply and divide method. Here is an example of how it works:

$$\frac{10}{100} = \frac{5}{?}$$

First, flip the proportion so the missing number is in the numerator. This makes it easier to solve.

$$\frac{?}{5} = \frac{100}{10}$$

Multiply diagonally as follows:

$$\frac{?}{5} = \frac{100}{10}$$

This yields:

$$? = \frac{100 \times 5}{10}$$
$$? = \frac{500}{10}$$
$$? = 50$$

Recall that when working with fractions, you can cross out zeros that appear at the end of the numerator and denominator. For example:

$$\frac{100}{10}$$

This would have made the calculation simpler:

$$? = \frac{10 \times 5}{1} = 50$$

Here is another example:

$$\frac{25.6}{?} = \frac{16}{100}$$

Flip the proportion:

$$\frac{?}{25.6} = \frac{100}{16}$$

Cross multiply and divide. Recall from Chapter 1 that when multiplying by 100, simply move the decimal point two positions to the right.

$$\frac{100 \times 25.6}{16} = ?$$
$$\frac{2,560}{16} = ?$$

$$16\overline{)2,5\,60}^{160}$$

The answer is 160.

Solve the following proportions.

1. $\dfrac{11}{44} = \dfrac{?}{100}$

2. $\dfrac{23}{115} = \dfrac{?}{10}$

3. $\dfrac{3}{12} = \dfrac{?}{62}$

Using Proportions to Convert Units of Measure

In your experience with medications, you will certainly notice that medications are measured in particular units, such as grams and milliliters. This section discusses how to convert one unit of measure to another. For reference, Table 5-1 lists the relationships of various units of measure to one another (also called conversion factors), and Table 5-2 lists the abbreviations used for each unit of measure.

Proportions can be used to convert from one unit of measure to another—something that often needs to be done in the field. Many medications are stored on the ambulance in units of measure that are larger than any patient requires. Having such a large vol-

Table 5-1   Conversion Factors for Units of Measure
16 oz = 1 lb
2.2 lb = 1 kg
1 kg = 1,000 g
1 g = 1,000 mg
1 g = 1,000,000 µg
1 mg = 1,000 µg
1 kg = 1,000 g = 1,000,000 mg = 1,000,000,000 µg
1 L = 1,000 mL

Table 5-2 Abbreviations for Units of Measure	
Abbreviation	Unit of Measure
g	gram
kg	kilogram
L	liter
mg	milligram
mL	milliliter
oz	ounce
lb	pound
µg	microgram

ume available is convenient if the medication might be administered in more than one way. But, in many cases, this means you will need to convert units, for example, when a medication is available in grams and the order is for milligrams. Clearly, being able to convert from one unit to another is essential for prehospital medication administration. It is also as easy as cross multiply and divide.

The examples in this section show how to convert medications from one unit of measure to another. Note that the labels of the unit of measure are kept beside each number in the ratios. Labeling units helps keep track of your goals, avoid mistakes, and check your math. For each calculation, remember to ask yourself, "Is my answer reasonable?" Changing from a smaller unit of measure to a larger unit of measure should make your numbers smaller (you need fewer of a larger unit), and vice versa.

$$2 \text{ g} = ? \text{ mg}$$

The first step is to set up the proportion to compare two things:

$$\frac{?}{?} = \frac{?}{?}$$

Table 5-1 shows that 1 g equals 1,000 mg. This information will help solve the equation.

Fill in what is known. The conversion factor is 1 g = 1,000 mg. Be sure to label all of the units.

$$\frac{1 \text{ g}}{2 \text{ g}} = \frac{1,000 \text{ mg}}{? \text{ mg}}$$

Note that the same units are on the same side of the equation.

Flip the equation.

$$\frac{2 \text{ g}}{1 \text{ g}} = \frac{? \text{ mg}}{1,000 \text{ mg}}$$

Now, cross multiply and divide:

$$(2 \text{ g} \times 1,000 \text{ mg}) \div 1 \text{ g} = 2,000 \div 1 = 2,000 \text{ mg}$$

Does the answer make sense? If 1 g equals 1,000 mg, then it makes sense that 2 g equals 2,000 mg.

Proportions can often be set up in more than one way. As long as like units are placed in the same relative place, on each side of the equal sign or in both numerators or both denominators, the answer will be the same because proportions compare two things with equal values expressed in different ways. If both proportions are flipped, the comparison does not change. If you get stuck trying to set up a proportion, use a very simple problem with an obvious answer as a model for setting up the more complex proportion.

Practice

1. 2 μg = ? mg

2. 253 lb = ? kg

3. 5 mg = ? μg

Concentrations of Common Prehospital Medications

Sometimes, a medication order from medical control is given in a unit of measure not supplied on the ambulance. What do you do? First, you must realize that the system of measurement for the desired dose is different from the unit of measure on hand. A conversion may need to be done to determine the correct amount of medication to administer.

Prehospital medications come in various intravenous drip concentrations. For example:

- The concentration of lidocaine is listed as mg/mL.
- The concentration of dopamine is listed as μg/mL.

If 1 g of lidocaine is added to a 250-mL bag of D_5W, what is the concentration? To begin the calculation, the grams need to be expressed as milligrams, so first convert the grams to milligrams, and then calculate the concentration:

$$1 \text{ g} = 1,000 \text{ mg}$$

$$\frac{1,000 \text{ mg}}{250 \text{ mL}} = \frac{4 \text{ mg}}{1 \text{ mL}}$$

Therefore, the concentration of the medication once you've added it to the bag is 4 mg/mL.

The concentration of lidocaine is listed as mg/mL. The concentration of dopamine is listed as μg/mL.

Likewise, for a dose on hand of 800 mg of dopamine in a 500-mL bag of D_5W and an order that is in micrograms, the conversion is as follows:

$$800 \text{ mg} \times \frac{1,000 \text{ μg}}{1 \text{ mg}} = 800,000 \text{ μg}$$

$$\frac{800,000 \text{ μg}}{500 \text{ mL}} = 1,600 \text{ μg/mL}$$

The concentration of the medication in the bag is 1,600 μg/mL.

Epinephrine commonly comes in two concentrations: 1:1,000 and 1:10,000. This means:

- 1:1,000 means there is 1 g per 1,000 mL
- 1:10,000 means there is 1 g per 10,000 mL

Therefore, when administering epinephrine, be sure to note the concentration of the medication on hand: 1:1,000 or 1:10,000.

Never add medication to a premixed bag! The medication has already been added.

Crossing Out Units

When you are cross multiplying and dividing, there is an easy way to keep track of the units you are converting to. The rule is this:

When the same units are in the numerator and denominator of a fraction, the units can be crossed out. They cancel each other out.

In the below example, with grams in the numerator and the denominator, the grams are canceled out. It is then clear that the only units left are milligrams, for which you are solving.

$$\frac{2 \text{ g} \times 1,000 \text{ mg}}{1 \text{ g}}$$

$$\frac{2 \times 1,000 \text{ mg}}{1} = 2,000 \text{ mg}$$

cccccccccccccccc

Units that appear in the numerator and denominator of a fraction can be crossed out.

Using Proportion Shorthand to Solve Calculations

Proportion shorthand means setting up an equation with a proportion on either side. This shorthand is used in health care to calculate many quantities, including one-time doses of medications. For example, it can be applied to the following calculation for $D_{50}W$.

Your patient will be given 12.5 g of $D_{50}W$ from an ampule containing 25 g of $D_{50}W$: in other words, 12.5 g of 25 g. The ampule contains 50 mL of $D_{50}W$. How much of the ampule (in mL) needs to be administered?

Write the problem using proportion shorthand, which consists of a simple equation. The equation is used to compare two quantities that are equal to each other, yet expressed differently:

1. Start by drawing the two lines and the equal sign.
2. Fill in the information you have, and place a question mark (or "X" or whatever suits you) in the space that represents the missing information. Keep the units in the two numerators the same (be sure to write out the units) and the units in the two denominators the same.
3. Cross multiply and divide to solve for the answer.

Here is how the calculations are done:

$$\frac{?}{?} = \frac{?}{?}$$

Math Hints

One key word in any word problem that compares information is "of." This word is a dead giveaway that you need to make a line, an equal sign, and another line to set up a quick and easy solution.

There is one exception to this rule: percentages. A word problem that says a percentage "of" something indicates multiplication.

In the original problem, the word "of" is a clue to some of the things needed in the proportion. The

problem reads "12.5 g $D_{50}W$ *of* 25 g $D_{50}W$," which is the amount in the 50-mL ampule.

$$\frac{12.5 \text{ g } D_{50}W}{25 \text{ g } D_{50}W} = \frac{?}{?}$$

The line in the fraction is another way to write anything expressed as part of the whole. In this case, 12.5 g is part of the whole, 25 g.

There has to be something to solve for, so one more piece of information is needed from the original problem. The missing piece must be the whole or a part of the whole, because the proportion includes another fraction. The original problem includes this question:

How much of the ampule needs to be administered?

This question really says:

How much of the (whole) ampule needs to be administered?

$$\frac{12.5 \text{ g } D_{50}W}{25 \text{ g } D_{50}W} = \frac{?}{?}$$

This problem is set up with the whole ampule (25 g) in the denominator of the fraction (that is, on the bottom of the ratio), so the second part of the proportion needs to be set up the same way, with the "part" in the numerator and the "whole" in the denominator. The question also indicates that:

The (whole) ampule contains 50 mL of $D_{50}W$.

By following the format set up in the first part of the proportion, this is the result:

$$\frac{12.5 \text{ g } D_{50}W}{25 \text{ g } D_{50}W} = \frac{?}{50 \text{ mL } D_{50}W}} \quad \begin{matrix} \leftarrow \text{(Parts)} \\ \leftarrow \text{(Wholes)} \end{matrix}$$

Only one piece of information is needed to complete the proportion and answer the original question. Including labels (that is, units of measure) in the proportion helps ensure that the numbers are in the right places and that the answer will make sense. In this case, grams is the unit of measure in the numerator and denominator of the left-hand ratio. In the right-hand ratio, a part of the whole will also be compared, so the units in the numerator and denominator of that ratio must also be the same (in this case, milliliters). The question asks us how much of the ampule should be administered to the patient, so having milliliters as the unit of measure for the answer makes sense.

Any symbol can be used to represent the unknown value in the right-hand ratio. Many traditional math books use the letter x for the unknown value. To avoid confusion with the times sign ($\times$), a question mark (?) is used in this book.

Now the problem reads as follows:

$$\frac{12.5 \text{ g D}_{50}\text{W}}{25 \text{ g D}_{50}\text{W}} = \frac{? \text{ mL}}{50 \text{ mL D}_{50}\text{W}} \quad \begin{matrix}\leftarrow \text{(Parts)} \\ \leftarrow \text{(Wholes)}\end{matrix}$$

Here is a review of the equation:

12.5 g of D_{50}W of the 25 g of D_{50}W in the ampule is indicated. I need ? (how many) milliliters of the 50 mL in the ampule.

At this point, ask, "Does my restatement of the problem make sense?" If it does, proceed with the calculation.

$$\frac{12.5 \text{ g D}_{50}\text{W}}{25 \text{ g D}_{50}\text{W}} = \frac{?}{50 \text{ mL D}_{50}\text{W}}$$

To solve the rest of the proportion, simply cross multiply and divide:

$$(12.5 \text{ g D}_{50}\text{W} \times 50 \text{ mL D}_{50}\text{W}) \div 25 \text{ g D}_{50}\text{W}$$

Hint: The unit for the "?" will be milliliters because milliliters is the unit of measure for the right side of the proportion, which compares the part and the whole volume.

Now use a calculator:

$$12.5 \times 50 = 625$$
$$625 \div 25 = 25$$

That completes the number crunching, but the number is meaningless without the unit of measure. The question asked for the number of milliliters, and the proportion indicated the answer would be given in milliliters.

The final step, as always, is to ask, "Does the answer make sense?" In this case, a full ampule containing 50 mL of D_{50}W was available. The patient

Proportions
Cross multiply and divide.

needs part of the whole, so the volume administered must be less than 50 mL. The total number of grams available is 25 g, and 12.5 g is the amount to be given, so the volume should be half of the total. The calculations indicated that 25 mL should be given, which is less than the total volume of the whole ampule and half the total number of grams in the ampule. Thus, the answer makes sense.

One more note for your math jump bag: To figure out how to solve a complicated math operation, set up a simple problem with small numbers and use it as a model. For example, construct a simple proportion that serves as a model for solving a more complicated problem.

Here is an example:

A 10-mL ampule contains 8 g of D_{50}W, and the order is for 4 g of D_{50}W.

In this problem, half of the D_{50}W is needed, and the math is easy and obvious, making this problem a great model for problems with larger numbers.

Parts: $\dfrac{?}{?} = \dfrac{?}{?}$
Wholes:

$$\frac{4 \text{ g D}_{50}\text{W}}{8 \text{ g D}_{50}\text{W}} = \frac{? \text{ mL}}{10 \text{ mL}}$$

The dose ordered, 4 g, is half of 8 g, the amount of D_{50}W available, so half of the volume of the ampule is half of 10 mL, or 5 mL.

This model can be used to work the problem by using the cross multiply and divide method:

$$(4 \text{ g} \times 10 \text{ mL}) \div 8 \text{ g D}_{50}\text{W} = ?$$
$$40 \div 8 = ? \text{ mL}$$

If you use your calculator to solve this equation, you should obtain an answer of 5 mL. You can now be sure you have an easy (and correct) model to follow.

Proportions can be used to solve for missing pieces of information in an astounding number of problems. Following the simple rules of comparing two things with the units in the correct places (as demonstrated earlier) and then cross multiplying and dividing allows you the freedom to leave any of the spaces in the proportion empty.

The following examples all use the following statement:

$$\frac{25 \text{ g D}_{50}\text{W}}{12.5 \text{ g D}_{50}\text{W}} = \frac{50 \text{ mL D}_{50}\text{W solution}}{25 \text{ mL D}_{50}\text{W solution}}$$

Both of the following statements are true regarding the above proportion:

- 25 g of $D_{50}W$ is present in 50 mL of solution, and 12.5 g of $D_{50}W$ is present in 25 mL of solution.
- 25 g of $D_{50}W$ divided by 12.5 g of $D_{50}W$ is equal to 50 mL of $D_{50}W$ solution divided by 25 mL of $D_{50}W$ solution.

Note that if both of the original fractions are flipped upside down, the two statements are still true. This type of comparison allows you to find any one piece of information missing from a proportion, no matter how the proportion is written, as long as the comparison is written correctly (the fractions must remain equal).

Practice

The math proves these statements true. Here are some examples for cross multiplying and dividing:

1. $\dfrac{25 \text{ g } D_{50}W}{12.5 \text{ g } D_{50}W} = \dfrac{50 \text{ mL } D_{50}W \text{ solution}}{?}$

2. $\dfrac{25 \text{ g } D_{50}W}{12.5 \text{ g } D_{50}W} = \dfrac{?}{25 \text{ mL } D_{50}W \text{ solution}}$

3. $\dfrac{25 \text{ g } D_{50}W}{?} = \dfrac{50 \text{ mL } D_{50}W \text{ solution}}{25 \text{ mL } D_{50}W \text{ solution}}$

4. $\dfrac{?}{12.5 \text{ g } D_{50}W} = \dfrac{50 \text{ mL } D_{50}W \text{ solution}}{25 \text{ mL } D_{50}W \text{ solution}}$

Converting Temperatures Between Fahrenheit and Centigrade

Converting temperature from Fahrenheit to centigrade, or vice versa, is a matter of plugging numbers into a formula. The formula for converting centigrade to Fahrenheit is:

$$\left(\frac{9}{5} \times {}^\circ C \right) + 32 = {}^\circ F$$

The formula for converting Fahrenheit to centigrade is:

$$\frac{5}{9} \times \left({}^\circ F - 32 \right) = {}^\circ C$$

Here is an example. Convert 98.6°F to centigrade.

$$\frac{5}{9} \times (98.6 - 32) = ?$$

$$\frac{5}{9} \times (66.6) = 37{}^\circ C$$

Now, convert 1°C to Fahrenheit.

$$\left(\frac{9}{5} \times 1 \right) + 32 = ?$$

$$\frac{9}{5} + 32 = ?$$

$$1.8 + 32 = 33.8{}^\circ F$$

Practice

Now, try some on your own.

1. Convert 50°C to Fahrenheit.

2. Convert 20°F to centigrade.

Concentration Percentages

Orders for medications are occasionally given as a percentage of a solution in which a certain amount of drug is suspended. For example, $D_{50}W$, also called 50% dextrose, is a percentage solution. A percentage solution describes the total amount of medication in a certain amount of solution.

There are three types of percentages that are used: weight/weight percentage, volume/volume percentage, and weight/volume percentage. The weight/weight percentage takes into account the weight of a solution and the weight of medication in the solution. It is the weight of the medication per 100 g of solution. The volume/volume percentage is the volume of medication per 100 mL of solution. The weight/volume percentage is the form most commonly used in calculations in the prehospital setting. It is the total weight of medication in 100 mL of solution.

Here is a closer look at some terms and definitions for dealing with problems about concentration percentages.

- Solution: a mixture consisting of a solute and a solvent
- Solute: a component dissolved in a solution, usually expressed as grams, milligrams, or micrograms
- Solvent: the liquid component of a solution to which a medication is added, usually expressed as milliliters
- Concentration: the amount of a solute present in a given volume, usually expressed as grams, milligrams, or micrograms per milliliter

Weight/Weight Percentage

Here is a closer look at weight/weight percentage (wt/wt).

If 3 g of sugar are mixed in 97 g of water, the total weight is 100 g. The weight/weight percentage is the number of grams of solute per number of grams of total solution. So, the weight/weight percentage for this solution is $\frac{3}{100}$, or 3%. Remember that weight/weight is the weight of the drug in 100 g of the solution or mixture.

The formula for calculating the weight/weight percentage is as follows:

$$\frac{\text{Grams of Solute}}{\text{Grams of Solution}} \times 100$$

$$= \text{Weight/Weight Percentage}$$

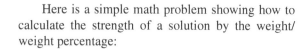

% wt/wt = Weight of Solute per 100 g of Solution

Here is a simple math problem showing how to calculate the strength of a solution by the weight/weight percentage:

You have 1,500 g of a solution and add 75 g of a drug. What is the weight/weight percentage of the solution?

The total weight of the solution is:

$$1,500 \text{ g} + 75 \text{ g} = 1,575 \text{ g}$$

Calculate the weight/weight percentage:

$$\frac{75 \text{ g}}{1,575 \text{ g}} \times 100 = 4.76\%$$

Try another one:

You add a 5-g cube of bouillon to 100 g of water. What is the percentage strength of the solution?

The total weight of the solution is:

$$100 \text{ g} + 5 \text{ g} = 105 \text{ g}$$

Calculate the weight/weight percentage:

$$\frac{5 \text{ g}}{105 \text{ g}} \times 100 = 4.76\%$$

Volume/Volume Percentage

Volume/volume percentage (vol/vol) describes the volume of solute (for example, liquid medication) in the total volume of the solution. For example, if a medication contains a volume/volume percentage of 10% vol/vol, there are 10 mL of medication per 100 mL of solution.

% vol/vol = Volume in mL of Solute per 100 mL of Solution

Here is the formula for finding volume/volume percentages.

$$\frac{\text{Volume of Solute}}{\text{Volume of Solution}} \times 100$$
$$= \text{Volume/Volume Percentage}$$

Here is an example.

What is the volume/volume percentage if 20 mL of vinegar is added to 300 mL of water?

The total volume is:

$$300 \text{ mL} + 20 \text{ mL} = 320 \text{ mL}$$

Calculate the volume/volume percentage:

$$\frac{20 \text{ mL}}{320 \text{ mL}} \times 100 = 6.25\%$$

Try another example.

There are 9 mL of mouthwash in a 25-mL solution. Express this as a volume/volume percentage.

The total volume is 25 mL because the 9 mL are already in the 25 mL. Calculate the volume/volume percentage:

$$\frac{9 \text{ mL}}{25 \text{ mL}} \times 100 = 36\%$$

One note: In the upcoming chapters, there are problems in which a small volume of medication is added to a bag of fluid. For example, 5 mL of medication may be added to a 250-mL bag of fluid. For practical purposes in the field, because the amount of medication is so small compared with the amount of fluid in a bag, the actual total volume of the bag is not calculated. Rather, the volume of the bag is used as the total volume, which makes the calculation easier and you still get the same answer as you would if you had calculated the total volume.

Math Hints

Whether you have a full vial, half a vial, a third of a vial, and so forth, the *concentration* does not change unless more medication or fluid is added to the vial.

Weight/Volume Percentage

Weight/volume percentage (wt/vol) is sometimes referred to as mass-volume percentage or percentage weight per volume. The weight/volume percentage describes the mass of the solute (usually in grams) per 100 mL of the resulting solution. For example, a weight/volume percentage of 10% means there are 10 g of medication in 100 mL of solution. Here are some examples of weight/volume percentage solutions:

10% calcium chloride wt/vol refers to 10 g of calcium chloride in 100 mL of solution (commonly normal saline solution).

A 50% dextrose solution in 100 mL refers to 50 g of dextrose per 100 mL of total solution.

% wt/vol = Weight of Solute per 100 mL of Solution

The formula used for the weight/volume percentage is:

$$\frac{\text{Weight of Solution (g)}}{\text{Volume of Solution (mL)}} \times 100$$
$$= \text{Weight/Volume Percentage}$$

Understanding what it really means when a solution of medication is expressed as a percentage allows you to write the shorthand version of the problem. Recall that percentages are actually shorthand for "parts per 100" or "part of 100." The "of" can be written as a line in a fraction—the same notation that you learned previously.

Here are some examples:

50% is the same as $\frac{50}{100}$, or 50 parts of a total 100 parts.

25% is the same as $\frac{25}{100}$, or 25 parts of a total 100 parts.

13.26783974% is the same as $\frac{13.26783974}{100}$.

When referring to medications present in a weight/volume percentage solution, it is important to realize that *the amount of medication, expressed as a percentage, is actually present in 100 mL of solution.* This means "parts of a total 100," but the units are understood to be the weight, such as grams, *in 100 mL of solution.*

Here is a problem.

A physician orders administration of D_5W. How many grams of dextrose are present in the solution after preparing a 1,000-mL solution?

D_5W is 5% dextrose in water, which means 5 g of dextrose in 100 mL of solution. The problem can be solved by using a proportion.

$$\frac{5 \text{ g}}{100 \text{ mL}} = \frac{? \text{ g}}{1,000 \text{ mL}}$$

$$\frac{5 \times 1,000}{100} = 50 \text{ g}$$

Here is another example. The following example demonstrates calculations related to orders from medical control. The order calls for only a portion of the dose on hand. A proportion is used to determine what "part of the whole" dose on hand must be administered.

Medical control orders administration of 300 mg of a 10% calcium chloride solution.

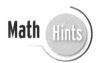

Math Hints

When a problem says to administer grams of a solution, "of" means "divide." In other words, 10 g of a 50% solution equals 10 divided by the 50% solution, or 10 divided by $\frac{50 \text{ g}}{100 \text{ mL}}$.

Hint: Convert grams of calcium chloride to milligrams.

Use proportions to solve this calculation:

$$10\% \text{ calcium chloride} = \frac{10 \text{ g}}{100 \text{ mL}} \text{ by definition.}$$

Set up the proportion:

$$\frac{10 \text{ g}}{100 \text{ mL}} = \frac{300 \text{ mg}}{? \text{ mL}}$$

Note that in the proportion, there is a problem. The numerators are not given in the same units (one is grams, and the other is milligrams). The units must be the same. Convert 300 mg to grams by using the conversion factor, which is 1 g per 1,000 mg:

$$\frac{? \text{ g}}{300 \text{ mg}} = \frac{1 \text{ g}}{1,000 \text{ mg}}$$

$$? \text{ g} = \frac{1 \text{ g} \times 300 \text{ mg}}{1,000 \text{ mg}}$$

$$? \text{ g} = \frac{300 \text{ g}}{1,000}$$

$$? \text{ g} = 0.3 \text{ g}$$

Insert this into the original equation:

$$\frac{10 \text{ g}}{100 \text{ mL}} = \frac{0.3 \text{ g}}{? \text{ mL}}$$

Flip the equation:

$$\frac{100 \text{ mL}}{10 \text{ g}} = \frac{? \text{ mL}}{0.3 \text{ g}}$$

$$(100 \times 0.3) \div 10 = 3 \text{ mL of calcium chloride solution}$$

Is the answer reasonable? Yes—3 mL is a very small part of the original 100 mL on hand; 0.3 g is a very small part of the original 10 g. Try an estimated answer.

Practice
Now for the last practice. Solve the following problems involving percentages.

1. Administer 50 g of a 50% dextrose solution. How many milliliters of solution will you administer?

2. Administer 200 mg of a 10% lactated Ringer's solution. How many milliliters of solution will you administer?

Diluting a Solution
As a prehospital provider, you may need to administer a medication in a concentration different from the one on hand. For example, you need to give $D_{25}W$ to a

child with diabetes, but you have only $D_{50}W$ on hand. How do you administer the medication?

$D_{50}W$ means that there are 50 g of dextrose for every 100 mL of solution. (It is usually packaged as 25 g of dextrose in 50 mL of solution.) The order for $D_{25}W$ means 25 g of dextrose for every 100 mL of solution. Therefore, you need to split the concentration of the $D_{50}W$ in half to obtain $D_{25}W$. To split the concentration in half and create $D_{25}W$, follow this simple process:

- Start with a prefilled syringe of 25 g/50 mL.
- Expel half of the contents. Because you started with 25 g/50 mL, you will now have half of that, or 12.5 g of dextrose in 25 mL of solution.
- Next, draw up 25 mL of normal saline into the syringe. Be sure to gently mix the solution, not shake it.

The result is a syringe containing 12.5 g of dextrose in 50 mL of solution, which is equivalent to $D_{25}W$. Check this mathematically to ensure that you have created $D_{25}W$.

$$\frac{12.5 \text{ g dextrose}}{50 \text{ mL total volume}} = \frac{? \text{ g}}{100 \text{ mL}}$$

$$\frac{12.5 \times 100}{50} = 25 \text{ g}$$

This answer is correct: 25 g/100 mL of solution is $D_{25}W$.

In a similar manner $D_{10}W$ can be made from $D_{50}W$ by following these steps:

- Start with a prefilled syringe of 25 g/50 mL.
- $D_{10}W$ (10 g in 100 mL) equals 5 g in 50 mL. To get 5 g of medication, how many milliliters should you expel from the syringe?

$$\frac{? \text{ mL}}{5 \text{ g}} = \frac{50 \text{ mL}}{25 \text{ g}}$$

$$? \text{ mL} = \frac{50 \text{ mL} \times 5}{25}$$

$$? \text{ mL} = 10 \text{ mL}$$

You need to keep 10 mL to have 5 g of medication. Therefore, expel 40 mL (50 mL − 10 mL = 40 mL).

- Because you started with 25 g/50 mL, you will now have one fifth of that, or 5 g of dextrose in 10 mL of solution.
- Next, draw up 40 mL of normal saline into the syringe. Be sure to stir the solution, not shake it.

The syringe contains 5 g of dextrose in 50 mL of solution, which is equivalent to $D_{10}W$. Check this mathematically to ensure that you have created $D_{10}W$.

$$\frac{5 \text{ g dextrose}}{50 \text{ mL total volume}} = \frac{? \text{ g}}{100 \text{ mL}}$$

$$\frac{5 \times 100}{50} = 10 \text{ g}$$

The answer is correct: 10 g/100 mL of solution is $D_{10}W$.

To make $D_{10}W$ from $D_{25}W$, the following easy approach gives a concentration relatively close to $D_{10}W$ but not an exact $D_{10}W$ concentration:

- Start with a syringe of 12.5 g/50 mL.
- Expel half of the contents to obtain half of that, or 6.25 g of dextrose in 25 mL of solution.
- Next, draw up 25 mL of normal saline into the syringe. Be sure to stir the solution, not shake it.

Does a syringe containing 6.25 g of dextrose in 50 mL of solution equal $D_{10}W$?

$$\frac{6.25 \text{ g dextrose}}{50 \text{ mL total volume}} = \frac{? \text{ g}}{100 \text{ mL}}$$

$$\frac{6.25 \times 100}{50} = 12.5 \text{ g}$$

For $D_{10}W$, the answer would be 10 g per 100 mL, but 12.5 g in 100 mL is the solution made. With this particular drug, dextrose, administering an amount that is slightly greater than needed will not harm the patient; however, with other drugs, slight differences in the dose could have harmful, even fatal, outcomes.

To make exactly $D_{10}W$ from $D_{25}W$, work backwards. Assume that $D_{25}W$ comes as 12.5 g in 50 mL. To make $D_{10}W$, 10 g per 100 mL, or 5 g per 50 mL, is needed. How many milliliters of $D_{25}W$ contain 5 g of medication? Set up a proportion:

$$\frac{50 \text{ mL}}{12.5 \text{ g}} = \frac{? \text{ mL}}{5 \text{ g}}$$

$$\frac{50 \times 5}{12.5} = 20 \text{ mL}$$

The calculation shows that 5 g of medication are present in 20 mL of solution. Therefore, the extra 30 mL need to be expelled from the 50-mL syringe (50 mL − 20 mL = 30 mL). The process is, therefore:

- Start with a syringe of 12.5 g/50 mL.
- Expel 30 mL, leaving 5 g/20 mL of solution.
- Next, draw up 30 mL of normal saline into the syringe. Be sure to stir the solution, not shake it.

The syringe contains 5 g of dextrose in 50 mL of solution, which is equal to $D_{10}W$ and is confirmed by the following calculation.

$$\frac{5 \text{ g dextrose}}{50 \text{ mL total volume}} = \frac{? \text{ g}}{100 \text{ mL}}$$

$$\frac{5 \times 100}{50} = 10 \text{ g}$$

A final note: Dextrose is sold as $D_{50}W$, $D_{25}W$, and $D_{10}W$, but if your ambulance does not carry all of these concentrations, you may need to know how to make them. Also, if you make different concentrations of dextrose, make the solution shortly before using it and do not store it, as it can deteriorate with exposure to temperatures above 77°F (25°C). Prepackaged dextrose solutions come with an expiration date, which of course you should always check before using.

Conclusion

You are moving beyond basic math skills and learning how to use math in the world of paramedic calculations. You have built on your fraction skills by learning the meaning of ratios and how to set up proportions and have learned new math skills such as how to cross multiply and divide, cross out units, and convert units of measure. Finally, you have been introduced to percentage solutions. These are some of the most invaluable skills for everyday paramedic calculations. As you practice, confirm that your answers make sense.

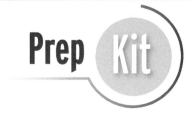

Math Vocabulary

concentration   A medication's weight per volume.

conversion factors   The numbers that represent the relationship between two numbers and that can be multiplied or divided to convert from one unit of measure to another.

cross multiply and divide method   A method in math in which the numerator (top number) of each side of the fraction is multiplied by the denominator (bottom part) of the opposite side of the fraction.

percentage solution   A solution that contains a medication and that is named using a percentage representing the amount of medication in 100 g or 100 mL of solution.

proportion   Two ratios that equal each other in value and are written with an equal sign separating the two ratios.

ratio   An expression in math that states a relationship between two numbers, written as two numbers separated by a colon (1:2).

solute   A component dissolved in a solution, usually expressed as grams, milligrams, or micrograms.

solution   A mixture consisting of a solute and a solvent.

solvent   The liquid component of a solution to which a medication is added, usually expressed as milliliters.

volume/volume percentage   A way of naming a solution that states the volume of medication per 100 mL of solution; abbreviated vol/vol.

weight/volume percentage   A way of naming a solution that states the weight of medication per 100 mL of solution; abbreviated wt/vol.

weight/weight percentage   A way of naming a solution that states the weight of medication per 100 g of solution; abbreviated wt/wt.

Practice Problems

Solve the following proportions. Hint: Remember to cross multiply and divide.

1. $\dfrac{3}{4} = \dfrac{?}{100}$

2. $\dfrac{50}{?} = \dfrac{1}{2}$

3. $\dfrac{?}{200} = \dfrac{3}{4}$

4. $\dfrac{32}{64} = \dfrac{4}{?}$

5. *Complete the table. Conversion factors have been provided for easy reference. Hint:* Use proportions.

Convert this number...	...to this unit of measure	Conversion factor
10 g	? mg	1,000 mg = 1 g
4 mL	? L	1,000 mL = 1 L
76 g	? kg	1,000 g = 1 kg
1,726 mg	? kg	1,000 mg = 1 g and 1,000 g = 1 kg

Use proportions to convert the following units of measure.

6. 750 mg = _____ g

7. 3.3 g = _____ mg

8. 25 mg = _____ μg

9. 500 μg = _____ mg

10. 1,000 mg = _____ μg

11. 33 mL = _____ L

12. 2.2 L = _____ mL

13. 7.4 mL = _____ L

14. 1,250 mL = _____ L

15. 0.05 L = _____ mL

16. 0.25 mg = _____ μg

17. 1.25 g = _____ mg

18. 800 mg = _____ μg

19. 1,600 μg = _____ g

20. 100 mL = _____ L

21. 0.005 L = _____ mL

22. 6.75 μg = _____ mg

23. 989 mg = _____ g

31. 0.5 kg = _____ g

24. 50 g = _____ µg

32. 79 mg = _____ µg

25. 1.001 mg = _____ µg

33. 5,000 µg = _____ g

26. 3.5 kg = _____ g

34. 400 mg = _____ µg

27. 0.75 kg = _____ g

35. 10 µg = _____ kg

28. 0.025 kg = _____ g

36. 7,500 mg = _____ kg

29. 86 g = _____ mg

37. 600 g = _____ kg

30. 7 kg = _____ g

38. 2,000 g = _____ kg

Convert the following temperatures.

39. Convert 105°F to °C.

40. Convert 100°F to °C.

41. Convert 38°C to °F.

42. Convert 36.5°C to °F.

43. Convert 32°F to °C.

Calculate the concentration in the following problems.

44. You mix 800 mg of dopamine in a 500-mL bag of D₅W. What is the concentration of 1 mL?

45. You mix 1 g of lidocaine in a 250-mL bag of D₅W. What is the concentration of 1 mL?

46. You mix 400 mg of dopamine in a 250-mL bag of D₅W. What is the concentration of 1 mL?

47. You have 2 g of lidocaine in a 500-mL bag of D₅W. How many milligrams are in 10 mL?

48. How many milligrams of epinephrine are there in 1 mL of a 1:1,000 ampule?

Calculate the amount to be administered in the following problems.

49. You receive an order to give 5 g of a 50% dextrose solution. There is a total of 50 mL in the prefilled syringe. How many milliliters will you administer?

50. You receive an order to give 5 g of a 50% dextrose solution. There is a total of 10 mL in the prefilled syringe. How many milliliters will you administer?

51. You place 1 g of a medication into 50 mL of solution. A physician orders that the patient be given 400 mg of the medication. How many milliliters do you administer?

52. You place 500 mg of a medication into 50 mL of solution. A physician orders you to give 175 mg of the medication. How many milliliters do you administer?

53. You receive an order to give 25 g of a 50% dextrose solution. There is a total of 50 mL in the prefilled syringe. How many milliliters will you administer?

54. You receive an order to give 4 g of a 10% dextrose solution. There is a total of 20 mL in the prefilled syringe. How many milliliters will you administer?

55. You receive an order to give 2.75 g of a 25% dextrose solution. There is a total of 50 mL in the prefilled syringe. How many milliliters will you administer?

56. You mix 2 g of lidocaine in 500 mL of D_5W. You are then instructed to give 3 mL per minute. How many milligrams will you administer with the 3 mL?

57. You have a 60% solution in a 50-mL prefilled syringe. You are instructed to give 6 g of the medication. How many milliliters will you administer?

58. You have an 80% solution in a 20-mL prefilled syringe. The physician orders you to give 8 g of the medication. How many milliliters will you administer?

59. You have a 50% dextrose solution, and the physician orders you to administer 10 g. How many milliliters of solution will you administer?

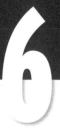

Rate-Dependent Calculations

Introduction

A medical director might order a medication to be administered with consideration for some or all of the following factors:

- As a single standard dose of medication
- As a dose of medication with consideration of rate (time)
- As a dose of medication with consideration for a patient's weight

The first item, a single standard dose of medication, is simply administered and does not require special problem solving to determine the dose. An example would be administering an EpiPen. There are no dose calculations involved. This chapter discusses a dose of medication that considers the rate (time). The next chapter discusses a dose of medication that considers the patient's weight.

Solving problems involving medication administered at a certain rate is one of the more challenging tasks in medical math. Some services have intravenous (IV) pumps that may calculate the rate; all you have to do is plug in the rate ordered by the physician or established by protocols. In many situations, however, this technology may not be available or may not be functioning properly—so you need to know how to perform the calculations.

Table 6-1 ▾ shows examples of drug doses with a time factor, or rate-based doses. Rate-based medication doses will be easy enough to calculate after working through the chapters of this text. By using ratios and the rate-based formula introduced in this chapter, you can solve any medication administration calculation. First, here is a brief discussion of IV solutions and administration sets to explain how the administration set affects the rate.

Intravenous Solutions

Chemically Prepared Solutions

There are two types of chemically prepared IV saline forms used in the prehospital care environment: crystalloids and colloids. A crystalloid solution contains electrolytes and nonelectrolytes that can diffuse into all body fluid compartments. The solution lacks many of the high-protein elements that its counterpart, colloid solution, has. A colloid solution contains many high-protein elements that are not easily passed through the circulatory system. Colloids are known to be volume expanders because they raise osmotic pressure within the circulatory system.

The most commonly used fluid is the crystalloid fluid better known as normal saline, a solution of sodium chloride at 0.9% concentration, which closely matches the concentration in the blood. Lactated Ringer's is another solution often used for large-volume fluid replacement. You will usually see EMS providers using this for trauma cases to replenish the patients' blood volume.

Another common crystalloid solution is 5% dextrose in water, sometimes called D_5W; it is often used to treat patients at risk for having low blood glucose levels or high sodium levels.

It is not uncommon to see paramedics, nurses, and other prehospital care providers using crystalloid or colloid solutions to treat hypovolemia, dehydration, and electrolyte imbalances, and to administer medication through the veins. Table 6-2 ▾ lists common IV solutions found in the prehospital environment.

There are basically three types of fluids used in prehospital care for IV infusions:

- D_5W, 5% dextrose and sterile water, given when the IV line is used to establish a lifeline or a medication route
- Normal saline (NS), which is 0.9% sodium chloride in sterile water, also used for irrigation of wounds

Table 6-1 Sample Drug Doses With Time Factor

Drug Dose	Reads As
2 mg/min	2 milligrams per minute
5 µg/kg/min	5 micrograms per kilogram per minute
5 mg/2 mL/min	5 milligrams per 2 milliliters per minute
1 mg/10 mL/min	1 milligram per 10 milliliters per minute

Table 6-2 Types of Common Intravenous Fluids

0.9% sodium chloride solution (NS)
0.45% sodium chloride solution (NS ½)
0.25% sodium chloride solution (NS ¼)
5% dextrose in H_2O (D_5W)
10% dextrose in H_2O ($D_{10}W$)
5% dextrose in 0.45% sodium chloride solution (D_5 ½)
Lactated Ringer's solution

- Lactated Ringer's, a solution of electrolytes that is isotonic (has an electrolyte content similar to that of blood so it does not destroy red blood cells when injected into the bloodstream) and that is used in trauma, burn, and hemorrhagic shock cases

Administration Sets

An administration set, or solution set as it is sometimes known in the field, is the tubing, drip chamber, and connectors used to move fluid from the IV bag into the patient's vascular system. There are different sizes of administration sets for different situations and patients. The administration set you select will depend on how much fluid will be administered. Each set delivers a certain number of drops per milliliter. This rate can be adjusted within a certain range, by using the roller clamp that is part of the set. Each administration set package lists the number of drops in every milliliter (Figure 6-1 ▾).

The unit of measure used on an administration set is gtt, which is short for guttae, meaning drops; gtt is the number of drops per milliliter an administration set is calibrated to deliver. For example, in a 10-gtt/mL administration set, 10 drops of fluid equal 1 mL of fluid. A 60-drop administration set provides 60 drops for every milliliter of solution infused into the patient.

An administration set includes a drip chamber in which fluid accumulates so that the tubing remains filled with fluid. Administration sets come in two primary sizes: microdrip and macrodrip. A microdrip set allows 60 gtt (drops)/mL through the small, needlelike orifice inside the drip chamber. Microdrip sets are ideal for medication administration or pedi-

Table 6-3	Common IV Tubing Drop Factors	
gtt/mL	Macrodrip vs Microdrip	Adult vs Pediatric
10	Macrodrip	Adult
15	Macrodrip	Adult
20	Macrodrip	Adult
60	Microdrip or minidrip	Adult and pediatric

atric fluid delivery because it is easy to control the fluid flow. A macrodrip set allows 10 to 20 gtt/mL through a large opening between the piercing spike and the drip chamber. Macrodrip sets are best used for rapid fluid replacement but can also be used for maintenance and keep-the-vein-open IV setups.

Many types of administration sets are available. Table 6-3 ▴ lists some common IV tubing drop factors. The most commonly used are 10-drop, 15-drop, and 60-drop sets. Some administration sets allow you to change the drip rate without changing the entire administration set. Consider a 10-drop set, which is calibrated to deliver 10 drops of medication for every milliliter of fluid. By contrast, a 60-drop set is calibrated to deliver 60 drops for every milliliter of fluid. Clearly, the 60-drop set uses much smaller drops of medication (Figure 6-2 ▾).

Infusion Rates

In prehospital care, IV pumps are not commonly available, so paramedics need to be able to do the calculations. The following terms need to be understood:

- The total volume, or milliliters to be infused
- The drop factor, also known as drops per milliliter (gtt/mL)

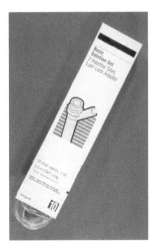

Figure 6-1 The number of drops equal to 1 milliliter is usually visible on the administration set packaging.

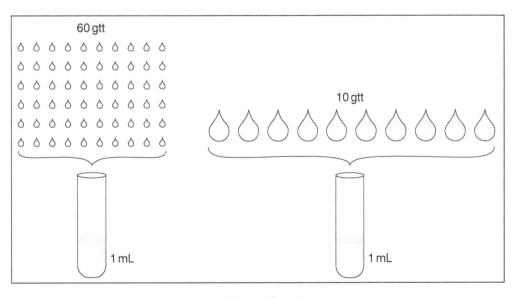

Figure 6-2 The larger the number of drops per milliliter (gtt/mL), the smaller the drops.

- The total time the medication is to be infused. Usually in prehospital care, infusions are based on minutes, not hours. But when getting an order, check to be sure you know what infusion rate the physician wants. Also check with your local protocols for standard infusion rates.

During your shift, you may be asked to perform many IV infusions. To administer IV fluids safely, you need to know how much fluid to give, the length of time to give it, what type of fluid to give, and what, if any, medications you need to add to the fluid. You will also need to select the right tubing, calculate the drip factor, and adjust the flow rate. Most ambulances carry two or three tubing sizes, such as a microdrip set and macrodrip set.

Fluid Volume Infusion

The fluid volume infusion refers to the number of milliliters of fluid to be infused during 1 hour (mL/h) or 1 minute (mL/min). IV fluids can be administered two ways: by intermittent infusion and by continuous infusion. A continuous flow infusion is usually used to replace electrolytes or improve fluid balance possibly owing to dehydration, vomiting, or hemorrhage. Intermittent infusion devices, such as a saline lock, are most commonly used to administer low-volume boluses of fluid without continuous infusions. The lock is attached to an IV catheter and filled with about 2 mL of saline to prevent blood clotting at the end of the catheter. It keeps the vein open for periodic administration of medication.

Prehospital Calculations

Part of your responsibility as a prehospital care provider is to apply the basic mathematical principles you learned in school or at the station to calculate medication and fluid doses before administering them to a patient. In the prehospital care setting, most medications are packaged in prefilled syringes, ampules, vials, or IV solution bags (eg, lidocaine). You will be required to learn to calculate the basic drug doses by using these three pieces of information:

- Desired dose
- Dose on hand
- Volume on hand

Desired Dose

What is a desired dose (DD)? It is the amount of drug or drug fluid ordered by the physician. Sometimes the order will include a time factor, as noted in the following examples. A dose that includes a time factor requires a rate-dependent calculation, the topic of this chapter.

There are several key ingredients to a problem involving a DD: How much medication did the physician order? What is the concentration of the drug, if applicable? And what is the unit of measurement? The following are examples of problems. See if you can identify the DD.

> You arrive at the scene with a patient experiencing an asthma attack. The online medical director orders 0.3 mg of epinephrine 1:1,000 SC (subcutaneously). You have on hand one ampule containing 1 mg in 10 mL of epinephrine 1:10,000. What is the DD?

The DD is exactly what the medical director ordered (0.3 mg). Here is another problem.

> According to your state protocols, you respond to a possible drug overdose and must administer 2 mg of naloxone (Narcan) IV. Your drug box includes a vial containing 2 mg in 2 mL. What is the DD?

The DD is the 2 mg indicated by your state's protocols.

Dose on Hand

The dose on hand (DOH) is literally that—the dose of medication that you have on hand. In the preceding examples, identify the dose on hand.

In the first example, the dose on hand is 1 mg/10 mL. In the second example, the dose on hand is 2 mg/2 mL.

All liquid medications are packaged as a concentration, which was discussed in Chapter 5—weight/volume percentage. A medication's concentration is the drug's weight per volume (for example, grams, milligrams, or micrograms per mL). From a concentration, you can determine the dose on hand and the volume on hand. For example, 50% dextrose in a prefilled syringe is 25 g of the drug in 50 mL of fluid, which, broken down, is a 25-g dose on hand and a 50-mL volume on hand.

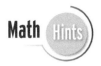

To calculate a concentration of a medication, divide the total number of milligrams by the total number of milliliters per container. Show the milligrams in the numerator (top) and the milliliters in the denominator (bottom) of the fraction. The formula for calculating a medication's concentration is as follows:

$$\frac{\text{Number of milligrams in container}}{\text{Number of milliliters in container}} = \text{mg/mL}$$

The following example calculates the concentration of a medication using dose on hand and volume on hand:

$$\frac{2 \text{ mg}}{2 \text{ mL}} = 1 \text{ mg/mL}$$

Some of the math problems might require you to convert milligrams (mg) to micrograms (μg). In this type of problem, you need to divide a larger number (the denominator) into a smaller number (numerator). This problem will produce a decimal fraction. For example, if you are calculating a dopamine drip and the desired dose is 5 μg/min but the dose on hand is in milligrams, you must convert the milligrams to micrograms by moving the decimal point three places to the right. Refer to Table 5-1 for conversion factors.

Here is an example of calculating a concentration in which units need to be converted.

> You have received an order to initiate a dopamine drip. You have one single-dose vial containing 400 mg of dopamine, one IV bag containing 250 mL of normal saline, and a 60-gtt/mL administration set. Once it is added to the 250-mL bag of fluid, what will be the concentration of dopamine, in micrograms?

First, convert the units from milligrams to micrograms.

$$400 \text{ mg} \times \frac{1,000 \text{ μg}}{\text{mg}} = 400,000 \text{ μg}$$

Then calculate the concentration.

$$\frac{400,000 \text{ μg}}{250 \text{ mL}} = 1,600 \frac{\text{μg}}{\text{mL}}$$

The answer is 1,600 μg/mL.

Table 6-4 ▶ shows common adult medications and their doses, concentrations, and routes.

Calculating Drip Rates

The Formula for Rate-Dependent Doses

Here is the formula for calculating rate-dependent doses:

$$\frac{\text{DD}}{\text{DOH}} \times \frac{\text{gtt}}{\text{mL}} = \text{Rate}$$

- **DD** represents the desired dose as ordered by protocol, medical director, or another physician.
- **DOH** represents the dose on hand in the medication container.
- **gtt/mL** represents the number of drops per milliliter as dictated by the administration set.
- Rate represents the number of drops per minute to which the administration set must be set to administer the dose ordered.

After a little more exploration of what the pieces of the formula mean, you will be ready to calculate any medication order.

The DD is whatever is ordered. It may be in grams, milligrams, milligrams per minute, micrograms per kilogram per minute, or another dose, but regardless of the units, the order is always the DD. The DD is often dictated in local protocols or stated over the phone by a physician. The dosing of the medication may be expressed as "Give 2 mg per minute," or "Administer 300 mg of a 10% solution over 10 minutes."

The preceding orders include a *time* during which the medication must be administered. That is a clue that you should use the rate-based formula to solve the problem.

The DOH is the amount of medication available. Some medications are premixed (the concentrated dose of medication has been added to a bag of solution, and the prepared concentration is indicated on the "premixed" bag), some come in prefilled syringes, and others consist of small volumes of liquid that need to be mixed into a larger volume of solution, such as normal saline.

Table 6-4   Common Adult Medications

Drug	Common Dose	Concentration	Route
2 g lidocaine (premixed)	1–4 mg/min	2 g/500 mL (4 mg/mL)	IV maintenance infusion
2% lidocaine	1–1.5 mg/kg	100 mg/5 mL	IV injection
Albuterol sulfate	2.5 mg	2.5 mg/3 mL	Nebulizer
Amiodarone	150 mg	50 mg/mL	IV injection
Atropine	0.5–1 mg	0.1 mg/mL	IV injection
Diltiazem	20–25 mg	5 mg/mL	IV injection
Diphenhydramine (Benadryl)	25–50 mg	50 mg/mL	IV or IM injection*
Dopamine (premixed)	2–20 µg/kg/min	800 mg/500 mL (1.6 mg/mL or 1,600 µg/mL)	IV maintenance infusion
Epinephrine	1 mg	1:10,000	IV injection
Epinephrine	0.3 mg	1:1,000	SC or IM injection*
Furosemide (Lasix)	40–80 mg	10 mg/mL (in a 10-mL prefilled syringe)	IV injection
Magnesium sulfate	1–2 g	0.5 g/mL	IV injection
Nitroglycerin	0.4 mg	0.4 mg/tablet or spray	Sublingual

*IM = intramuscular; SC = subcutaneous

Many of the medications carried on your ambulance will be present in volumes larger than 1 mL. In such cases, the math becomes much simpler if you figure out how much medication is found in 1 mL of the solution. For example, performing calculations with 20 g of medication in 10 mL of solution means more work than performing calculations with 2 g of medication in 1 mL of solution.

The rate in this formula is expressed as drops per minute. It takes into consideration the dose ordered, the time during which the dose should be administered, the type of medication available, and the administration set that will be used to deliver the medication.

Calculating the rate with the preceding formula will allow you to give the medication without the benefit of technology to calculate the amount to give. The final result, expressed in drops per minute, will enable you to confirm that your patient is receiving the correct dose. You do this by looking at the drip chamber of your administration set, glancing at the second hand on your watch, and turning the wheel on the clamp to adjust the flow to the correct number of drops per minute.

Solving Rate-Dependent Problems by Using the Number 1

Before practicing with some examples, reconsider the formula for solving rate-dependent problems once more—this time with the units represented. The units shown are not the only units of measure that will be

Math Hints
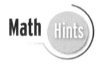

Make a list of the information you need. Eliminate distractions by making an organized list of the information that is available—including the question.

used while performing calculations for medication delivery by using this formula, of course. Rather, they are shown simply to illustrate why this formula works so well.

This formula is derived in the following manner (using milligrams in this example):

Desired dose (DD) = mg/min

Dose on hand (DOH) = mg/mL

gtt/mL = drops/mL (or cc, which is interchangeable with mL)

$$\frac{\frac{mg}{min}}{\frac{mg}{mL}} \times \frac{gtt}{mL} = \text{rate}$$

To solve problems of this sort, follow these steps:
1. Understand that the line in each fraction means "divided by."

2. Follow the rule for dividing two fractions: invert and multiply.

Thus, the formula is rewritten as follows:

$$\frac{mg}{min} \times \frac{mL}{mg} \times \frac{gtt}{mL} = rate\ (gtt/min)$$

When the fraction is reduced (that is, when like units in the numerators and denominators on opposite sides of the formulas are crossed out), the unit of measure for the rate becomes "gtt/min."

"**mg**" can be crossed out in the numerator and denominator.

$$\frac{\cancel{mg}}{min} \times \frac{mL}{\cancel{mg}} \times \frac{gtt}{mL} = rate\ (gtt/min)$$

"**mL**" can also be crossed out in the numerator and denominator.

$$\frac{\cancel{mg}}{min} \times \frac{\cancel{mL}}{\cancel{mg}} \times \frac{gtt}{\cancel{mL}} = rate\ (gtt/min)$$

The unit of measure left in the equation is "gtt/min."

$$\frac{\cancel{mg}}{min} \times \frac{mL}{\cancel{mg}} \times \frac{\cancel{gtt}}{mL} = rate\ (gtt/min)$$

Now, take advantage of the number 1. If a certain dose of medication is provided in a volume of solution larger than 1 mL, find out how much medication is present in 1 mL. All of the calculations become easier when all denominators are 1. The best method is to first convert the DD to units expressed in terms of "1 minute," the DOH in terms of "1 mL" (or some other unit of measure), and the administration set in terms of "gtt/1 mL."

Math Hints

Pay attention to the units of measure. Be sure that you use *like* units of measure in your calculations. Change the units of measure in the problem, if necessary, to the units you will be administering to the patient.

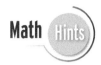

Math Hints

Calculations are easier when the denominators are all 1. Therefore:

- If a dose is provided in a volume of solution larger than 1 mL, find out how much medication is present in 1 mL.
- If the medication should be given during a period longer than 1 minute, figure out the amount of medication needed in 1 minute.

Here are a few problems:

The physician orders a lidocaine drip for a patient being transported by ground (inclement weather prevents air transport) to a facility a long distance away. The orders are given by phone, and you are required to give 2 mg/min. After you repeat the order to the online medical control physician, you open the medication drawer in the ambulance and find that the lidocaine in your service is stocked in 250-mL bags containing 1 g of lidocaine, and a microdrip administration set is already in use for the patient.

You need to determine how to administer the medication to your patient. First, write out the formula:

$$\frac{DD}{DOH} \times \frac{gtt}{mL} = rate\ (gtt/min)$$

Next, you plug in the pieces of information. First, plug in the number of drops per milliliter of the administration set. In this case, the patient has a 60-gtt/mL set (a microdrip set) hooked up to the IV catheter, which means that the administration set will deliver 60 drops per milliliter (60 gtt/mL). There is no reason to do anything with this number because the fraction already has 1 as the denominator, which is the simplest form of the fraction.

$$\frac{DD}{DOH} \times \frac{60\ gtt}{1\ mL} = rate\ (gtt/min)$$

Next, plug in the DD—the amount of medication ordered by the physician, or 2 mg/min.

$$\frac{2\ mg/1\ min}{DOH} \times \frac{60\ gtt}{mL} = rate\ (gtt/min)$$

Now, only two pieces are missing in the formula. One missing piece is the rate. The DOH is 1 g of lidocaine in a 250-mL bag of normal saline.

The formula now looks like this:

$$\frac{2 \text{ mg}/1 \text{ min}}{1 \text{ g}/250 \text{ mL}} \times \frac{60 \text{ gtt}}{\text{mL}} = \text{rate (gtt/min)}$$

First, convert the grams of lidocaine into milligrams of lidocaine: 1 g is equal to 1,000 mg.

$$\frac{\dfrac{2 \text{ mg}}{1 \text{ min}}}{\dfrac{1{,}000 \text{ mg}}{250 \text{ mL}}} \times \frac{60 \text{ gtt}}{\text{mL}} = \text{rate (gtt/min)}$$

The fraction "1,000 mg lidocaine/250 mL NS" would be easier to use in the formula if 1 mL were in the denominator instead of 250 mL. So, change 250 to 1. Proportions are the appropriate tool in your math jump bag.

$$\frac{1{,}000 \text{ mg}}{250 \text{ mL}} = \frac{? \text{ mg}}{1 \text{ mL}}$$

Solve the proportion using cross multiply and divide.

$$(1{,}000 \text{ mg} \times 1 \text{ mL}) \div 250 \text{ mL} = 4 \text{ mg}$$

You have determined that the 1 g of lidocaine in 250 mL of normal saline is equal to 4 mg of lidocaine in 1 mL, which is the concentration.

Now, insert this value into the formula:

$$\frac{\dfrac{2 \text{ mg}}{1 \text{ min}}}{\dfrac{4 \text{ mg}}{1 \text{ mL}}} \times \frac{60 \text{ gtt}}{\text{mL}} = \text{rate (gtt/min)}$$

Or

$$\frac{2 \text{ mg}}{1 \text{ min}} \times \frac{1 \text{ mL}}{4 \text{ mg}} \times \frac{60 \text{ gtt}}{\text{mL}} = \text{rate (gtt/min)}$$

We've mentioned that calculations are always easier when the denominators are 1. There is currently a 4 in the denominator. We can change this to 1 by "using the number one" in the form of $\frac{4}{4}$ as follows (divide the 4 and the 60 by 4):

$$\frac{2 \text{ mg}}{1 \text{ min}} \times \frac{1 \text{ mL}}{4 \text{ mg}} \times \frac{\overset{15}{\cancel{60 \text{ gtt}}}}{\text{mL}} = \text{rate (gtt/min)}$$

We've also crossed out like units (mg and mL).

Now you have simplified the formula by changing all of the denominators to 1. Finding the rate is as easy as:

$$2/\text{min} \times 15 \text{ gtt} = \text{rate (gtt/min)}$$
$$30 \text{ gtt/min} = \text{rate}$$

Remember: Your answer using a 60-gtt/mL infusion set is 30 gtt/min, so adjust the drops to 30 gtt/min by using the "wheel" on the IV tubing, and count the drops.

Use the same administration set used in your calculation. If you calculated with a 60-gtt/mL set, do not use a 10-gtt/mL set.

Every minute, 30 drops of solution must drip into the chamber of the administration set (and, therefore, the patient). Another way to look at this is that 1 drop of medication should drip every 2 seconds.

$$30 \text{ gtt}/1 \text{ min} = 30 \text{ gtt}/60 \text{ s}$$

Reduce the fraction:

$$\frac{30 \text{ gtt}}{60 \text{ s}} = \frac{1 \text{ gtt}}{2 \text{ s}}$$

Here is another example.

The medical control physician orders 1 g/min of medication for the patient. Your ambulance stocks 100-mL bags containing 10 g of the prescribed medication. A microdrip administration set is available.

Begin by plugging in the drops per milliliter of the administration set. Because it is a microdrip set, the value is 60 gtt/mL. Next, plug in the DD, which is 1 g/min. Finally, plug in the DOH, or 10 g/100 mL:

$$\frac{1 \text{ g/min}}{10 \text{ g}/100 \text{ mL}} \times \frac{60 \text{ gtt}}{1 \text{ mL}} = \text{rate (gtt/min)}$$

By using proportions, convert the DOH so that the denominator will be 1. Note that the denominator will actually be the grams, since the equation looks like this once broken out:

$$\frac{1\text{ g}}{\text{min}} \times \frac{100\text{ mL}}{10\text{ g}} \times \frac{60\text{ gtt}}{1\text{ mL}} = \text{rate (gtt/min)}$$

Set up the proportion:

$$\frac{10\text{ g}}{100\text{ mL}} = \frac{1\text{ g}}{?\text{ mL}}$$

Flip the equation:

$$\frac{100\text{ mL}}{10\text{ g}} = \frac{?\text{ mL}}{1\text{ g}}$$

Solve the proportion by using cross multiply and divide.

$$(100\text{ mL} \times 1\text{ g}) \div 10\text{ g} = 10\text{ mL}$$

Plug this value into the original formula:

$$\frac{1\text{ g/min}}{1\text{ g/10 mL}} \times \frac{60\text{ gtt}}{1\text{ mL}} = \text{rate (gtt/min)}$$

Now that the fractions have 1 as the denominators, solve the formula:

$$\frac{1\text{ g}}{\text{min}} \times \frac{10\text{ mL}}{1\text{ g}} \times \frac{60\text{ gtt}}{\text{mL}} =$$

$$\frac{600\text{ gtt}}{1\text{ min}} = 600\text{ gtt/min}$$

Practice

1. You are asked to administer a procainamide infusion at 3 mg/min. You have on hand 1 g of the drug in 250 mL of dextrose and water (D₅W). Your infusion set is a 60 gtt/mL set. How many drops per minute will you give?

2. You respond to a 9-1-1 call for a 70-year-old woman complaining of sweating, shortness of breath, and tightness in the chest. When you arrive on scene, your patient states she has a history of black lung disease and in the past has "felt her heart jumping out of her chest." Now she says it feels "different;" she feels light-headed and cannot catch her breath. While your EMT partner is giving the patient oxygen, you decide to apply the cardiac monitor and run a 12-lead strip. You notice on the electrocardiograph monitor that the patient has a sinus rhythm with some multifocal premature ventricular contractions and some short runs of ventricular tachycardia. Per your protocol you administer two doses of lidocaine. The patient seems to respond well to the treatment, and the monitor shows occasional irregularities. You decide that the patient needs a lidocaine drip, which you start at 3 mg/min. You have 2 g of lidocaine in a 500-mL bag of normal saline on hand and a 60-gtt/mL administration set. How many drops per minute must this drip run?

Dimensional Analysis

The approach discussed in the previous section is actually called dimensional analysis. Most prehospital care providers prefer the dimensional analysis approach (also known as factor analysis). One advantage of using this approach is the ability to consolidate several arithmetic steps into a single equation. With dimensional analysis, you can set up problems with fractions so that like units cancel out, and you keep the units you want. In addition, in the previous section, the number 1 was used to change the denominators to ones, simplifying the calculation.

Here are a few more examples, this time without using the number 1. Dimensional analysis is a good, easy way to approach calculating drug doses because you need only one equation to find the answer. Also, to make it easier, make sure you round your answer (gtt/min) to the nearest whole number.

A physician orders 2 mg/min of lidocaine to be administered to a patient experiencing chest discomfort. A vial containing 1 g of lidocaine in 5 mL of solution is on hand. Your unit carries only 250-mL bags of D₅W. You have a microdrip administration set. How many drops per minute should you administer?

Write out the information:
- DD: 2 mg lidocaine/min IV
- DOH: 1 g lidocaine/5 mL
- Volume on hand: 250 mL D$_5$W
- Administration set: 60 gtt/mL
- How many gtt/min?

By using the formula, write out the problem and solve it. The formula is:

$$\frac{DD}{DOH} \times \frac{gtt}{mL} = \text{rate (gtt/min)}$$

As always, the DD is what the physician ordered: 2 mg/min of lidocaine. The DOH is what you have: 1 g/5 mL of lidocaine.

The next step will be to plug the numbers into the formula. The DD is 2 mg/min. The DOH is 1 g of lidocaine in a 5-mL vial, and a 250-mL bag of D$_5$W is available. The vial of lidocaine will be added to the bag of D$_5$W to make a bag of fluid containing the medication, which will be the actual DOH.

The vial contains 5 mL, and the bag contains 250 mL. Therefore, when the contents of the 5-mL vial are added to the 250-mL bag, the total volume becomes 255 mL. However, as a general rule, when the volume of the vial is less than 10% of the volume of the bag, it is not necessary to consider the added volume in the calculation. In this case, 10% of the volume of the bag would be 25 mL. Because 5 mL is less than 25 mL, the 5 mL can be ignored and 250 mL used as the total volume.

Therefore, the DOH in this case will be 1 g lidocaine/250 mL D$_5$W.

First, convert the grams to milligrams.

$$1 \text{ g} \times \frac{1,000 \text{ mg}}{1 \text{ g}} = 1,000 \text{ mg}$$

Plug the numbers into the formula:

$$\frac{2 \text{ mg/min}}{1,000 \text{ mg/250 mL}} \times \frac{60 \text{ gtt}}{mL} = ? \text{ gtt/min}$$

Restated, this is:

$$\frac{2 \text{ mg}}{\text{min}} \times \frac{250 \text{ mL}}{1,000 \text{ mg}} \times \frac{60 \text{ gtt}}{mL} = ? \text{ gtt/min}$$

$$\frac{2 \times 250 \times 60}{1,000} = ? \text{ gtt/min}$$

$$\frac{2 \times 25 \times 6}{10} = \frac{300}{10}$$

Reduce the fraction:

$$\frac{300}{10} = \frac{30}{1}$$

The answer is a rate of 30 gtt/min.

In the next sections are other types of problems that can be solved by using dimensional analysis.

Calculating the Number of Milliliters to Administer
Here is another type of problem that can be solved with dimensional analysis.

> You have orders to give 0.3 mg of epinephrine IM. You have 1 mg in a 1-mL ampule. How much medication do you draw up to give the correct amount?

In this example you want to calculate the amount to draw up, or the number of milliliters. Set up the problem so that when units are canceled out, milliliters are left:

$$0.3 \text{ mg} \times \frac{1 \text{ mL}}{1.0 \text{ mg}} = ? \text{ mL}$$

$$0.3 \div 1 = 0.3 \text{ mL}$$

The answer is 0.3 mL.

Here is another example in which units need to be converted so that all of the units are the same.

> The patient needs 400 µg of a medication. The DOH is 2 mg in a 10-mL prefilled syringe. How much will you administer?

First, convert milligrams to micrograms. Refer to Table 5-1 for the conversion factor.

$$2 \text{ mg} \times \frac{1,000 \text{ µg}}{\text{mg}} = ? \text{ µg}$$

$$2 \times 1,000 = 2,000 \text{ µg}$$

Set up the problem so that milliliters are the units.

$$\frac{10 \text{ mL}}{2,000 \text{ µg}} \times 400 \text{ µg} = ? \text{ mL}$$

$$\frac{10 \times 400}{2,000} = 2 \text{ mL}$$

The answer is 2 mL.

Calculating How Long It Will Take The next problem asks how many minutes it will take to administer a medication.

> You need to administer 2 mg/min of a medication. The total amount of medication to give is 68 mg. How long will it take to give the medication?

Set up the problem so that when the units cancel out, minutes are left.

$$68 \text{ mg} \times \frac{1 \text{ min}}{2 \text{ mg}} = ? \text{ min}$$

$$68 \div 2 = 34 \text{ min}$$

The answer is 34 minutes.

Calculating the Drip Rate Here is one more example. This example revisits setting up the problem to result in the rate, or gtt/min.

> You are asked to give 100 mL to a patient during the next 2 hours. You have established an IV line with microdrip tubing (60 gtt/mL). What rate is needed to give the correct amount?

First, convert hours to minutes so the units in the answer will be in the usual gtt/min.

$$2 \text{ hours} \times \frac{60 \text{ min}}{h} = ? \text{ min}$$

$$2 \times 60 = 120 \text{ min}$$

Next, set up the problem so the units are gtt/min.

$$\frac{60 \text{ gtt}}{mL} \times \frac{100 \text{ mL}}{120 \text{ min}} = \frac{? \text{ gtt}}{min}$$

$$\frac{60 \times 100}{120} = \frac{50 \text{ gtt}}{min}$$

The answer is a rate of 50 gtt/min.

In some problems, more information is given than is needed to solve it. Figure out what is needed and what is not important.

> The physician orders that a 200-mL fluid bolus be given during 20 minutes to a patient with hypotension. On hand is a 500-mL bag of normal saline and macrodrip tubing (10 gtt/mL). What is the correct drip rate?

It is nice to know that a 500-mL bag of normal saline is available because it means there is enough

fluid on hand to administer the requested 200 mL. However, knowing that 500 mL is available is not required to solve the problem. Set up the problem the same way as the others, with the units resulting in the rate, or gtt/min.

$$\frac{200 \text{ mL}}{20 \text{ min}} \times \frac{10 \text{ gtt}}{mL} = ? \text{ gtt/min}$$

$$\frac{200 \times 10}{20} = 100 \text{ gtt/min}$$

The answer is a rate of 100 gtt/min.

Here's one last example.

> The medical control physician orders an IV infusion of 250 mL of normal saline running to keep the vein open for 90 minutes. Your administration set is for 10 gtt/mL. How many drops per minute should be administered?

The formula for this simple IV infusion rate problem is:

$$DD \times \frac{gtt}{mL} = gtt/min$$

The DD, in this case, is 250 mL for 90 minutes. Therefore, the units in the formula will be:

$$\frac{mL}{min} \times \frac{gtt}{mL} = gtt/min$$

Plugging the numbers from the scenario into the formula gives:

$$\frac{250 \text{ mL}}{90 \text{ min}} \times \frac{10 \text{ gtt}}{mL} = 27.8 \text{ gtt/min}$$

Round the answer to the nearest whole number, or 28 gtt/min. Therefore, you need to administer approximately 28 gtt/min (7 drops every 15 seconds).

Here are some problems for practice.

Practice
1. You are given orders to give a patient 10 mg of morphine sulfate. You have a multidose vial that contains 50 mg in 5 mL. What is the correct amount of medication to administer?

2. You are instructed to give 1.75 mg/min of a medication. The total amount of medication to give is 63 mg. How long will it take to give the medication?

3. You are asked to give 100 mL to a patient during the next 2 hours. You have inserted an IV line and used macrodrip tubing (10 gtt/mL). What rate will you need to establish to give the correct amount?

4. You have been ordered to administer 50% dextrose at 100 mL/h. Your unit has a 500-mL IV bag on board and a 10-gtt/mL administration set. How many drops per minute should be given?

5. The medical control physician ordered administration of 120 mL of normal saline per hour. Your ambulance carries a 1,000-mL bag. By using a 20-gtt/mL administration set, how many drops per minute should be given?

The Clock Method

Calculating drip rates has been the cause of much anxiety among EMS providers. To help reduce the anxiety of calculating drip rates, there is another method used to solve drip rate problems: the clock method.

With the clock method, you envision a clock divided into quarters. Each quarter has two numbers, an inside number representing a certain number of drops and an outside number representing the amount of drug delivered in that many drops.

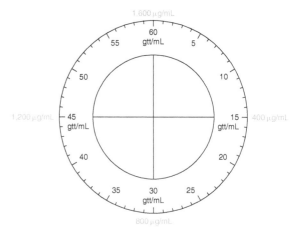

Figure 6-3 A sample clock using a 60-gtt/mL administration set and a maximum concentration of 1,600 µg/mL.

Note that the clock method only applies to a microdrip (60 gtt/mL) administration set. It cannot be used with a macrodrip administration set.

To construct a clock, first, inside the clock, write the gtt/mL from the administration set at the 12 o'clock position. For example, for a microdrip administration set, write "60 gtt/mL" at the 12 o'clock position. Then write progressive quarter amounts of the total number of drops per minute at each quarter interval. For example, write 15 gtt/mL at the 3 o'clock position, 30 gtt/mL at the 6 o'clock position, and 45 gtt/mL at the 9 o'clock position. The clock method can be used for any medication being administered with a 60-gtt/mL administration set.

Next, outside the clock, write the maximum concentration at 12 o'clock and then subsequent quarters at the 3, 6, and 9 o'clock positions. For example, if the concentration is 1,600 µg/mL, write 1,600 µg/mL at the 12 o'clock position, 400 µg/mL at the 3 o'clock position, 800 µg/mL at the 6 o'clock position, and 1,200 µg/mL at the 9 o'clock position. Figure 6-3 shows the completed clock just described.

The figure shows how to set up a clock but not how to use it. The next sections cover the concept behind the clock and how to use such a clock.

You can set up a clock for any drug or solution administered with a 60-gtt/mL administration set.

The Rule of Fours   The rule of fours is a method for determining the flow rate when the desired dose is rate-based. When using this method, a clock is created with the drops per milliliter written inside the clock at four points and the concentration written outside the clock at the same four points.

To understand this method, consider drops per milliliter and concentration. An administration set delivers a certain number of drops per milliliter. For example, a 60-gtt/mL administration set delivers 60 drops per milliliter. Meanwhile, concentration indicates the weight (g, mg, or μg) per milliliter. For example, a concentration of 5 mg/mL means that there are 5 mg in 1 mL.

Because both of the amounts are per 1 mL, the amount of medication delivered in the number of drops listed on the administration set can be deduced. In other words, continuing with the example, because there are 60 gtt/mL and 5 mg/mL, 60 drops contain 5 mg of medication:

$$\frac{60 \text{ gtt}}{\text{mL}} = \frac{5 \text{ mg}}{\text{mL}}$$

The rule of fours uses this concept by setting up a clock that compares the drops per milliliter with the concentration. Two examples of clocks follow—lidocaine and dopamine—because these are the most frequently used drips.

Lidocaine Clock   Here is an example.

> The medical control physician orders administration of 1 mg/min of lidocaine. The DOH is a vial containing 1 g of lidocaine in 5 mL. Also on hand are 500-mL bags of D_5W and a microdrip administration set. How many drops per minute should you administer?

Step 1: Calculating the Concentration   Use the same information as in the dimensional analysis problem, but this time the concentration is also needed. The concentration indicates how much drug is in the IV solution (for example, mg/mL).

How is the concentration calculated? The key is to calculate the "per milliliter" concentration. The following is a simple formula. You may recall this formula from the section on DOH.

$$\frac{\text{Solute (g or mg of drug)}}{\text{Solvent (mL or L of volume)}} = ?$$

You have on hand 1 g of lidocaine and an IV bag of 500 mL, or 1 g/500 mL. (Because 10% of 500 mL is 50 mL, the 5 mL from the vial does not need to be considered in the total volume.) To solve this problem, first an answer in milligrams is needed because the physician's order is for milligrams. To convert the grams to milligrams, recall from Table 5-1 that 1 g equals 1,000 mg. After converting to milligrams, divide the number of milligrams by the total number of milliliters to determine the concentration.

$$1 \text{ g} = 1,000 \text{ mg}$$
$$\frac{1,000 \text{ mg}}{500 \text{ mL}} = 2 \text{ mg/mL}$$

Therefore, the concentration is 2 mg/mL, or 2 mg/1 mL, of solution. This means that for every 1 mL there are 2 mg of lidocaine.

Step 2: Setting Up the Clock   To set up the clock, start at 12 o'clock. Because a microdrip administration set is being used, place 60 gtt on the inside and 2 mg on the outside of the clock. Move to the right quarter, and mark the 15-minute position with 15 gtt inside and 0.5 mg outside. Move to the right another quarter, and mark the 30-minute position with 30 gtt and 1 mg. Continue another quarter, and mark the 45-minute position with 45 gtt and 1.5 mg. Figure 6-4 ▶ shows this clock.

How does the clock help determine how many drops are needed to give the DD? Find the DD on the clock—the corresponding number of drops (gtt) will deliver the DD.

Because the physician ordered 1 mg/min, you will need an administration set that can drip 30 gtt/min. Because administration sets are adjustable, a 60-gtt/mL administration set could be adjusted to administer 30 drops per minute.

The physician's order was to administer 1 mg/min of lidocaine. The clock reveals that 30 gtt corresponds to 1 mg. You may administer 30 drops a minute with a 60-drop administration set.

One note: Sometimes, based on protocols, you may give an initial dose of a medication IV push, or by simple injection, and then follow up with a drip. This initial injection does not factor into the calculations for the drip.

Dopamine Clock   Another common clock used in prehospital care is the dopamine clock. Note that dopamine doses are weight-based. Weight-based calculations are covered in Chapter 7, but the clock is discussed briefly here. Here is an example.

> The medical director orders 10 μg/kg/min of dopamine via IV. The drug vial on hand contains 200 mg of dopamine in 10 mL of solution. The patient weighs 60 kg. You have 250-mL bags of D_5W and a microdrip administration set. How many drops per minute are needed for correct administration of dopamine?

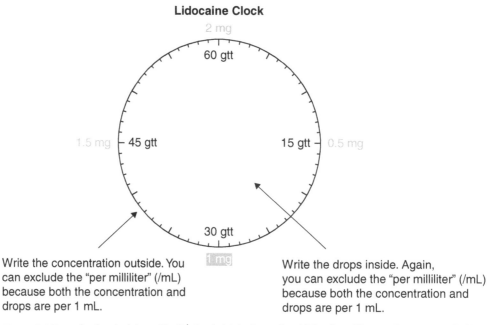

Lidocaine Clock

Write the concentration outside. You can exclude the "per milliliter" (/mL) because both the concentration and drops are per 1 mL.

Write the drops inside. Again, you can exclude the "per milliliter" (/mL) because both the concentration and drops are per 1 mL.

Figure 6-4 Example of a clock for a 60-gtt/mL administration set and lidocaine with a maximum concentration of 2 mg/mL.

Set up the problem the same way as for lidocaine.

Revisit the steps: Calculate the concentration, and set up the clock. After these two steps is a third step: Factor in the patient's weight, which is necessary because dopamine doses are weight-based.

Step 1: Calculating the Concentration   First, calculate the concentration available. Convert 200 mg into micrograms (µg). Dopamine uses micrograms for measurement. There are 1,000 µg in 1 mg.

$$200 \text{ mg} \times \frac{1,000\,\mu g}{\text{mg}} = 200,000\,\mu g$$

$$\frac{200,000\,\mu g}{250 \text{ mL}} = \frac{800\,\mu g}{\text{mL}}$$

Therefore, the total concentration is 800 µg/mL.

Step 2: Setting Up the Clock   Figure 6-5 ▶ shows the setup of a dopamine clock using the 800-µg/mL concentration and a 60-gtt/mL administration set (microdrip).

Step 3: Factoring in the Patient's Weight   As mentioned earlier, with dopamine and other weight-based medications, before using the clock the patient's weight needs to be factored in.

At this point, with the lidocaine clock, you would simply look at the clock and determine the drops per minute that will give the DD. However, with dopamine, the clock cannot be used until the DD has been

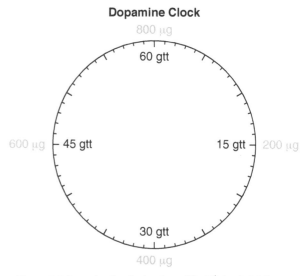

Dopamine Clock

Figure 6-5 Example of a clock using a 60-gtt/mL administration set and dopamine with a maximum concentration of 800 µg/mL.

adjusted to factor in the patient's weight. To adjust the DD, multiply the DD (in µg/kg/min) by the patient's weight in kilograms, as shown in this formula:

$$\text{Patient weight (kg)} \times \text{DD}\left(\frac{\mu g}{\text{kg/min}}\right) = \frac{\mu g}{\text{min}}$$

In this example, the patient weighs 60 kg and the DD is 10 µg/kg/min. Plugging these numbers into the formula gives the adjusted DD:

$$60 \text{ kg} \times \frac{10 \text{ µg}}{\text{kg/min}} = 600 \frac{\text{µg}}{\text{min}}$$

Now you have the information needed to use the clock. Refer to the dopamine clock. You need to administer 600 µg/min, and the clock shows that with 800 µg/mL as the concentration, 45 gtt/min will deliver the adjusted DD.

Other Clocks   Other clocks can be created for other medications according to the concentration available and the administration set that will be used. The following are examples with the information shown in tables in addition to the clocks. Check your local protocols for the doses used in your system.

Epinephrine   Figure 6-6 ▾ shows a clock for epinephrine based on a concentration of 4 µg/mL. For example, you would get this concentration by mixing 1 mg of 1:10,000 epinephrine in 250 mL of D₅W.

$$1 \text{ mg} = 1,000 \text{ µg}$$
$$\frac{1,000 \text{ µg}}{250 \text{ mL}} = 4 \text{ µg/mL}$$

You can administer a dose between 2 and 10 µg/min by using a microdrip set (60 gtt/mL).

Because the clock shows only a maximum dose of 4 µg, Table 6-5 ▸ shows flow rates for larger doses.

Magnesium Sulfate   Figure 6-7 ▸ shows a clock for magnesium sulfate based on a concentration of 4 mg/mL. For example, you would get this concentration

Table 6-5 Epinephrine Flow Rate for a Concentration of 4 µg/mL Using a 60-gtt/mL Administration Set	
Dose (µg/min)	Flow Rate (gtt/min)
1	15
2	30
3	45
4	60
5	75
6	90
7	105
8	120
9	135
10	150

by mixing 1 g of magnesium sulfate in 250 mL of D₅W.

$$1 \text{ g} = 1,000 \text{ mg}$$
$$\frac{1,000 \text{ mg}}{250 \text{ mL}} = 4 \text{ mg/mL}$$

By using a 60-gtt/mL administration set, you can administer a dose between 2 and 4 mg/min. Table 6-6 ▸ shows the flow rates as well.

Nitroglycerin   Figure 6-8 ▸ shows a clock for nitroglycerin based on a concentration of 50 µg/mL. For example, you would get this concentration by mixing 5 mg of nitroglycerin in 100 mL of D₅W.

Epinephrine Clock

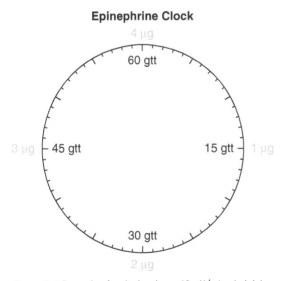

Figure 6-6 Example of a clock using a 60-gtt/mL administration set and epinephrine with a maximum concentration of 4 µg/mL.

Magnesium Sulfate Clock

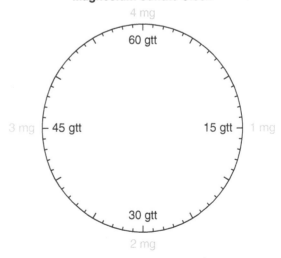

Figure 6-7 Example of a clock using a 60-gtt/mL administration set and magnesium sulfate with a maximum concentration of 4 mg/mL.

Table 6-6 Magnesium Sulfate Flow Rate for a Concentration of 4 mg/mL Using a 60-gtt/mL Administration Set	
Dose (mg/min)	Flow Rate (gtt/min)
1	15
2	30
3	45
4	60

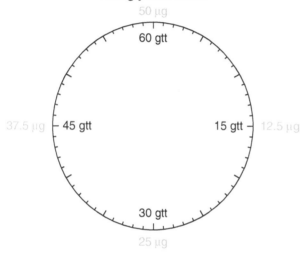

Figure 6-8 Example of a clock using a 60-gtt/mL administration set and nitroglycerin with a maximum concentration of 50 µg/mL.

Table 6-7 Nitroglycerin Flow Rate for a Concentration of 50 µg/mL Using a 60-gtt/mL Administration Set	
Dose (µg/min)	Flow Rate (gtt/min)
5	6
6	7
7	8
8	10
13	16
17	20
20	24

$$5 \text{ mg} = 5,000 \text{ µg}$$

$$\frac{5,000 \text{ µg}}{100 \text{ mL}} = 50 \text{ µg/mL}$$

By using a 60-gtt/mL administration set, you can administer a dose between 5 and 20 µg/min. Table 6-7 shows the flow rates in whole numbers.

Procainamide   Figure 6-9 shows a clock for procainamide based on a concentration of 4 mg/mL. For example, you would get this concentration by mixing 1,000 mg of procainamide in 250 mL of D_5W.

$$\frac{1,000 \text{ mg}}{250 \text{ mL}} = 4 \text{ mg/mL}$$

By using a 60-gtt/mL administration set, you can administer 1 to 4 mg/min. Table 6-8 shows the flow rates as well. You may also notice that this clock is the same as the clock for magnesium sulfate because the concentration and administration set for these two examples are the same.

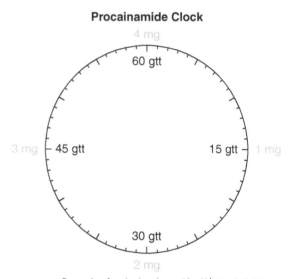

Figure 6-9 Example of a clock using a 60-gtt/mL administration set and procainamide with a maximum concentration of 4 mg/mL.

Table 6-8 Procainamide Flow Rate for a Concentration of 4 mg/mL Using a 60-gtt/mL Administration Set	
Dose (mg/min)	Flow Rate (gtt/min)
1	15
2	30
3	45
4	60

Practice

1. You place 2 g of lidocaine in a 500-mL bag of D_5W with microdrip tubing. The physician orders 4 mg/min to control cardiac irregularities. What drip rate will you establish?

2. The medical control physician orders dopamine for a 175-pound patient. On hand, you have two 200-mg vials of the drug. You mix them into a 250-mL bag of D_5W. The dose ordered is 5 µg/kg/min. How many drops per minute will you administer with a 60-gtt/mL administration set?

Adjusting Flow Rates

Sometimes you may be asked to adjust a flow rate during transport because the fluid being administered through the vein is too much (possibly resulting in edema) or too little (and inadequate to treat dehydration). Adjusting the flow rate helps avoid overdosing or underdosing the patient. Prehospital care providers need to know the prescribed dose, concentration of the dose in 1 mL of solution, and the drops per milliliter given by the administration set. During administration of IV fluids, with or without medication added, it is essential to monitor the drops per minute being given and, if necessary, adjust the flow if the rate becomes too slow or too fast. However, do not adjust the flow rate without a physician's order if the ordered rate is being maintained. Some medications produce negative or deleterious effects such as nausea and vomiting, dizziness, or heart palpitations if pushed too fast. Other medications need to be given fast because their life in the body is short. Be sure to administer the medication at the rate ordered. It is also essential to monitor the effects of the fluids and medication on the patient's condition and to seek further orders from medical control if a problem is encountered. For example, if a patient's respirations become labored during IV infusion, the rate might be too fast, and medical control should be consulted.

Here is an example.

The medical control physician orders administration of an infusion of normal saline to a patient at 100 mL during 20 minutes using a 10-gtt/mL infusion set. What is the correct rate?

The formula and calculation are as follows:

$$\text{DD} \times \frac{\text{gtt}}{\text{mL}} = \text{gtt/min}$$

In this case, the desired dose is 100 mL/20 min. Plugging in the numbers gives:

$$\frac{100\,\text{mL}}{20\,\text{min}} \times \frac{10\,\text{gtt}}{1\,\text{mL}} = \text{gtt/min}$$

$$\frac{100}{20\,\text{min}} \times \frac{10\,\text{gtt}}{1} = 50\,\text{gtt/min}$$

The answer is 50 gtt/min. The 10-gtt/mL administration set can be adjusted to the correct number of drops per minute by using the wheel on the IV set and counting the drops per minute. To avoid having to count drops for 60 seconds, calculate the number of drops needed in 15 seconds by dividing the number of drops per minute by 4 (because 60 seconds ÷ 15 seconds = 4). Fifty drops divided by 4 equals 12.5 drops.

$$\frac{50\,\text{drops}}{60\,\text{seconds}} \div \frac{4}{4} = \frac{12.5\,\text{drops}}{15\,\text{seconds}}$$

To administer 50 gtt/min, about 13 drops should be given in 15 seconds.

Conclusion

This chapter has covered some background information on IV solutions and administration sets and the DD, DOH, volume on hand, and concentration. This chapter introduced the formula for calculating the rate of flow for IV solutions (gtt/min) and showed how to simplify the calculation by using the number 1. Dimensional analysis was explained as a way to calculate the number of milliliters to draw up, determine the amount of time it will take to administer a given amount of solution, and calculate the correct rate (gtt/min). In addition, the chapter showed how to set up a clock and use the rule of fours, an alternative method for calculating the rate of flow.

Solidify your knowledge by completing the practice problems at the end of this chapter.

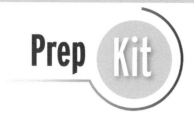

Math Vocabulary

administration set   The drip chamber and tubing used to move fluid from an IV bag into a patient's vascular system.

clock method   A method for calculating drip rates that uses a clock divided into quarters representing the number of drops provided by the administration set and the maximum concentration of the medication to be administered.

colloid solution   A solution that contains many high-protein elements used to expand the blood volume because it increases the osmotic pressure within the circulatory system.

continuous infusion   An infusion that is given for a relatively long period, such as hours or days, at a consistent rate (as opposed to an intermittent infusion); usually used to replace electrolytes or improve fluid balance.

crystalloid solution   A solution that contains electrolytes and nonelectrolytes but not high-protein elements.

desired dose (DD)   The amount of medication ordered by protocol or a physician.

dimensional analysis   A method of calculation in which fractions are set up and like units in the numerators and denominators are cancelled out, resulting in the desired units; for example, mg/min × mL/mg × gtt/mL results in gtt/min.

dose on hand (DOH)   The medication available and how it is packaged.

drip chamber   The part of an administration set in which the fluid accumulates so that the tubing remains filled with fluid.

drop factor   The number of drops per milliliter, or gtt/mL, that an administration set delivers.

gtt   The unit of measure listed on an administration set, which is short for guttae, meaning drops; when written with milliliters on an administration set, represents the number of drops the set delivers per milliliter.

intermittent infusion   An infusion that is given for a relatively short period, such as minutes or hours; commonly used to administer low-volume boluses, for example, a small dose repeated every 3 to 5 minutes, such as diazepam to treat a seizure or morphine for pain management. See also continuous infusion and saline lock.

IV push   An IV injection given directly into a vein, through a port in IV tubing, or through an infusion device such as a saline lock; used when a dose is needed quickly.

macrodrip set   A type of administration set that allows 10 to 20 gtt/mL through a large opening between the piercing spike and the drip chamber.

microdrip set   A type of administration set that allows 60 gtt/mL through the orifice inside the drip chamber.

rate   The number of drops per minute to which the administration set must be set to accomplish the dose ordered.

rule of fours   A method for determining the flow rate when the desired dose is rate-based; gtt/mL and concentration are written on a "clock" divided into quarters and compared to facilitate determining how much medication is contained in a certain number of drops.

saline lock   A device used to aid in the process of administering medication quickly into the body; often used to provide an intermittent infusion and to give chemotherapy drugs for cancer treatment.

total time   The total amount of time during which a medication is to be infused; EMS infusions are usually in minutes.

total volume   The amount of fluid in consideration; includes the amount of fluid in an IV bag and the amount of fluid in a vial of medication that is being added to the bag.

Practice Problems

Solve the following problems to determine the amount of medication to draw up.

1. You receive an order to give 100 µg of fentanyl IV push (IVP). You have 150 µg/3 mL of the medication in a prefilled syringe. What is the correct amount of medication to administer?

2. You have orders to administer 5 mg of valium. You have 10 mg/2 mL ampules. How much will you administer?

3. You have orders to administer 8 mg of valium. You have 10 mg/2 mL ampules. How much will you administer?

4. You need to administer 100 mg of a medication. You have 250 mg in 10 mL of fluid. How much medication will you administer?

5. You need to give 5 mg of medication. You have 40 mg in 20 mL of fluid. How much will you draw up into the syringe?

6. Your patient needs to receive 400 mg of a medication. You have 1 g in a 10-mL prefilled syringe. How much will you administer?

7. You need to give 65 mg of medication. You have 100 mg in 50 mL of fluid. How much will you draw up into the syringe?

8. You need to give 0.2 mg of medication. You have 4 mg in 2 mL of fluid. How much will you draw up into the syringe?

9. Your patient needs to receive 0.05 mg of a medication. You have 1 mg in a 10-mL prefilled syringe. How much will you administer?

10. Your patient needs to receive 0.5 μg of a medication. You have 5 μg in a 10-mL prefilled syringe. How much will you administer?

11. Your patient needs to receive 4 mg of a medication. You have 12 mg in a 5-mL prefilled syringe. How much will you administer?

12. You are given orders to give 1.0 mg of a medication. You have a multidose vial that contains 50 mg in 20 mL of fluid. What is the correct amount of medication to administer?

13. You are given orders to give 250 μg of a medication. You have a multidose vial that contains 5.0 mg in 5 mL of fluid. What is the correct amount of medication to administer?

Solve the following problems using dimensional analysis to determine the amount of time it will take to give a medication.

14. You are instructed to give 4.5 mg/min of a medication. The total amount of medication to give is 252 mg. How long will it take to give the medication?

15. You are instructed to give 100 μg/min of a medication. The total amount of medication to give is 5 mg. How long will it take to give the medication?

16. You are instructed to give 10 μg/min of a medication. The total amount of medication to give is 0.45 mg. How long will it take to give the medication?

17. You are instructed to give 1,000 μg/min of a medication. The total amount of medication to give is 75 mg. How long will it take to give the medication?

18. You are instructed to give 1.25 g/min of a medication. The total amount of medication to give is 30 g. How long will it take to give the medication?

19. You are instructed to give 0.75 mg/min of a medication. The total amount of medication to give is 45 mg. How long will it take to give the medication?

20. You are instructed to give 0.1 mg/min of a medication. The total amount of medication to give is 10 mg. How long will it take to give the medication?

21. You need to administer 12 mg/min of a medication. The total amount of medication to give is 175 mg. How long will it take to give the medication?

22. You need to administer 0.2 mg/min of a medication. The total amount of medication to give is 60 mg. How long will it take to give the medication?

23. You are instructed to give 18 mg/min of a medication. The total amount of medication to give is 350 mg. How long will it take to give the medication?

24. You are instructed to give 37 mg/min of a medication. The total amount of medication to give is 1.3 g. How long will it take to give the medication?

25. You are instructed to give 11 mg/min of a medication. The total amount of medication to give is 1.67 g. How long will it take to give the medication?

Solve the following word problems involving how many milliliters to administer.

26. You are ordered to give 50 mg of diphenhydramine to a patient who is having an allergic reaction. You have a multidose vial that contains 200 mg in 10 mL of fluid. How much medication will you draw up into the syringe?

27. Your patient has a slow heart rate, and the physician has ordered 0.5 mg of atropine by IVP. On your ambulance is a prefilled syringe of 1.0 mg in 10 mL of fluid. How much medication will you administer?

28. You respond to a patient who has a low blood glucose level. Your protocols call for you to administer 25 g of dextrose IV. You have a 50% solution of dextrose that comes prepackaged as 0.5 g/mL, and you have a 50-mL syringe. How much will you administer?

29. You have a patient in atrial flutter. The medical control physician has ordered 5 mg of atenolol by IVP, slowly over 5 minutes. Your ambulance carries this medication in a multidose vial of 25 mg in 10 mL of fluid. How much medication will you administer?

30. You respond to a pregnant patient who is experiencing eclampsia. The physician has ordered 1 g of magnesium sulfate. Your ambulance carries a 4-g solution of magnesium sulfate in 10 mL of fluid. How much medication will you give?

31. You have a patient in cardiac arrest. CPR is in progress when you arrive on scene. Your partner is able to quickly insert an IV line. The first medication to give per your protocol is 1.0 mg of epinephrine 1:10,000. You have a prefilled syringe that contains 2.5 mg/10 mL. How much medication will you give?

32. You and your partner are called to the aid of a driver alongside a road. The driver is conscious and complaining of severe pain in his chest. Your patient is moved to the back of the ambulance, and you give him oxygen. You apply the cardiac monitor, which shows that the rhythm is normal. You insert an IV line. You administer aspirin and give the patient sublingual nitroglycerin spray. You determine that the patient needs to receive 5 mg of morphine sulfate to help relieve the chest pain. You open the narcotic box and find a vial of morphine sulfate that contains 15 mg in 2 mL of fluid. How much medication do you administer to this patient?

The following problems provide dose information for two patients and ask you to determine which patient is receiving more medication. Use dimensional analysis to calculate the amount of medication that will be given to each patient, and indicate which patient receives more.

33. One patient receives 4 mg/min of a medication for 34 minutes. A second patient receives 5 mg/min for 27 minutes. Which patient receives the most medication? Calculate the totals for both patients.

34. One patient receives 0.5 mg/min of a medication for 2.6 hours. A second patient receives 4 mg/min for 20 minutes. Which patient receives the most medication? Calculate the totals for both patients.

35. One patient receives 40 µg/min of a medication for 3.3 hours. A second patient receives 0.2 mg/min for 45 minutes. Which patient receives the most medication? Calculate the totals for both patients.

36. One patient receives 300 µg/min of a medication for 6.5 hours. A second patient receives 0.5 mg/min for 187 minutes. Which patient receives the most medication? Calculate the totals for both patients.

37. One patient receives 7 mg/min of a medication for 4.2 hours. A second patient receives 14 mg/min for 150 minutes. Which patient receives the most medication? Calculate the totals for both patients.

Use dimensional analysis to solve the following problems, converting mL/h to gtt/min.

38. You are asked to give 300 mL to a patient during the next 6 hours. An IV line is inserted, and a microdrip administration set (60 gtt/mL) is used. What rate is needed to give the correct amount?

39. You are asked to give 1,000 mL to a patient during the next 5 hours. An IV line is inserted, and a macrodrip administration set (10 gtt/mL) is used. What rate is needed to give the correct amount?

40. You are asked to give 650 mL to a patient during the next 3 hours. An IV line is inserted, and a macrodrip administration set (10 gtt/mL) is used. What rate is needed to give the correct amount?

41. Your patient needs to receive 2 L of normal saline during the next 18 hours. An IV line is inserted, and a macrodrip administration set (10 gtt/mL) is used. How many drops per minute will you set the IV to run?

42. Your patient needs to receive 1 L of normal saline during the next 2.5 hours. An IV line is inserted, and a macrodrip administration set (10 gtt/mL) is used. How many drops per minute will you set the IV to run?

43. Your patient needs to receive 400 mL of normal saline during the next 90 minutes. An IV line is inserted, and a macrodrip administration set (10 gtt/mL) is used. How many drops per minute will you set the IV to run?

44. Your patient needs to receive 1,200 mL of normal saline during the next 4 hours. An IV is inserted, and a macrodrip administration set (10 gtt/mL) is used. How many drops per minute will you set the IV to run?

45. Your patient needs to receive 900 mL of normal saline during the next 10 hours. An IV line is inserted, and a macrodrip administration set (10 gtt/mL) is used. How many drops per minute will you set the IV to run?

Solve the following word problems involving rate (gtt/min).

46. Your ambulance responds to a motor vehicle crash in which the driver was ejected from the vehicle. You find a man lying on the ground 50 feet from an overturned vehicle. The police estimate the vehicle was traveling 60 mph when the crash occurred. The patient is unconscious and has the following vital signs: blood pressure, 40 mm Hg/palpation; pulse, 110 beats/min; and respirations, 6 breaths/min. You secure the airway and begin assisting ventilations with a bag-valve device and 100% oxygen. The medical control physician has ordered two 250-mL fluid boluses during 15 minutes. You insert two IV lines and hang a 1,000-mL bag of normal saline with each IV using a macrodrip administration set (10 gtt/mL). What rate will you establish for each IV?

47. You need to insert an IV line and give 1,000 mL during the next 3 hours. You place a macrodrip administration set (10 gtt/mL) on a 1,000 mL of lactated Ringer's. What will the rate need to be to give the correct amount of fluid in the proper time frame?

48. The physician orders a 250-mL fluid bolus during 30 minutes. You have a 500-mL bag of normal saline and a macrodrip administration set (10 gtt/mL). What is the correct rate?

49. You place 2 g of lidocaine in a 500-mL bag of D$_5$W and use a microdrip administration set. The physician orders 4 mg/min to control cardiac irregularities. What rate will you establish?

50. The physician orders a 400-mL fluid bolus during 15 minutes. You have a 500-mL bag of normal saline and a macrodrip administration set (10 gtt/mL). What is the rate?

51. The physician orders a 100-mL fluid bolus during 18 minutes. You have a 500-mL bag of normal saline and a macrodrip administration set (10 gtt/mL). What is the correct rate?

52. You place 1 g of lidocaine in a 250-mL bag of D$_5$W and use a microdrip administration set. The physician orders 3 mg/min to control cardiac irregularities. What rate will you establish?

Solve the following problems by using the clock method to determine the rate of flow.

53. Your rescue captain advises you to administer lidocaine per orders from hospital staff. An initial dose is to be given by IVP, followed by a lidocaine drip to be run at 2 mg/min. You reach into the drug box and pull out two vials of lidocaine containing 1 g each, a 500-mL bag of normal saline, and a microdrip administration set. How many drops per minute will you give to achieve a lidocaine drip at 2 mg/min?

54. The medical control physician ordered 7 μg/kg/min of dopamine to a 220-lb patient. You have a 60-gtt/mL administration set, a 250-mL bag of D$_5$W, and two vials each containing 200 mg of dopamine. How many gtt/min will you give?

55. The physician orders a dopamine IV drip at 5 μg/kg/min. You carry a vial of 200 mg/10 mL, a 250-mL IV bag of normal saline, and a microdrip administration set. The patient weighs 80 kg. At how many drops per minute will you set the IV?

7 Weight-Based Calculations

Introduction

Problems that involve time but do not consider the patient's weight can be solved by using the rate-based formula discussed in Chapter 6. But when the patient's weight needs to be factored into the dose, a weight-based calculation is needed.

Dopamine calculations are the usual example instructors introduce for calculating medication based on a patient's weight. It is worthwhile to work through some calculations and master the process before a real need occurs.

In some areas, many calls involve pediatric patients. Most medications administered to children and infants are weight-based. Some medications for adults are also weight-based. Most require conversion from pounds to kilograms. The method outlined here is simple and easy to memorize.

Calculating a Weight-Based Dose

For an order in milligrams per kilograms, part of solving the math problem is to convert the patient's weight from pounds to kilograms and then adjust the dose to account for the weight. This calculation does not involve a rate in drops per minute, so it is quite simple. Keep the following in mind when solving this type of problem:

- The amount of drug to be given
- The amount of drug to administer per kilogram

Most of the problems solved in this section require the use of dimensional analysis.

The medical control physician orders administration of a 1-mg/kg lidocaine bolus to a person with stable ventricular tachycardia. The person weighs 110 lb. How many milligrams will you administer to your patient?

First, convert pounds to kilograms. Because 1 kg equals 2.2 lb, divide 110 lb by 2.2.

$$110 \text{ lb} \div 2.2 \text{ lb/kg} = 50 \text{ kg}$$

So, 110 lb equals 50 kg.

Because the desired dose (DD) is 1 mg/kg and the patient's weight is 50 kg, calculate the dose to be administered as follows:

$$\frac{1 \text{ mg}}{\text{kg}} \times 50 \text{ kg} = 50 \text{ mg}$$

Therefore, the dose you will give to a 110-lb patient is 50 mg.

To convert pounds to kilograms, divide the weight in pounds by 2.2.

Practice

1. Use the conversion factor for kilograms and pounds and determine how many kilograms a 185-lb patient weighs.

2. Convert 52 lb to kilograms.

3. If 2.2 lb equals 1 kg, how many pounds does a 75-kg patient weigh?

Calculating a Rate for a Weight-Based Medication

Here is another example that takes into account the patient's weight.

An order for a dopamine drip according to protocols is received from online medical control for a man having blood pressure problems. The physician hangs up before you can ask that the number of drops per minute be repeated.

You confirm that your standard operating procedures state to administer 10 µg/kg/min of dopamine. The ambulance medication drawer has 200 mg of dopamine in a 10-mL vial. You have 250-mL bags of normal saline on hand to mix medications, and a microdrip administration set.

Because this much information can be overwhelming, organize your thoughts by sifting through what you need to know and what you can push aside.

Most medication calculations can be done with simple proportions (cross multiply and divide) unless a rate (time) is involved. The standard operating procedures direct you to give 10 µg/kg/*min*. Because this problem involves time, use the same formula as for rate-based medication calculations:

$$\frac{DD}{DOH} \times \frac{gtt}{mL} = \text{rate (gtt/min)}$$

Make a list of what you know:

DD: The DD according to standard operating procedures is 10 µg/kg/min.

DOH: The dose on hand (DOH) is 200 mg of dopamine in a 10-mL vial.

Administration set: A microdrip administration set delivers 60 gtt/mL.

Other: 250-mL bags of normal saline are available to mix the dopamine.

Plug this information into the rate-based formula:

$$\frac{10 \text{ µg/kg/min}}{200 \text{ mg/10 mL}} \times \frac{60 \text{ gtt}}{mL} = \text{rate (gtt/min)}$$

A few areas in this equation need refinement. First, the dose needs to take into account the patient's weight. Second, the rate is in drops per minute, but the units will not cancel out that way, as shown when the equation is rearranged:

$$\frac{10 \text{ µg}}{kg/min} \times \frac{10 \text{ mL}}{200 \text{ mg}} \times \frac{60 \text{ gtt}}{mL} = ?$$

Converting Pounds to Kilograms

As stated, the patient's weight has not been factored in. The numbers consider only a patient weighing 1 kg. The dose needs to be changed to reflect the weight of *your* patient: The 10 µg/kg/min needs to be changed.

Also, the math is more complicated than necessary. The math needs to be simplified.

The patient's weight is needed in kilograms. You estimate his weight to be 176 lb. To convert this to kilograms, set up a proportion: 2.2 lb for every 1 kg is the conversion factor. Because no time is involved in this part of the problem, a ratio gives a quick and easy calculation:

$$\frac{1 \text{ kg}}{2.2 \text{ lb}} = \frac{? \text{ kg}}{176 \text{ lb}}$$

Cross multiply and divide to solve.

$$(1 \text{ kg} \times 176 \text{ lb}) \div 2.2 \text{ kg} = ?$$
$$? = 80 \text{ kg}$$

The revised list of information is as follows:

DD: 10 µg/kg/min

DOH: 200 mg of dopamine in a 10-mL vial

Administration set: 60 gtt/mL

Other: 250-mL bags of normal saline available to mix the dopamine

Patient weight: 80 kg

Adjusting the DD for the Patient's Weight

Now that you know the patient's weight in kilograms, you can take the patient's weight into consideration. You know you need 10 µg of dopamine for every kilogram of the patient's body weight every minute. Now, calculate how many micrograms of dopamine should be administered for an 80-kg patient every minute. Because time is not mentioned, a simple proportion can be set up:

$$\frac{10 \text{ µg}}{1 \text{ kg/min}} = \frac{? \text{ µg}}{80 \text{ kg}}$$

Cross multiply and divide to solve:

$$\frac{10 \text{ µg} \times 80 \text{ kg}}{1 \text{ kg/min}} = ?$$
$$10 \text{ µg} \times 80 \text{ kg} \times \frac{1}{1 \text{ kg /min}} = 800 \text{ µg/min}$$

Therefore, the 80-kg patient needs 800 µg of dopamine every minute. The revised list of information is now as follows:

DD: The desired dose was initially 10 µg/kg/min. With the patient's weight factored in, it is now 800 µg/min.

DOH: 200 mg of dopamine in a 10-mL vial

Administration set: 60 gtt/mL

Other: 250-mL bags of normal saline available to mix the dopamine

Patient weight: 80 kg

Simplifying the DOH

The last piece to deal with is the DOH of dopamine, which is 200 mg of dopamine in a 10-mL vial. There are 250-mL bags of intravenous (IV) normal saline available in which to mix the medication. Therefore, you have:

$$\frac{200 \text{ mg}}{250 \text{ mL}}$$

This is the DOH. However, the calculation will be easier if the denominator is 1. Use a proportion to convert the denominator to 1:

$$\frac{200 \text{ mg}}{250 \text{ mL}} = \frac{? \text{ mg}}{1 \text{ mL}}$$

Cross multiply and divide to solve:

$$\frac{200 \text{ mg}}{250 \text{ mL}} \times 1 \text{ mL} = 0.8 \text{ mg}$$

The answer is that there is 0.8 mg of dopamine in every 1 mL of normal saline.

The DD is in micrograms. But the calculation gave milligrams, so the dopamine DOH needs to be converted to micrograms. By referring to Table 5-1, you confirm that there are 1,000 µg for every 1 mg. Because there is no time in this calculation, set up another simple proportion.

$$\frac{1,000 \text{ µg}}{1 \text{ mg}} = \frac{? \text{ µg}}{0.8 \text{ mg}}$$

Cross multiply and divide:

$$\frac{1,000 \text{ µg}}{1 \text{ mg}} \times 0.8 \text{ mg} = 800 \text{ µg}$$

The calculations show that 1 mL of normal saline contains 800 µg of dopamine.

Solving the Calculation With the Revised Numbers

Here is an updated list of information:

DD: The DD was initially 10 µg/kg/min. The estimated patient's weight of 176 lb was converted to 80 kg. By factoring in the patient's weight in kilograms, the DD became 800 µg/min.

DOH: 200 mg of dopamine in a 10-mL vial, added to a 250-mL bag of normal saline. Adjusting the numbers to make the denominator 1 resulted in 800 µg of dopamine per 1 mL of normal saline.

Administration set: 60 gtt/mL

All of the information has been simplified and can be plugged into the rate-based formula to determine how many drops per minute to administer.

Here is the formula:

$$\frac{\text{DD}}{\text{DOH}} \times \frac{\text{gtt}}{\text{mL}} = \text{rate (gtt/min)}$$

Plug in the revised numbers:

$$\frac{800 \text{ µg/min}}{800 \text{ µg/mL}} \times \frac{60 \text{ gtt}}{\text{mL}} = \text{gtt/min}$$

$$\frac{800 \text{ µg}}{\text{min}} \times \frac{\text{mL}}{800 \text{ µg}} \times \frac{60 \text{ gtt}}{\text{mL}} = ? \text{ gtt/min}$$

$$800 \div 800 = 1$$

$$1 \times 60 \text{ gtt/min} = \text{rate}$$

$$60 \text{ gtt/min} = \text{rate}$$

Working Through a Problem

Here is another example.

> You need to administer 5 µg/kg/min of dopamine to a patient who has low blood pressure and is symptomatic. The patient weighs 113 lb. You place 400 mg of dopamine in a 250-mL bag of D₅W with a microdrip administration set. What will be the rate of administration for this patient?

This problem can be solved in the same way as the previous problem. Here is the information available:

DD: 5 µg/kg/min

DOH: 400 mg in a 250-mL bag of D_5W

Administration set: 60 gtt/mL

Patient weight: 113 lb

First, convert pounds to kilograms.

$$113 \text{ lb} \div 2.2 \text{ lb/kg} = 51.36 \text{ kg}$$

Next, adjust the dose to take the patient's weight into account.

$$\frac{5\ \mu g}{kg\ /min} \times 51.36\ kg\ =\ 256.8\ \mu g/min$$

Revise the information as follows:

DD: 256.8 μg/min

DOH: 400 mg in a 250-mL bag of D₅W

Administration set: 60 gtt/mL

Convert milligrams to micrograms.

$$400\ mg\ \times\ \frac{1,000\ \mu g}{mg}\ =\ 400,000\ \mu g$$

Simplify the dose on hand.

$$\frac{400,000\ \mu g}{250\ mL}\ =\ \frac{?\ \mu g}{1\ mL}$$

$$\frac{400,000\ \mu g}{250\ mL}\ \times\ 1\ mL\ =\ 1,600\ \mu g\ in\ 1\ mL\ of\ fluid$$

Update the information again, as follows:

DD: 256.8 μg/min

DOH: 1,600 μg/mL

Administration set: 60 gtt/mL

All of the information is simplified. Plug it into the formula:

$$\frac{DD}{DOH}\ \times\ \frac{gtt}{mL}\ =\ gtt/min$$

$$\frac{256.8\ \mu g/min}{1,600\ \mu g/mL}\ \times\ \frac{60\ gtt}{mL}\ =\ ?\ gtt/min$$

$$\frac{256.8\ \mu g}{min}\ \times\ \frac{mL}{1,600\ \mu g}\ \times\ \frac{60\ gtt}{mL}\ =\ 9.63\ gtt/min$$

Round to the nearest whole number, or 10 gtt/min.

If you have a calculator, you do not need to simplify all of the numbers first, and the process is shorter. Simply convert the units as needed (patient's weight from pounds to kilograms and micrograms to milligrams), and plug all of the numbers into the formula.

Convert the patient's weight to kilograms:

$$\frac{113\ lb}{2.2}\ =\ 51.36\ kg$$

Convert the milligrams to micrograms:

$$400\ mg\ \times\ \frac{1,000\ \mu g}{mg}\ =\ 400,000\ \mu g$$

Plug the numbers into the formula, and include the patient's weight:

$$\frac{5\ \mu g/kg/min}{400,000\ \mu g/250\ mL}\ \times\ 51.36\ kg\ \times\ 60\ gtt/mL$$

$$=\ ?\ gtt/min$$

$$\frac{5\ \mu g}{kg\ /min}\ \times\ \frac{250\ mL}{400,000\ \mu g}\ \times\ 51.36\ kg\ \times\ 60\ gtt/\ mL$$

$$=\ 9.63\ gtt/min$$

Round to the nearest whole number, or 10 gtt/min. Whether the numbers are simplified ahead of time or not, the answer is the same.

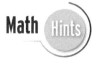

Math Hints

You might have noticed that for dopamine, when the dose on hand is:
- 400 mg in 250 mL or
- 800 mg in 500 mL,

the concentration is 1,600 μg/mL.

Practice

1. A patient who weighs 201 lb needs a dopamine drip at 20 μg/kg/min to help raise the blood pressure. You add 800 mg of dopamine to a 500-mL IV bag of D₅W. You have a microdrip administration set. What is the rate to give the proper amount of medication?

2. You need to give 12 μg/kg/min of dopamine to a patient who has low blood pressure and is symptomatic. The patient weighs 224 lb. You add 400 mg of dopamine to a 250-mL bag of D₅W and use a microdrip administration set. What will be the rate?

3. You are dispatched to an unconscious patient. Upon arrival you find a 65-year-old man who is awake but confused. He reports losing consciousness after exercising this morning. You check his vital signs and find a blood pressure of 60/40 mm Hg, a pulse of 132 beats/min, and respirations of 24 breaths/min. He denies chest pain and shortness of breath. He does not appear dehydrated and has a normal blood glucose level. His lung sounds are clear bilaterally. The medical control physician orders a fluid bolus of 250 mL of normal saline and, if the blood pressure does not increase, to start a dopamine drip at 10 μg/kg/min. The patient weighs 175 lb. After the fluid bolus, the blood pressure is 50/30 mm Hg. You add 800 mg of dopamine to a 500-mL bag of D₅W. You have a microdrip administration set. What is the concentration of 1 mL, and what rate will you establish for this patient?

Calculating Drug Doses for Children and Infants

Two methods are used for calculating pediatric drug doses. The first is based on body weight and the second on body surface area (BSA). Of the two methods, the BSA is the most accurate. However, using the BSA method requires calculating square meters on a device called a nomogram. This device is rarely used in the field. Instead, a method that converts milligrams to kilograms is frequently used. When solving a milligram-to-kilogram problem, μg/kg might be cited when very small amounts of medication are required.

Estimating Body Weight

Sometimes in the field you will be unable to determine an adult's body weight, let alone a child's weight.

For pediatric weight estimates, most paramedics rely on some form of published estimates, protocols, or the Broselow Tape to help determine a patient's weight and the appropriate weight-based drug dose.

Units of Measurement in Kilograms

When dealing with pediatric patients, you will be asked to administer a drug based on the patient's weight. Almost always you will be converting grams, milligrams, micrograms, and so forth into kilograms.

To convert pounds to kilograms, divide the patient's weight in pounds by 2.2. Here are some examples:

- 25 lb ÷ 2.2 = 11.36 kg, or 11 kg
- 120 lb ÷ 2.2 = 54.55 kg, or 55 kg
- 200 lb ÷ 2.2 = 90.91 kg, or 91 kg

Note: You can round off all body weights in kilograms to the nearest whole number.

To convert a patient's weight in kilograms to pounds, multiply the weight in kilograms by 2.2. For example:

- 10 kg × 2.2 = 22 lb
- 50 kg × 2.2 = 110 lb
- 85 kg × 2.2 = 187 lb

To solve a conversion problem that involves converting grams to milligrams, take the DD in grams and multiply it by 1,000 to get milligrams. Remember that for every gram, there are 1,000 milligrams. Here are some examples:

- 2.5 g × 1,000 = 2,500 mg
- 2 g × 1,000 = 2,000 mg
- 10 g × 1,000 = 10,000 mg
- 0.010 g × 1,000 = 10 mg
- 0.0010 g × 1,000 = 1.0 mg

Calculating a Pediatric Weight-Based Dose

Here is an example of a physician's order based on a pediatric patient's weight.

The medical director has ordered 10 mg/kg of medication for a child. Calculate the dose of this drug for a 44-lb child.

First, convert 44 lb to kilograms.

$$44 \text{ lb} \div 2.2 \text{ lb/kg} = 20 \text{ kg}$$

Multiply the weight by the dose.

$$20 \text{ kg} \times \frac{10 \text{ mg}}{\text{kg}} = 200 \text{ mg}$$

Therefore, the dose is 200 mg. Note that this is the same method described at the beginning of this chapter.

Practice

1. Convert 50 lb to kilograms.

2. How many pounds does a 15-kg patient weigh?

3. The medical director has ordered 10 mg/kg of medication to a child. Calculate the dose of drug for a 20-lb child.

Calculating a Rate for a Pediatric Weight-Based Medication

To calculate a drip rate for a pediatric weight-based medication, follow the same steps for calculating a drip rate for an adult weight-based medication.

> The patient weighs 37 kg. You have determined that you need to start a dopamine drip at 10 µg/kg/min to help raise the patient's blood pressure. You place 800 mg of dopamine in a 500-mL IV bag of D_5W. You have a microdrip administration set. What is the rate (gtt/min) to give the proper amount of medication?

Start by listing the information:

DD: 10 µg/kg/min

DOH: 800 mg in a 500-mL bag of D_5W

Administration set: 60 gtt/mL

Patient weight: 37 kg

Because this problem gives the patient's weight in kilograms, conversion from pounds to kilograms is not necessary.

Adjust the DD to account for the patient's weight:

$$\frac{10\ \mu g}{kg/min} \times 37\ kg = 370\ \mu g/min$$

Convert and simplify the DOH, otherwise known as calculating the concentration. As usual for dopamine, it is 1,600 µg/mL.

$$800\ mg \times \frac{1,000\ \mu g}{mg} = 800,000\ \mu g$$

$$\frac{800,000\ \mu g}{500\ mL} = \frac{?\ \mu g}{1\ mL}$$

$$\frac{800,000\ \mu g}{500\ mL} \times 1\ mL = 1,600\ \mu g\ in\ 1\ mL\ of\ fluid$$

Plug into the formula:

$$\frac{370\ \mu g/min}{1,600\ \mu g/mL} \times \frac{60\ gtt}{mL} = ?\ gtt/min$$

$$\frac{370\ \mu g}{min} \times \frac{mL}{1,600\ \mu g} \times \frac{60\ gtt}{mL} = 13.88\ gtt/min$$

Round to the nearest whole number, or 14 gtt/min.

Practice

1. The medical director orders administration of a drug at 6 µg/kg/min via IV. The drug is supplied as 200 mg/5 mL vial. You have a 250-mL IV bag of D_5W and a microdrip administration set. The patient weighs 165 lb. What is the correct rate for the IV?

2. You receive an order to administer 5 mg/kg during 40 minutes. The drug is supplied as 500 mg/10 mL. The patient weighs 170 lb. You have on hand a 250-mL IV bag and a 10-gtt/mL administration set. How many drops per minute will you run the IV?

Rate-Dependent vs Weight-Based Calculations

When you receive a medication order, the physician will not tell you what type of calculation is needed (rate-dependent vs weight-based). Rather, you will need to recognize which type of calculation is required. The first clue to figuring out whether a calculation is rate-dependent or weight-based is to look at the units in the dose ordered. Orders to give the medication during a period of time (such as 2 mg/*min*) are rate-dependent. Orders that involve kilograms (for example, 5 µg/kg/min) are solely weight-based if a period for administration is not indicated.

The following are a rate-dependent problem and a weight-based problem.

> You start an IV of normal saline and want to give 500 mL of fluid during 75 minutes. You have on hand a 1,000-mL bag and a 10-gtt/mL administration set. How many drops per minute will you run the IV?

> The medical control physician ordered a dopamine drip at 5 µg/kg/min. You place 800 mg of dopamine in a 500-mL bag of D₅W and attach a microdrip administration set. The patient weighs approximately 100 lb. What is the correct rate?

In the first problem, the DD is 500 mL of fluid during 75 minutes. There is no mention of weight in the DD. Therefore, this problem is rate-dependent.

In the second problem, the desired dose is 5 µg/kg/min. Because this dose includes kilograms, the problem is weight-based.

Review the following problems, and determine whether they are rate-dependent or weight-based. Then work them out using what you have learned in this chapter.

Practice

1. As a member of an air-rescue team you are transporting a 175-lb patient from the East Coast to the West Coast. You have been instructed to administer 1,000 mL of normal saline fluid during a 6-hour period. With an IV administration set that delivers 10 gtt/mL, how many drops per minute should be given to the patient?

2. You are preparing a standard dose of dopamine solution containing 400 mg in a 250-mL bag of D₅W. With a microdrip administration set, what would be the infusion rate in milliliters per hour for a 150-pound patient, based on 5 µg/kg/min?

3. You are administering the first dose of diltiazem to a patient. Your protocol calls for 0.25 mg/kg for the first dose. The patient weighs 154 lb. How many milligrams should be given to the patient?

4. The patient needs to receive 500 mL of normal saline during the next 75 minutes. The IV is established with a macrodrip administration set (10 gtt/mL). How many drops per minute will you set the IV to run?

Conclusion

In this chapter, you have calculated the answer to one of the most challenging types of medication administration problems for paramedics. The math involved simple proportions and one rate-based formula.

With a strong foundation of simple math principles and a couple of formulas, medication calculations can be simplified and done quickly. Skills stay sharp with practice. Medication administration is one of the paramedic skills that needs to be practiced often so you remain ready to treat patients effectively and minimize chances of error. More rate-dependent calculations are provided on the next few pages to provide additional practice.

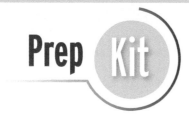

Math Vocabulary

weight-based calculation A medication calculation that takes the patient's weight into consideration; for example, if a dose is ordered per kilogram, the dose must be adjusted to correspond to the patient's weight in kilograms.

Practice Problems

By using the desired dose and the patient's weight, calculate the dose you will administer.

1. A patient is having multifocal premature ventricular contractions (PVCs) at a rate of 20/min. Per protocol, you are directed to administer lidocaine, 1.5 mg/kg to control the PVCs. The patient weighs 150 lb. You have 100 mg of lidocaine in a 10-mL prefilled syringe. What is the dose (adjusted for weight), and how much medication will you administer?

2. You have a patient who needs cardioversion, and, per protocol, you need to administer etomidate, 0.3 mg/kg, for sedation. The patient weighs 122 lb. You have 50 mg of etomidate in a 5-mL vial. What is the adjusted dose, and how much medication will you administer?

3. A 65-year-old patient is in cardiac arrest. During the resuscitation, you receive orders for 1 mEq/kg of sodium bicarbonate. The patient weighs 128 lb. On hand you have 60 mEq of sodium bicarbonate in 50 mL of solution. What volume will you administer?

4. A female patient takes phenytoin for seizures, and, by protocol, you need to administer 15 mg/kg of the medication to help control seizures. You determine that the patient weighs 130 lb. You have 1 g of phenytoin in a 20-mL vial. What is the adjusted dose, and how much medication will you administer to this patient?

5. A patient is having cardiac problems. An electrocardiogram shows a rapid atrial flutter with a rate of 150 beats/min. The medical control physician orders diltiazem, 0.25 mg/kg. The patient weighs 185 lb. You have 25 mg of diltiazem in a 10-mL vial. What is the adjusted dose, and how much medication will you give?

6. The physician has ordered ketamine, 1 to 2 mg/kg during 1 minute, to help control a patient's pain. The patient weighs 142 lb. You decide to administer 2 mg/kg. You have 150 mg of ketamine in 10 mL of solution. How much medication will you administer to this patient?

7. A 51-year-old man is complaining of a severe headache and, after several minutes, becomes unconscious. You attempt intubation, and because of difficulty, the physician gives you an order for rapid-sequence intubation. After a successful intubation and owing to a lengthy transport time, the physician also gives you an order for 0.1 mg/kg of vecuronium to maintain the paralysis of this patient. The patient weighs 174 lb. You have 10 mg of the medication in 10 mL of solution. What is the adjusted dose, and how much medication will you give?

8. The ambulance you are riding on responds to a call for a cardiac patient. The patient is a 75-year-old woman complaining of chest pain and shortness of breath. You apply the monitor and find tachycardia and multifocal PVCs at a rate of 12/min. Per protocol, you are directed to administer lidocaine, 1.0 mg/kg, to control the PVCs. The patient weighs 170 lb. You have 100 mg of lidocaine in a 10-mL prefilled syringe. How much medication will you administer?

9. You respond to a patient suspected of taking an overdose of medications. The patient has shallow and slow respirations, and you attempt to provide an airway but are unable to intubate. The medical control physician gives permission to administer succinylcholine, 0.8 mg/kg. You determine the patient weighs 114 lb. You have on hand 100 mg of succinylcholine in a 2-mL vial. How much medication will you administer?

10. Your ambulance responds to a patient complaining of chest pain. You find a 47-year-old woman complaining of a heavy feeling in her chest and shortness of breath. Your partner gives the patient oxygen, applies the cardiac monitor, and inserts an IV line. When you look at the monitor, you find that the patient needs cardioversion, and, per protocol, you need to administer etomidate, 0.3 mg/kg, for sedation before the delivery of the shock. Your patient weighs 157 lb. You have 50 mg of etomidate in a 5-mL vial. What is the correct dose, and how much medication will you administer?

11. A patient is having multifocal PVCs at a rate of 10/min. Per protocol, you are directed to administer lidocaine, 1.0 mg/kg, to control the PVCs. The patient weighs 208 lb. You have 100 mg of lidocaine in a 10-mL prefilled syringe. How much medication will you administer?

12. A patient is having cardiac problems. Examination shows uncontrolled atrial fibrillation with an irregular rate of 140 beats/min. The medical control physician orders diltiazem, 0.25 mg/kg. The patient weighs 133 lb. You have 20 mg of diltiazem in a 10-mL vial. What is the adjusted dose, and how much medication will you give?

13. You have a patient who needs cardioversion, and, per your protocol, you need to administer etomidate, 0.3 mg/kg, for sedation. The patient weighs 290 lb. You have 50 mg of etomidate in a 5-mL vial. What is the adjusted dose, and how much medication will you administer?

14. The physician ordered ketamine, 1-2 mg/kg during 1 minute, to help control pain. The patient weighs 175 lb. You decide to administer 1 mg/kg. You have 100 mg of ketamine in 10 mL of solution. How much medication will you administer?

15. A patient is having major motor seizures, and, by protocol, you need to administer 15 mg/kg of phenytoin to help control the seizures. You determine that the patient weighs 138 lb. You have 1 g of phenytoin in a 20-mL vial. What is the adjusted dose, and how much medication will you administer?

16. Your patient is in cardiac arrest. During resuscitation, you receive orders for 1 mEq/kg of sodium bicarbonate. The patient weighs 200 lb. In your drug box you have an ampule of 50 mEq of sodium bicarbonate in 50 mL of solution. What volume will you administer?

17. A patient with a head injury is having difficulty breathing, but you are unable to intubate. The medical control physician orders succinylcholine, 0.8 mg/kg. You determine the patient weighs 184 lb. You find 100 mg of succinylcholine in a 2-mL vial. How much medication will you administer?

18. A patient is having multifocal PVCs at a rate of 15/min. Per protocol, you are directed to administer lidocaine, 1.5 mg/kg, to control the PVCs. Your patient weighs 118 lb. You have 100 mg of lidocaine in a 10-mL prefilled syringe. How much medication will you administer?

19. A patient is complaining of a "heavy feeling" in his chest and shortness of breath. The examination shows uncontrolled atrial fibrillation with an irregular rate of 123 beats/min. The medical control physician orders diltiazem, 0.25 mg/kg. The patient weighs 163 lb. You have 20 mg of diltiazem in a 10-mL vial. What is the adjusted dose, and how much medication will you give?

20. A patient is having major motor seizures, and, by protocol, you need to administer 15 mg/kg of phenytoin to help control the seizures. You determine that the patient weighs 105 lb. You have 1 g of phenytoin in a 20-mL vial. What is the adjusted dose, and how much medication will you administer?

21. You are attempting to perform rapid-sequence intubation, and, per your protocol, you need to administer etomidate, 0.3 mg/kg, for sedation. Your patient weighs 200 lb. You have 50 mg of etomidate in a 5-mL vial. What is the adjusted dose, and how much medication will you administer?

22. You have a patient with difficulty breathing and who is unconscious, but you cannot maintain an airway. The medical control physician orders succinylcholine, 0.8 mg/kg. You determine the patient weighs 144 lb. You have 100 mg of succinylcholine in a 2-mL vial. How much medication will you administer?

23. A patient is having multifocal PVCs at a rate of 8/min. Per protocol, you are directed to administer lidocaine, 1.0 mg/kg, to control the PVCs. Your patient weighs 100 lb. You have 100 mg of lidocaine in a 10-mL pre-filled syringe. How much medication will you administer?

24. You have a patient who takes phenytoin for seizures, and, by protocol, you need to administer 15 mg/kg of the medication to help control the seizures. You determine that the patient weighs 190 lb. You have 1 g of phenytoin in a 20-mL vial. What is the adjusted dose, and how much medication will you administer?

25. A patient is in cardiac arrest. During the resuscitation, you receive orders for 1 mEq/kg of sodium bicarbonate. The patient weighs 115 lb. In your drug box, you have 50 mEq of sodium bicarbonate in 50 mL of solution. How much medication and what volume will you administer?

26. A patient is having frequent multifocal PVCs. Per protocol, you are directed to administer lidocaine, 1.5 mg/kg, to control the PVCs. Your patient weighs 289 lb. You have 100 mg of lidocaine in a 10-mL prefilled syringe. How much medication will you administer?

27. A patient is having multifocal PVCs, as shown on the cardiac monitor. You receive an order to administer 1.5 mg/kg of lidocaine. The patient weighs approximately 200 lb. You have 150 mg/10 mL of lidocaine in a prefilled syringe. What is the adjusted dose, and how much lidocaine will you administer?

Solve the following word problems involving rate- and weight-based medications.

28. You need to give 20 µg/kg/min of dopamine to a patient who has extremely low blood pressure and is symptomatic. The patient weighs 289 lb. You place 800 mg of dopamine in a 500-mL bag of D_5W and use a microdrip administration set. What is the rate?

29. You need to give 20 µg/kg/min of dobutamine to a patient who has extremely low blood pressure and is symptomatic. The patient weighs 169 lb. You place 800 mg of dobutamine in a 500-mL bag of D_5W and use a microdrip administration set. What is the rate?

30. A patient weighs 198 lb, and you need to give 18 µg/kg/min of dopamine for treatment of very low blood pressure and the presence of symptoms. You place 400 mg of dopamine in a 250-mL bag of D_5W and use a microdrip administration set. What is the rate?

31. You have a 77-year-old patient in congestive heart failure who has low blood pressure. It seems that the patient may be having an acute myocardial infarction, and the physician does not want to increase the patient's heart rate while trying to raise his blood pressure. He has ordered 10 µg/kg/min of dobutamine. The patient weighs 135 lb. You have a prefilled syringe of 32 mL of dobutamine that contains 12.5 mg/mL. You place the entire amount into a 250-mL bag of D_5W and use a microdrip administration set. What is the correct rate?

32. You need to give 5 µg/kg/min of dobutamine to a patient who has extremely low blood pressure and is symptomatic. The patient weighs 80 kg. You place 400 mg of dobutamine in a 250-mL bag of D_5W and use a microdrip administration set. What is the rate?

33. The patient weighs 150 kg. You have determined you need to start a dopamine drip at 15 µg/kg/min to help raise the patient's blood pressure. You place 800 mg of dopamine in a 500-mL IV bag of D_5W. You have a microdrip administration set. What is the rate to give the proper amount of medication?

34. You respond to a call for a patient with cardiac problems. On arrival, you find a 47-year-old woman experiencing chest pain. Her weight is 120 lb. You apply the cardiac monitor and determine that she is having multifocal PVCs at a rate of 10/min. Per protocol, you give an initial dose of lidocaine by IV push, which controls the PVCs. You then need to start a lidocaine drip at 1 mg/min. You place 1 g in a 250-mL bag of D_5W and use a microdrip administration set. At how many drops per minute will you set the rate?

35. You need to give 2 µg/kg/min of dopamine to a patient who is symptomatic and has low blood pressure. The patient weighs 79 kg. You place 400 mg of dopamine in a 250-mL bag of D_5W and use a microdrip administration set. What is the rate?

36. You need to give 14 µg/kg/min of dopamine to a patient who is symptomatic and has low blood pressure. The patient weighs 129 kg. You place 800 mg of dopamine in a 500-mL bag of D_5W and use a microdrip administration set. What is the rate?

37. The physician orders a dopamine drip at 10 µg/kg/min for a patient who is symptomatic and has low blood pressure. The patient weighs 188 lb. On the ambulance you have 400 mg of dopamine in a 5-mL prefilled syringe, a 250-mL bag of fluid, and a microdrip administration set. What rate will you establish?

38. You have a patient in congestive heart failure, and the medical control physician has ordered 12 µg/kg/min of dobutamine. The patient weighs 45 kg. You place 800 mg of dobutamine into a 500-mL bag of D$_5$W and attach a microdrip administration set. What rate will you establish?

39. The physician orders a dopamine drip at 15 µg/kg/min for a patient who is complaining of general weakness and has a blood pressure of 72/50 mm Hg. The patient weighs 238 lb. On the ambulance, you have 800 mg of dopamine in a 5-mL prefilled syringe. You have a 500-mL bag of D$_5$W and a microdrip administration set to set up the dopamine drip. What rate will you establish?

40. You have a patient in congestive heart failure, and the medical control physician ordered 20 µg/kg/min of dobutamine. The patient weighs 160 lb. You place 800 mg of dobutamine into a 500-mL bag of D$_5$W and attach a microdrip administration set. What rate will you establish?

Calculate the following for a dopamine drip using 800 mg in a 500-mL IV bag of D$_5$W and using a microdrip administration set.

41. 10 µg/kg/min for a patient who weighs 193 lb.

42. 3 µg/kg/min for a patient who weighs 269 lb.

43. 7 µg/kg/min for a patient who weighs 243 lb.

44. 5 µg/kg/min for a patient who weighs 153 lb.

45. 14 µg/kg/min for a patient who weighs 177 lb.

46. 20 µg/kg/min for a patient who weighs 71 kg.

47. 15 µg/kg/min for a patient who weighs 41 kg.

48. 11 μg/kg/min for a patient who weighs 50 kg.

49. 4 μg/kg/min for a patient who weighs 111 kg.

50. 8 μg/kg/min for a patient who weighs 62 kg.

Calculate the following for a dobutamine drip using 400 mg in a 250-mL IV bag of D₅W and a microdrip administration set.

51. 5 μg/kg/min for a patient who weighs 173 lb.

52. 10 μg/kg/min for a patient who weighs 113 lb.

53. 6 μg/kg/min for a patient who weighs 256 lb.

54. 12 μg/kg/min for a patient who weighs 300 lb.

55. 18 μg/kg/min for a patient who weighs 225 lb.

56. 3 μg/kg/min for a patient who weighs 32 kg.

57. 2 μg/kg/min for a patient who weighs 124 kg.

58. 17 μg/kg/min for a patient who weighs 145 kg.

59. 13 μg/kg/min for a patient who weighs 106 kg.

60. 20 μg/kg/min for a patient who weighs 65 kg.

By using the desired dose and the patient's weight, calculate the pediatric dose.

61. You respond to a call for a pediatric patient who is unresponsive. On arrival, you find a 2-year-old boy who responds to painful stimuli. Examination shows a heart rate of 35 beats/min and a blood pressure of 50 mm Hg by palpation. The child has a history of cardiac problems. The medical control physician orders 0.01 mg/kg of epinephrine 1:10,000. You establish an intraosseous (IO) line and determine the patient weighs approximately 30 lb. You have a pediatric dose of epinephrine 1:10,000 that contains 1.0 mg in 10 mL of fluid. What is the correct dose and amount to administer?

62. Your ambulance is called to a day-care center for a sick child. On arrival, you find a 4-year-old girl complaining that her chest hurts. You begin your exam and apply the cardiac monitor, which shows a rapid narrow-complex paroxysmal supraventricular tachycardia. The medical control physician confirms you should give the patient adenosine, 0.1 mg/kg. You determine the patient weighs 44 lb. On hand you have adenosine in a 6 mg/1 mL vial. What is the correct dose and amount to administer?

63. The initial dose of adenosine does not seem to be effective in the preceding case, and the physician orders a dose of adenosine, 0.2 mg/kg. What is the correct dose and amount to administer?

64. You are in the ambulance stopped at a stoplight when a mother pulls up next to your vehicle, gets out, and requests your help for her sick child. She was en route to the child's physician when the baby suddenly slumped in his car seat. You move the child to the back of the ambulance and begin your assessment. The mother advises you the boy is 15 months old and was born prematurely. You find an unresponsive boy who appears to be grunting. You give him oxygen and begin assisting his respirations with a bag-mask device. You apply the cardiac monitor and determine that the heart rate is 28 beats/min. The child weighs approximately 25 lb. The medical control physician advises you to establish IO access and give atropine, 0.02 mg/kg. On hand you have a pediatric dose of atropine that contains 1 mg in 10 mL of solution. What is the correct dose and amount to administer?

65. You are called to assist a 7-year-old girl having a tonic-clonic seizure. Her skin feels warm, and the mother advises that the patient has had a fever for the past 3 hours; her last temperature was 103°F. The child weighs approximately 60 lb. You are unable to establish IV access because of the seizure movement, and the medical control physician advises you to administer diazepam, 0.5 mg/kg, rectally. On the ambulance you have a multidose vial of diazepam that contains 20 mg in 5 mL of solution. What is the correct dose and amount to administer?

66. You respond to a call for a child with an allergic reaction. The 10-year-old girl is complaining of severe itching and has a localized rash on both arms and her chest. She weighs about 75 lb. You receive an order to administer intramuscular (IM) diphenhydramine, 1 mg/kg, once to this patient. On hand you have 50 mg/1 mL vial. What is the correct dose and amount to administer?

67. Your ambulance responds to a Little League baseball field. You find an 8-year-old boy with an obviously fractured humerus. The patient appears to be in significant pain, and the medical control physician authorizes administration of morphine, 0.1 mg/kg, for pain. You establish IV access and determine that the patient weighs approximately 80 lb. You have 10 mg in a 1-mL ampule. What is the correct dose and amount to administer?

68. You respond to a call about an accidental overdose. A 3-year-old boy took several narcotic medications that were in open bottles in the parent's bathroom. The patient is unconscious with snoring, shallow respirations. You maintain his airway and begin assisting respirations with a bag-mask device. You establish IV access with an IO needle. The medical control physician advises you to administer naloxone, 0.1 mg/kg. The patient weighs 41 lb. The dose on hand is 2.0 mg in a 2-mL ampule. What is the correct dose and amount to administer?

69. A 14-year-old patient is complaining of a heavy feeling in her chest and being dizzy. You give the patient oxygen. The cardiac monitor shows multifocal PVCs at a rate of 10/min. The medical control physician advises you to administer lidocaine, 1 mg/kg. The patient weighs 150 lb. You have 100 mg in a 10-mL prefilled syringe. What is the correct dose and amount to administer?

70. You respond to a call about an unresponsive pediatric patient. The parents inform you that their 9-year-old daughter has diabetes and has been sick for several days with vomiting and diarrhea. They had given her a normal dose of insulin and tried to have her keep some food down, but she vomited her last meal. The girl appears to be dehydrated, and several attempts to establish IV access fail. The medical control physician advises you to administer glucagon, 0.03 mg/kg IM. You determine her weight to be 74 lb. You have on hand 1.0 mg in 1 mL of solution. What is the correct dose and amount to administer?

71. Your ambulance responds to a high school weight room for a 16-year-old boy complaining of back pain. The patient was lifting weights when a sudden onset of severe back pain and spasms occurred. The patient has no history of back problems and is not taking any medications. He is in obvious distress, and the medical control physician gives permission to administer fentanyl, 1 µg/kg. He weighs 179 lb. You have in your drug box fentanyl, 100 µg/mL. What is the correct dose and amount to administer?

72. You respond to a call from a physician's office for a patient with special needs who has an anxiety disorder. The patient is 10 years old and appears to be anxious and upset. Her physician would like you to insert an IV line and give lorazepam, 0.05 mg/kg, to help calm the patient. You quickly establish IV access and determine she weighs 72 lb. You have a vial of lorazepam that contains 2 mg in 2 mL of solution. What is the correct dose and amount to administer?

73. You respond to a call from a preschool for a patient with seizures. On arrival, you find a 4-year-old boy having a seizure. You protect his head and give him oxygen. Your partner is able to establish IV access. The medical control physician advises you to administer diazepam, 0.3 mg/kg. The patient appears to weigh about 45 lb. In the drug box is 10 mg/mL of diazepam. What is the correct dose and amount to administer?

74. Your ambulance is called to a middle school for a patient complaining of severe flank pain. On arrival, you find a very anxious 13-year-old boy complaining of intense pain in his right flank. He reports the pain started in his groin and moved to his side during the past hour. He relates this pain as similar to when he had a kidney stone last year. He has vomited and is unable to lie or sit down. You attempt to calm him and advise him you need to start an IV line to give him something for the pain. Your partner quickly establishes IV access, and you receive an order from medical control to give the patient morphine, 0.1 mg/kg. He tells you he weighs 160 lb. You have on hand 10 mg/mL. What is the correct dose and amount to administer?

75. You respond to a call for a pediatric patient having a seizure. On arrival, you find an 18-month-old girl who is warm to the touch having a seizure. You give her oxygen and look for a site for IV access. She has an infection on both legs, and the parents advise that she has had a fever for the past 24 hours. You advise medical control and request to administer midazolam rectally to this patient. You receive an order for 0.4 mg/kg. The parents tell you that the baby weighs 27 lb. You have 5 mg/mL in a vial of midazolam. What is the correct dose and amount to administer?

76. You have given several medications to a pediatric patient for an allergic reaction. The medical control physician advises you to administer methylprednisolone to enhance the effects of the other medications. You receive an order for 2 mg/kg. The patient is a 15-year-old boy who weighs 148 lb. The medication is carried as 250 mg/5 mL. What is the correct dose and amount to administer?

77. You respond to a call about an accidental overdose. A 4-year-old boy ingested his grandparent's calcium channel blocker medication. The patient is symptomatic, and the medical control physician advises you to establish IV access and administer 7 mg/kg of a 10% calcium chloride solution. The patient weighs 39 lb. On the ambulance is a prefilled syringe of 1 g in 10 mL. What is the correct dose and amount to administer?

78. You have been attempting resuscitation for more than 20 minutes of a 5-year-old girl who was found unconscious in a swimming pool. The medical control physician advises you to give sodium bicarbonate, 1 mEq/kg, followed by 0.5 mEq/kg every 10 minutes. The girl weighs approximately 40 lb. The prefilled pediatric syringe contains 25 mEq of sodium bicarbonate in 10 mL of solution. What is the correct dose and amount to administer? What is the correct dose and amount to administer in 10 minutes?

80. An 11-year-old patient has unexplained low blood pressure. You have determined that it is not due to hypovolemia. The patient weighs approximately 105 lb. The medical control physician has ordered a dopamine drip at 2 μg/kg/min. You place 800 mg of dopamine in a 500-mL bag of D_5W and attach a microdrip administration set. What is the correct rate?

Solve the following word problems involving pediatric rate- and weight-based medication doses.

79. A 12-year-old patient has unexplained low blood pressure. You have determined that it is not due to hypovolemia. The patient weighs approximately 135 lb. The medical control physician has ordered a dopamine drip at 2 μg/kg/min. You place 400 mg of dopamine in a 250-mL bag of D_5W and attach a microdrip administration set. What is the correct rate?

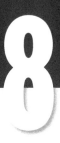
This chapter is a collection of problems representing each chapter of this book. Use it to test yourself, and when you get one wrong, go back to the chapter to refresh your memory.

Chapter 1: The Language of Math: Fractions, Percentages, and Decimals

Calculate the following fraction conversions.

1. Convert $\dfrac{22}{8}$ to a decimal fraction and a percentage.

2. Convert $\dfrac{14}{32}$ to a decimal fraction and a percentage.

3. Convert $\dfrac{35}{54}$ to a decimal fraction and a percentage.

Estimate the answers. Practice rounding off the answer into multiples of 2, 5, and 10 for quick calculating. Complete the function indicated. Check your estimated answers with the calculated answer in the back of the book.

4. $85 + 95 =$

5. $54 + 26 + 138 =$

Solve the following calculations by moving the decimal point.

6. $0.3 \times 10 =$

7. $0.3 \div 10 =$

8. $1.2 \times 100 =$

9. $1.2 \div 100 =$

10. $45.6 \times 1{,}000 =$

11. $45.6 \div 1{,}000 =$

Practice restating calculations using 10, 5, and 2. Follow the pattern in the example, leaving the first number as stated in the original calculation and restating the second number. Answers in the back of the text represent one possible answer.
Example:

$$18 \times 2 =$$
$$9 \times 2 \times 2 =$$
$$2 \times 2 = 4$$
$$\text{So, } 4 \times 9 = 36$$

12. $15 \times 14 =$

13. $88 \times 12 =$

14. $125 \div 25 =$

15. $38 \div 16 =$

Answer the following word problems.

16. When you draw up the medication in a syringe, you only have $\frac{12}{13}$ of the amount you need to give. Even though you do not have the full amount, the physician gives the order to administer. To correctly chart the amount given, what percentage and decimal fraction of the medication did you administer?

17. A patient is being given a medication in $\frac{1}{8}$ amounts of the supplied dose in one vial. In one day, the patient receives the medication 12 times. What is the total percentage and decimal fraction of the number of vials you will need to have on hand each day to give the proper amount of medication?

18. You are in the field without a calculator or writing materials. You need to give one medication to a patient at 2.5 times the normal dose. The usual amount to be given each time is 3.03 mg. Use estimation to determine which of the following you should give.
   A. 6.0
   B. 8.0
   C. 15
   D. 6.015

19. When responding to a multicasualty incident, you have two groups of patients. In the green group are 16 patients, and in the yellow group, there are 29. To quickly determine the total number of patients in both groups, calculate by rounding off.

20. You need to give 3 mg of a medication 20 times in the next hour. Determine the total number of milligrams needed by multiplying or dividing by 10.

Chapter 2: Back to the Basics: Adding, Subtracting, Multiplying, and Dividing

Solve the following addition problems.

21.   89
        $\underline{+\ 43}$

22.   37
        $\underline{+\ 79}$

23. 159
        $\underline{+\ 73}$

24.   58
        $\underline{+\ 39}$

Solve the following subtraction problems.

25. 160
        $\underline{-\ 15}$

26. 311
        $\underline{-\ 33}$

Solve the following multiplication problems.

27. 17
        $\underline{\times\ 6}$

28.   47
        $\underline{\times\ 69}$

29. 150
        $\underline{\times\ 61}$

30.   328
        $\underline{\times\ 256}$

Solve the following division problems.

31. $38 \div 5 =$

32. $112 \div 54 =$

33. $172 \div 8 =$

34. $248 \div 32 =$

35. $202 \div 4 =$

36. $4,108 \div 13 =$

Solve the following problems involving the addition of decimal fractions.

37.   8.3
      $+\ 4.9$

38.   434.69
      $+\ 57.934$

39.   1.1
      $+\ 9.7$

40.   974.2
      $+\ 13.5$

Solve the following problems involving the subtraction of decimal fractions.

41.   692.55
      $-\ 222.225$

42.   343.51
      $-\ 294.93$

43.   5.3
      $-\ 2.8$

44. 3102.4
      $-\ 4.043$

Solve the following calculations. (Hint: Remember "order of operations.")

45. $2 \times (20 - 5) + 12 \div 2 =$

46. $(50 \times 2) - 4 + 10 + 21 \div 3 =$

47. $10 \times 3 \times 14 \div 2 - 1 + 8 =$

48. Solve the following problems quickly by following the first example and then completing the table below.

	Estimate	Break it up	Calculate the answer	Check against your estimate
274 + 324	275 + 325 = 600	270 + 4 + 300 + 20 + 4	270 + 20 = 290 4 + 4 = 8 + 300 = 598	**Estimate = 600** **Answer = 598**
108 – 31				Estimate = Answer =
77 × 5				Estimate = Answer =

Solve the following word problems.

49. A patient takes 6.75 mg of a medication 5 times per day. What is the total amount of medication taken in one day? What is the total amount taken in one week?

50. Your supervisor ordered 22 cases of intravenous (IV) fluid. Ten cases are 1,000-mL bags, and there are 8 bags in each case. The remaining 12 cases are 500-mL bags, and there are 15 bags per case. You have been asked for an inventory of the total number of bags received.

51. Your agency responded to 4,200 calls last year. You were on duty 261 days. About how many calls did you respond to?

52. There are a possible 250 points on your paramedic final exam. As a joke, your instructor did not calculate your score, so you get to test your math skills one last time. In Part I, you missed 11 points. In Part II, you missed 15.5 points. In Part III, you missed 8.2 points. What was the total number of points you earned, and what was your score (percentage of correct answers)?

Chapter 3: Using the Number 1 With Fractions

Simplify the following problems by using more than one expression of the number 1.

53. $\dfrac{420}{12} =$

54. $\dfrac{300}{15} =$

Convert each of the following to a decimal fraction.

55. $\dfrac{4}{16}$

56. $\dfrac{4}{32}$

57. $\dfrac{16}{128}$

58. $\dfrac{11}{4}$

59. $\dfrac{22}{5}$

60. $\dfrac{62}{11}$

61. $\dfrac{65}{85}$

62. $\dfrac{87}{62}$

63. $\dfrac{19}{58}$

64. $\dfrac{74}{47}$

65. $\dfrac{13}{53}$

66. $\dfrac{8}{9}$

67. $\dfrac{10}{25}$

68. $\dfrac{33}{100}$

Simplify each of the following challenges by filling in the blanks.

69. $\dfrac{150}{120} \div \dfrac{2}{2} = \dfrac{?}{60} \div \dfrac{2}{2} = \dfrac{37.5}{?}$

70. $\dfrac{212}{20} \div \dfrac{2}{2} = \dfrac{106}{?} \div \dfrac{2}{2} = \dfrac{?}{5}$

71. $\dfrac{?}{25} \div \dfrac{5}{5} = \dfrac{110}{5} \div \dfrac{5}{5} = \dfrac{?}{1}$

Simplify the following fractions by using the number 1. Follow the first example.

$$\frac{6 \times 4 \times 8}{2 \times 2 \times 2} = \frac{3 \times \cancel{2} \times \cancel{2} \times \cancel{2} \times 2 \times 4}{\cancel{2} \times \cancel{2} \times \cancel{2}}$$

$$= 3 \times 2 \times 4 = 24$$

72. $\dfrac{3 \times 35 \times 16}{14 \times 4 \times 3}$

73. $\dfrac{1,200 \times 250}{400 \times 50}$

Simplify the following problems by reducing the fractions. Each example can be divided by the number 1 expressed as a fraction. Do not solve the equations here.

74. $\dfrac{2}{8} \times \dfrac{8}{10} =$

75. $\dfrac{14}{28} \times \dfrac{15}{20} =$

Convert the following fractions to decimal fractions (carrying out two decimal places) and/or percentages as requested.

76. Your service transported 3,540 patients last year. Of the patients, 1,989 were male and 1,551 were female. What percentage were male?

77. In your community there are 27,843 residents. If 18,930 are female and 8,913 are male, what percentage is female?

78. Your child's baseball team has won 33 of 46 games. What is the team's winning percentage?

79. You play 45 games of dominoes and win 28. What is your winning percentage?

Simplify the following word problems by reducing the fractions. Do not solve the equations, just simplify them.

80. Multiply 48 times 55 times 6, divided by 12 times 11 times 36.

81. Multiply 10 times 4 times 50, divided by 30 times 20 times 100.

82. Multiply 36 times 9 times 14, divided by 3 times 81 times 7.

83. Multiply 11.4 times 26.4 times 28, divided by 5.7 times 3.2 times 7.

84. Multiply 12.3 times 45.6 times 78.9 divided by 36.9 times 91.2 times 236.7.

Chapter 4: Fun With Fractions

Write the shorthand for the following examples.

85. On the exam, 26 of 40 answers were correct.

86. You administer 15 mg of the 25 mg of medication.

87. You used 11 of 45 vials this week.

Multiply the following fractions.

88. $\dfrac{5}{3} \times \dfrac{7}{2} =$

89. $\dfrac{18}{10} \times \dfrac{2}{22} =$

Divide the following fractions.

90. $\dfrac{18}{12} \div \dfrac{22}{10} =$

91. $\dfrac{55}{12} \div \dfrac{7}{2} =$

Simplify the following fractions.

92. $\dfrac{\dfrac{5}{6} \times \dfrac{4}{8}}{\dfrac{3}{2}} =$

93. $\dfrac{\dfrac{1}{2} \times \dfrac{8}{14}}{\dfrac{1}{3}} =$

Find the common denominators. Hint: There are several possibilities, but the smallest common denominator is usually the easiest to use in solving calculations.

94. $\dfrac{2}{10} + \dfrac{8}{5} =$

95. $\dfrac{7}{2} + \dfrac{18}{13} =$

Solve the following calculations. Hint: Find a common denominator first.

96. $\dfrac{1}{6} + \dfrac{5}{4} =$

97. $\dfrac{3}{8} + \dfrac{10}{22} =$

Chapter 5: Ratios and Proportions: Finding the Missing Piece

Solve the following proportions. Hint: Remember to cross multiply and divide.

98. $\dfrac{15}{11} = \dfrac{?}{20}$

99. $\dfrac{2}{34} = \dfrac{?}{18}$

Complete the following table. Conversion factors have been provided for easy reference. Hint: Use proportions.

100.

Convert this number	to this unit of measure	Conversion factor
100 g	? mg	1 g = 1,000 mg
8 mL	? L	1,000 mL = 1 L
55 g	? kg	1,000 g = 1 kg
924 mg	? kg	1,000 mg = 1 g and 1,000 g = 1 kg

Use proportions to convert the following units of measure.

101. 8,420 mg = _____ g

102. 4.1 g = _____ mg

103. 46 mg = _____ µg

104. 50 µg = _____ mg

105. 10,000 mg = _____ µg

Convert the following temperatures.

106. Convert 33.5°C to °F.

107. Convert 85°F to °C.

Calculate the concentration in the following problems.

108. You mix 200 mg of dopamine in a 250-mL bag of D_5W. What is the concentration of 1 mL?

109. You mix 0.5 g of lidocaine in a 250-mL bag of D_5W. What is the concentration of 1 mL?

110. You place 1 g of a medication into 100 mL of fluid. A physician orders 350 mg of the medication for a patient. How many milliliters do you administer?

111. You place 500 mg of a medication into 10 mL of fluid. A physician orders 175 mg of the medication for a patient. How many milliliters do you administer?

112. You place 1 mg of a medication into 5 mL of fluid. A physician orders 275 µg of the medication for a patient. How many milliliters do you administer?

113. You place 5 mg of a medication into 1 mL of fluid. A physician orders 50 µg of the medication for a patient. How many milliliters do you administer?

Solve the following problems. Note that you will be using percentages in the calculations.

114. What is $\dfrac{4}{15}$ of 1,489?

115. What is $\dfrac{3}{8}$ of 114?

116. What is $\dfrac{9}{100}$ of 51?

117. What $\dfrac{13}{45}$ of 660?

Solve the following problem involving a percentage solution.

118. To administer 5 g of a 50% dextrose solution, how many milliliters of solution will you administer?

Chapter 6: Rate-Dependent Calculations

Solve the following problems to determine the amount of medication (number of milliliters) to draw up in a syringe.

119. You have orders to give 0.2 mg of epinephrine by the intramuscular (IM) route. You have 1.0 mg in a 1.0-mL ampule. How much medication do you draw up to give the correct amount?

120. You are given orders to give a patient 15 mg of morphine sulfate. You have a multidose vial that contains 50 mg in 5 mL. What is the correct amount of medication to administer?

121. You receive an order to give a patient 125 μg of fentanyl by IV push. You have 150 μg/3 mL of the medication in a prefilled syringe. What is the correct amount of medication to administer?

122. You have orders to administer 6 mg of diazepam. You have 10 mg/2-mL ampules. How much will you administer?

123. You have orders to administer 14 mg of diazepam. You have 20 mg/2-mL ampules. How much will you administer?

124. You need to administer 140 mg of a medication. You have 250 mg in 10 mL of fluid. How much medication will you administer?

125. You need to give 5 mg of medication. You have 30 mg in 20 mL of fluid. How much will you draw up into the syringe?

126. Your patient needs 700 mg of a medication. You have 1 g in a 10-mL prefilled syringe. How much will you administer?

127. You have an order to give 50 mg of diphenhydramine to a patient who is having an allergic reaction. You have a multidose vial that contains 100 mg in 5 mL. How much medication will you draw up into the syringe?

128. You have a patient in atrial flutter. The medical control physician has ordered 5 mg of atenolol by IV push slowly during 5 minutes. Your ambulance carries this medication in a multidose vial of 20 mg in 10 mL of fluid. How much medication will you administer?

Solve the following problems by using dimensional analysis to determine the amount of time it will take to give a medication.

129. You are instructed to give a medication at 8 mg/min to a total of 600 mg. How long will it take to give the total amount of medication?

130. You are instructed to give a medication at 3.2 mg/min to a total of 412 mg. How long will it take to give the total amount of medication?

131. You are instructed to give a medication at 12 mg/min to a total of 20,000 µg. How long will it take to give the total amount of medication?

132. You are instructed to give a medication at 0.75 mg/min to a total of 160 mg. How long will it take to give the total amount of medication?

133. You are instructed to give a medication at 1.5 mg/h to a total of 80 mg. How long will it take to give the total amount of medication?

Solve the following problems by using the clock method to determine the amount of time it will take to give a medication.

134. You have an order for administration of lidocaine from a premixed bag in your rescue unit. You are to administer 2 mg/min. You have a drug concentration of 4 mg/mL and a 60-gtt/mL administration set. How many drops per minute should you give?

135. You have an order for administration of a lidocaine drip at 3 mg/min. You have on hand a vial containing 1 g of drug, a 250-mL bag of normal saline, and a microdrip administration set. How many drops per minute will you administer?

Solve the following problems converting milliliters per hour to drops per minute.

139. You need to give 750 mL of IV fluid during the next 5 hours. The IV is established with a microdrip administration set (60 gtt/mL). What rate is needed to give the correct amount?

136. You have an order for administration of a dopamine drip at 8 μg/kg/min. You have on hand a vial containing 400 mg of the drug, a 250-mL bag of normal saline, and a microdrip administration set. The patient weighs 145 lb. How many drops per minute would you give?

140. You need to give 1,800 mL of IV fluid during the next 25 hours. The IV is established with a microdrip administration set (60 gtt/mL). What rate is needed to give the correct amount?

137. You have an order for administration of a dopamine drip at 2 μg/kg/min. You have on hand a 400-mg vial, a 500-mL bag of normal saline, and a 60-gtt/mL administration set. The patient weighs 188 lb. How many drops per minute will you give?

141. You need to give 100 mL of IV fluid during the next 3.5 hours. The IV is established with a microdrip administration set (60 gtt/mL). What rate is needed to give the correct amount?

142. You need to give 1,200 mL of IV fluid during the next 3.5 hours. The IV is established with a macrodrip administration set (10 gtt/mL). What rate is needed to give the correct amount?

138. You have an order for administration of a dopamine drip at 5 μg/kg/min. The patient weighs 200 lb. You have on hand two ampules each containing 200 mg, a 250-mL bag of normal saline, and a 60-gtt/mL administration set. How many drops per minute will you give?

143. You need to give 500 mL of IV fluid during the next 4.2 hours. The IV is established with a microdrip administration set (60 gtt/mL). What rate is needed to give the correct amount?

Solve the following word problems involving rate.

144. The physician orders a 200-mL fluid bolus to be given during 30 minutes to a patient who is slightly hypotensive. You have a 500-mL bag of normal saline and a macrodrip administration set (10 gtt/mL). What is the correct rate?

145. The physician orders a 100-mL fluid bolus to be given during 15 minutes to a patient who is hypotensive. The patient weighs 166 lb. You have a 500-mL bag of normal saline and a macrodrip administration set (10 gtt/mL). What is the correct rate?

146. A patient needs 400 mL of normal saline during the next 75 minutes. The IV is established with a macrodrip administration set (10 gtt/mL). How many drops per minute will you set the IV to run?

147. A patient needs 1,000 mL of normal saline during the next 10 hours. The IV is established with a macrodrip administration set (10 gtt/mL). How many drops per minute will you set the IV to run?

148. You are asked to give 500 mL of a fluid to a patient during the next 3.3 hours. The IV is established with a macrodrip administration set (10 gtt/mL). What rate is needed to give the correct amount?

149. A patient needs 1,250 mL of normal saline during the next 4.6 hours. The IV is established with a macrodrip administration set (10 gtt/mL). How many drops per minute will you set the IV to run?

Chapter 7: Weight-Based Calculations

By using the desired dose and the patient's weight, calculate the correct dose to administer.

150. Your ambulance responds to a call for a cardiac patient. The rhythm on the ECG is irregular with a rate of 120 beats/min, and the patient is having multifocal premature ventricular contractions (PVCs) at a rate of 10 per minute. Per protocol, you are directed to administer lidocaine, 1.0 mg/kg, to control the PVCs. The patient weighs 228 lb. You have 100 mg of lidocaine in a 10-mL prefilled syringe. How many milliliters will you administer to this patient?

151. You respond to a nursing home for a patient with an unknown problem. On arrival, you find the patient is having cardiac problems. The cardiac monitor shows uncontrolled atrial fibrillation with an irregular rate of 143 beats/min. The medical control physician orders diltiazem, 0.25 mg/kg. The patient weighs 153 lb. You have 20 mg in a 10-mL vial. What is the dose to give, and how many milliliters will you give?

152. You are treating a patient complaining of chest pain and shortness of breath. The cardiac monitor indicates that the patient needs cardioversion. According to your protocols, you need to administer etomidate, 0.3 mg/kg, for sedation before the cardioversion. Your patient weighs 200 lb. You have 50 mg of etomidate in a 5-mL vial. What is the dose to give, and how many milliliters will you administer?

153. Your ambulance has responded to a construction site. You have a patient with a head injury who is unconscious and has difficulty breathing. You are unable to intubate him. The medical control physician authorizes administration of succinylcholine, 0.8 mg/kg. You determine the patient weighs 160 lb. You find 100 mg of succinylcholine in a 2-mL vial. How many milliliters will you administer?

Solve the following word problems involving rate- and weight-based medication administration.

154. You need to give 15 μg/kg/min of dobutamine to a patient who has extremely low blood pressure and is symptomatic. The patient weighs 159 lb. You place 800 mg of dobutamine in a 500-mL bag of D_5W and use a microdrip administration set (60 gtt/mL). What is the correct rate?

155. The physician orders a dopamine drip at 20 μg/kg/min for a patient who is symptomatic and has low blood pressure. During your assessment, you rule out that the patient may be hypovolemic. Your patient weighs 176 lb. On hand you have 400 mg of dopamine in a 5-mL prefilled syringe that you place into a 250-mL IV bag of D_5W; you also have a microdrip administration set. What is the correct rate?

156. The medical control physician orders a dopamine drip at 14 μg/kg/min for a patient who is complaining of "not feeling well." Her blood pressure is 72/50 mm Hg, and she weighs 213 lb. On hand you have 800 mg of dopamine in a 5-mL prefilled syringe. You have a 500-mL bag of D_5W and a microdrip administration set. What is the correct rate?

Calculate the following for giving a dopamine drip using 800 mg in a 500- mL IV bag of D_5W and a microdrip administration set.

157. 15 μg/kg/min to a patient who weighs 194 lb.

158. 16 µg/kg/min to a patient who weighs 229 lb.

159. 19 µg/kg/min to a patient who weighs 143 lb.

160. 8 µg/kg/min to a patient who weighs 79 kg.

161. 4 µg/kg/min to a patient who weighs 24 kg.

162. 11 µg/kg/min to a patient who weighs 55 kg.

By using the desired dose and the patient's weight, calculate the pediatric dose you will administer.

163. Your ambulance is called to a home baby-sitter center for a sick child. You find a 6-year-old girl complaining that her chest hurts. The cardiac monitor shows rapid, narrow-complex paroxysmal supraventricular tachycardia. The medical control physician confirms that you should give adenosine, 0.1 mg/kg. You determine the patient weighs 54 lb. On hand you have adenosine, 6 mg /1-mL vial. What is the correct dose and amount to administer?

164. You are called to assist a 5-year-old boy having a tonic-clonic seizure. His skin feels warm, and the mother advises that the patient has had a fever for the past 6 hours; the last temperature was 104°F. The child weighs approximately 45 lb. You are unable to establish an IV because of the seizure movement, and the medical control physician advises you to administer diazepam, 0.5 mg/kg, rectally. On hand you have a multidose vial of diazepam that contains 20 mg in 5 mL of solution. What is the correct dose and amount to administer?

165. You respond to a call for an 11-year-old child with an allergic reaction. The patient is complaining of severe itching and has a localized rash on both arms and her chest. She weighs about 65 lb. You receive an order to administer diphenhydramine, 1 mg/kg IM, once. On hand you have 50 mg/1-mL vial. What is the correct dose and amount to administer?

166. Your ambulance responds to a softball field. You find an 8-year-old girl with an obviously fractured leg. The patient appears to be in significant pain, and the medical control physician authorizes administration of morphine, 0.1 mg/kg, for pain. You establish IV access and determine that the patient weighs approximately 60 lb. You have 10 mg of morphine in a 1-mL ampule. What is the correct dose and amount to administer?

167. You respond to an unresponsive female patient. The parents inform you their 7-year-old daughter has diabetes and has been sick for several days with vomiting and diarrhea. They gave her a normal dose of insulin 4 hours ago and tried to have her keep some food down, but she vomited her last meal approximately

30 minutes ago. The patient appears to be dehydrated, and several attempts to establish IV access fail. The medical control physician advises you to administer glucagon, 0.03 mg/kg IM. You determine her weight to be 54 lb. You have on hand 1.0 mg in 1 mL of fluid. What is the correct dose and amount to administer?

Solve the following word problems involving pediatric rate- and weight-based medication administration.

168. A 14-year-old boy has unexplained low blood pressure. You have determined that the low blood pressure is not due to hypovolemia. *(In the case of hypovolemia, this medication would not be administered.)* The patient weighs approximately 140 lb. The medical control physician ordered a dopamine drip at 2 µg/kg/min. You place 400 mg of dopamine in a 250-mL bag of D_5W and attach a microdrip administration set (60 gtt/mL). What is the correct rate?

169. A 9-year-old girl has unexplained low blood pressure. You have ruled out hypovolemia. The patient weighs approximately 100 lb. The medical control physician has ordered a dopamine drip at 5 µg/kg/min. You place 800 mg of dopamine in a 500-mL bag of D_5W and attach a microdrip administration set. What is the correct rate?

170. Your ambulance responds to a call about a sick child at home. As you enter the bedroom, you find a 6-year-old boy lying in bed. He does not look up at you or acknowledge your presence. You begin your examination and obtain a history from the parents. They advise that there

have been no recent injuries or illnesses. Today, it was difficult to wake him up, and he is unable to move. When you check his vital signs, you find unexplained low blood pressure. The medical control physician asks you to establish IV access and administer a fluid challenge. After that is complete, the blood pressure remains unchanged and the physician orders a dopamine drip at 6 µg/kg/min. The patient appears to weigh approximately 60 lb. You place 400 mg of dopamine in a 250-mL bag of D_5W and attach a microdrip administration set (60 gtt/mL). What is the correct rate?

171. You respond to a physician's office for a call about a sick child. You are met by the physician who reports that the patient is a 13-year-old girl with low blood pressure. He would like a dopamine drip started, but his office does not stock the medication. The physician checks with your medical control base and has his orders confirmed by the medical control physician. The medical control physician advises you to proceed with the dopamine drip before transport and to start the drip at 10 µg/kg/min. The patient weighs 124 lb. You place 400 mg of dopamine in a 250-mL bag of D_5W and attach a microdrip administration set (60 gtt/mL). What is the correct rate?

172. At 3:00 AM, your ambulance is called to a high-rise hotel to treat a sick child. As you enter the hotel room, you find a 3-year-old boy lying on the bed. After receiving your report, the medical control physician advises you to establish a dopamine drip at 12 µg/kg/min. The patient weighs 33 lb. You place 400 mg of dopamine in a 250-mL bag of D_5W and attach a microdrip administration set (60 gtt/mL). What is the correct rate?

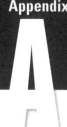

Conversion Factors, Abbreviations, and Useful Formulas

Table A-1   Conversion Factors for Units of Measure

16 oz = 1 lb
2.2 lb = 1 kg
1 kg = 1,000 g
1 g = 1,000 mg
1 g = 1,000,000 µg
1 mg = 1,000 µg
1 kg = 1,000 g = 1,000,000 mg = 1,000,000,000 µg
1 L = 1,000 mL

Table A-2   Abbreviations for Units of Measure

Abbreviation	Unit of Measure
g	gram
kg	kilogram
L	liter
mg	milligram
mL	milliliter
oz	ounce
lb	pound
µg	microgram

The "Cross Multiply and Divide Method"

$$\frac{A}{B} \diagup\!\!\!\diagdown \frac{C}{D}$$

$$A \times D = C \times B$$

Table A-3   Solving with the Cross Multiply and Divide Method

Written in Fraction Format	Written With Math Symbols
$A = \dfrac{C \times B}{D}$	$(C \times B) \div D = A$
$B = \dfrac{D \times A}{C}$	$(D \times A) \div C = B$
$C = \dfrac{A \times D}{B}$	$(A \times D) \div B = C$
$D = \dfrac{B \times C}{A}$	$(B \times C) \div A = D$

Converting From Centigrade to Fahrenheit

$$\left(\frac{9}{5} \times {}^{\circ}C\right) + 32 = {}^{\circ}F$$

Converting From Fahrenheit to Centigrade

$$\frac{5}{9} \times ({}^{\circ}F - 32) = {}^{\circ}C$$

Calculating Milliliters to Administer

Convert units if necessary. Then use dimensional analysis. The below example uses mg.

$$mg \times \frac{mL}{mg} = ?\,mL$$

Calculating How Long a Drip Will Take

Convert units if necessary. Then use dimensional analysis. The below example uses mg.

$$mg \times \frac{min}{mg} = ?\ min$$

Calculating an Infusion Rate

Convert hours to minutes if necessary. Convert units if necessary. Then use dimensional analysis.

$$\frac{gtt}{mL} \times \frac{mL}{min} = ?\ gtt/min$$

The Formula for Rate-Dependent Doses

$$\frac{DD}{DOH} \times \frac{gtt}{mL} = rate$$

- DD represents the desired dose—including time, such as mg/min.
- DOH represents the dose on hand once prepared, such as mg/mL.
- gtt/mL represents the number of drops per milliliter as dictated by your administration set.
- Rate represents the number of drops per minute to which you must set your administration set to accomplish the dose ordered. It is usually in gtt/min.

Approach to Solving Rate-Dependent Problems

1. List out the following:
   - DD (including weight and time)
   - DOH (concentration)
   - Administration set

2. If necessary, convert units. For example:

$$g \times \frac{1,000\ mg}{g} = ?\ mg$$

3. If necessary, convert hours to minutes.

$$h \times \frac{60\ min}{h} = ?\ min$$

4. Simplify the dose on hand. For example:

$$\frac{mg}{mL} = \frac{?\ mg}{1\ mL}$$

5. Plug into the formula. For example:

$$\frac{mg/min}{mg/mL} \times \frac{gtt}{mL} = ?\ gtt/min$$

$$\frac{mg}{min} \times \frac{mL}{mg} \times \frac{gtt}{mL} = ?\ gtt/min$$

6. Round to the nearest whole number.

Clock Approach to Rate-Dependent Problems

1. List out the following:
   - DD (including time)
   - DOH (concentration)
   - Administration set

2. If necessary, convert units. For example:

$$g \times \frac{1,000\ mg}{g} = ?\ mg$$

3. If necessary, convert hours to minutes.

$$h \times \frac{60\ min}{h} = ?\ min$$

4. Simplify the dose on hand (concentration). For example:

$$\frac{mg}{mL} = \frac{?\ mg}{1\ mL}$$

5. Set up the clock using 60 gtt/mL and the concentration. Figure A-1 ▶ shows an example.

6. Find where the desired dose falls on the clock. Estimate the corresponding gtt. This is your rate.

7. To confirm that your estimate is correct, you can set up a proportion comparing numbers on the clock to your desired dose. For example, using the clock in Figure A-1:

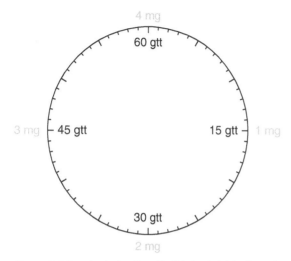

Figure A-1 Sample clock with a 60 gtt/mL administration set and a concentration of 4 mg/mL.

$$\frac{15 \text{ gtt}}{1 \text{ mg}} = \frac{? \text{ gtt}}{\text{Desired dose (mg)}}$$

Round to the nearest whole number.

Approach to Solving Weight-Based Problems

1. List out the following:
   - DD (including weight and time)
   - DOH (concentration)
   - Administration set
   - Patient weight

2. Convert pounds to kilograms.

$$\frac{\text{lb}}{2.2} = ? \text{ kg}$$

3. Adjust the desired dose to account for the patient's weight. For example:

$$\frac{\mu g}{\text{kg/min}} \times \text{Patient weight (kg)} = ? \mu g/\text{min}$$

4. Convert and simplify the dose on hand. For example:

$$\text{mg} \times \frac{1{,}000 \ \mu g}{\text{mg}} = \mu g$$

$$\frac{\mu g}{\text{mL}} = \frac{? \ \mu g}{1 \text{ mL}}$$

5. Plug into the formula. For example:

$$\frac{\mu g/\text{min}}{\mu g/\text{mL}} \times \frac{\text{gtt}}{\text{mL}} = ? \text{ gtt/min}$$

$$\frac{\mu g}{\text{min}} \times \frac{\text{mL}}{\mu g} \times \frac{\text{gtt}}{\text{mL}} = ? \text{ gtt/min}$$

6. Round to the nearest whole number.

Clock Approach to Weight-Based Problems

1. List out the following:
   - DD (including time)
   - DOH (concentration)
   - Administration set
   - Patient's weight

2. If necessary, convert units. For example:

$$\text{mg} \times \frac{1{,}000 \ \mu g}{\text{mg}} = ? \ \mu g/\text{mg}$$

3. If necessary, convert hours to minutes.

$$\text{h} \times \frac{60 \text{ min}}{\text{h}} = ? \text{ min}$$

4. Simplify the dose on hand (concentration). For example:

$$\frac{\mu g}{\text{mL}} = \frac{? \ \mu g}{1 \text{ mL}}$$

5. Set up the clock using 60 gtt/mL and the concentration. Figure A-2 ▶ shows an example.

6. Convert the patient's weight to kg:

$$\frac{\text{lb}}{2.2} = ? \text{ kg}$$

7. Adjust the desired dose to accommodate the patient's weight:

$$\frac{\mu g}{\text{kg/min}} \times \text{Patient's weight (kg)} = ? \ \mu g/\text{min}$$

Round to the nearest whole number.

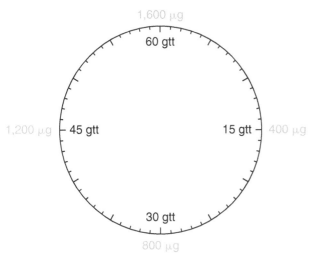

$$\frac{15 \text{ gtt}}{400 \text{ μg}} = \frac{? \text{ gtt}}{\text{Desired dose (μg)}}$$

Round to the nearest whole number.

Shortcut Formula for Dopamine

The following formula assumes a concentration of 1,600 μg/mL (400 mg/250 mL, or 800 mg/500 mL).

$$\frac{\text{μg/kg/min}}{1,600 \text{ μg/mL}} \times \text{Patient's weight (kg)} \times \frac{\text{gtt}}{\text{mL}}$$

$$= ? \frac{\text{gtt}}{\text{min}}$$

Restated showing how units cancel out:

$$\frac{\text{μg}}{\text{kg/min}} \times \frac{\text{mL}}{1,600 \text{ μg}} \times \text{Patient's weight (kg)} \times \frac{\text{gtt}}{\text{mL}}$$

$$= ? \frac{\text{gtt}}{\text{min}}$$

Figure A-2 Sample clock with a 60 gtt/mL administration set and a concentration of 1,600 μg/mL.

8. Find where the adjusted desired dose falls on the clock. Estimate the corresponding gtt. This is your rate.

9. To confirm that your estimate is correct, you can set up a proportion comparing numbers on the clock to your desired dose. For example, using the clock in Figure A-2:

Collected Hints and Notes

Chapter 1

Math

A multiple of 10 is a number that can be reached when you multiply 10 × 10 enough times. For example:

$$10 \times 10 = 100$$
$$10 \times 10 \times 10 = 1{,}000$$
$$10 \times 10 \times 10 \times 10 = 10{,}000$$

These numbers—100, 1,000, and 10,000—are multiples of 10.

The multiple of 10 used in the denominator will have the same number of zeros as the number of places to the right of the decimal point. If the number with decimals is 1.345, the number written with a fraction will be $\frac{345}{1{,}000}$, with 1,000 having three zeros.

The decimal point in whole numbers is presumed to be positioned after the whole number. Such a number may or may not be written with a zero to make the decimal place obvious. In other words, if the number is "12," the decimal point is assumed to follow the "2," as in 12.0.

Notice the pattern: When multiplying or dividing by multiples of 10, the decimal point moves one place for 10 (which has one zero), two places for 100 (which has two zeros), and three places for 1,000 (which has three zeros). You can predict correctly that the decimal point will move four places when multiplying or dividing by 10,000, and so forth.

Is the answer reasonable?
How precise does the math need to be?

The decimal point moves to the left for division.
The decimal point moves to the right for multiplication.

Chapter 2

Math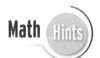

Sometimes it is difficult to keep the numbers aligned. Here's a trick. When multiplying the tens number of the multiplier times the foundation number, you can place a zero in the ones place, to "hold" the place. This will remind you not to accidentally place the tens number in the ones place.

```
    1
    36
×   12
    72
+ 360    A zero holds the "ones" place so you don't
  432    accidentally misalign numbers.
```

Keep your work neat! This will help you avoid mis-aligning numbers, resulting in inaccurate calculations.

Remember to align your work when multiplying in manual mode.

To figure out the number of times a number will go into another, figure out the largest number that you can multiply the divisor by without exceeding the value of the number you are dividing into. See the following example:

$$3\overline{)527}^{\,?}$$

Here, the maximum number of times 3 can be divided into 5 is just 1 (3 × 2 = 6, which is greater than 5, so 2 cannot be used. The 1 must be used because 3 × 1 = 3, which is less than 5).

Another example:

$$2\overline{)862}^{\,?}$$

This is an easy one: 2 goes into 8 exactly 4 times because 2 × 4 = 8. Because the value of 8 was not exceeded, 4 can be used.

In division, the first zero that holds the place can be "dropped" (no longer written) when the calculation is complete. It does not have any numeric value and is only written to keep the numbers properly aligned during the calculation.

For every number after the decimal point in the original problem, place the decimal point that many spaces to the left in your answer.

If your problem has one number after the decimal point, your answer will have one number after the decimal point. If your problem has two numbers after the decimal point, your answer will have two numbers after the decimal point, and so forth.

In prehospital medication calculations, rounding off a number to the nearest tenth (1 decimal place to the right) is as specific as necessary (see the note on clinical significance at the end of this chapter).

Is your answer reasonable?

Chapter 3

Math Hints

Instead of going through the motions of dividing the numerator and denominator by 10, recall how you learned to divide by 10 in Chapter 1: Simply move the decimal point one place to the left. An easier way to see this is to cross out the zeros:

$$\frac{32\cancel{0}}{64\cancel{0}}$$

Any time you have zeros holding the same place in a number (here, they are both in the tens place), they can be omitted.

Rule of multiplication: When all numbers are being multiplied, the order in which they are multiplied does not matter; the numbers can be rearranged with no change in the answer.

Chapter 4

Remember that whole numbers can be expressed as fractions. (Recall using the number 1 from Chapter 3).

Fractions
Multiply: Multiply the numerators, and then multiply the denominators.
Divide: Invert the second fraction, and then multiply.
Add or subtract: Find a common denominator, and then add or subtract the numerators.

Chapter 5

One key word in any word problem that compares information is "of." This word is a dead giveaway that you need to make a line, an equal sign, and another line to set up a quick and easy solution.

    There is one exception to this rule: percentages. A word problem that says a percentage "of" something indicates multiplication.

Whether you have a full vial, half a vial, a third of a vial, and so forth, the *concentration* does not change unless more medication or fluid is added to the vial.

When a problem says to administer grams of a solution, "of" means "divide." In other words, 10 g of a 50% solution equals 10 divided by the 50% solution, or 10 divided by $\dfrac{50 \text{ g}}{100 \text{ mL}}$.

Numerators and denominators can be moved around by cross multiplying with the opposite side of the equation.

The concentration of lidocaine is listed as mg/mL. The concentration of dopamine is listed as μg/mL.

According to the cross multiply and divide method, with the following equation as a basis:

$$\frac{A}{B} = \frac{C}{D}$$

any of the following equations are true:

$$(A \times D) \div B = C$$
$$(D \times A) \div C = B$$
$$(B \times C) \div A = D$$
$$(C \times B) \div D = A$$

Never add medication to a premixed bag! The medication has already been added.

Units that appear in the numerator and denominator of a fraction can be crossed out.

Proportions
Cross multiply and divide.

% wt/wt = Weight of Solute per 100 g of Solution

% vol/vol = Volume in mL of Solute per 100 mL of Solution

% wt/vol = Weight of Solute per 100 mL of Solution

Chapter 6

Math Hints

Remember, when a medication is named with a weight/volume percentage, the percentage indicates the weight of the medication in 100 mL of solution.

Make a list of the information you need. Eliminate distractions by making an organized list of the information that is available—including the question.

Pay attention to the units of measure. Be sure that you use *like* units of measure in your calculations. Change the units of measure in the problem, if necessary, to the units you will be administering to the patient.

Calculations are easier when the denominators are all 1. Therefore:
- If a dose is provided in a volume of solution larger than 1 mL, find out how much medication is present in 1 mL.
- If the medication should be given during a period longer than 1 minute, figure out the amount of medication needed in 1 minute.

You can set up a clock for any drug or solution administered with a 60-gtt/mL administration set.

Use the same administration set used in your calculation. If you calculated with a 60-gtt/mL set, do not use a 10-gtt/mL set.

Chapter 7

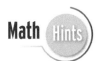
Math Hints

You might have noticed that for dopamine, when the dose on hand is:
- 400 mg in 250 mL or
- 800 mg in 500 mL,
the concentration is 1,600 µg/mL.

To convert pounds to kilograms, divide the weight in pounds by 2.2.

Answer Key

Chapter 1
Chapter Problems

Table 1-10	Practicing Multiplying and Dividing by 10, 100, and 1,000	
Multiply × 10	**Multiply × 100**	**Multiply × 1,000**
4 × 10 = 40	4 × 100 = 400	4 × 1,000 = 4,000
1,893 × 10 = 18,930	1,893 × 100 = 189,300	1,893 × 1,000 = 1,893,000
2.6 × 10 = 26	2.6 × 100 = 260	2.6 × 1,000 = 2,600
0.07 × 10 = 0.7	0.07 × 100 = 7	0.07 × 1,000 = 70
Divide by 10	**Divide by 100**	**Divide by 1,000**
4 ÷ 10 = 0.4	4 ÷ 100 = 0.04	4 ÷ 1,000 = 0.004
1,893 ÷ 10 = 189.3	1,893 ÷ 100 = 18.93	1,893 ÷ 1,000 = 1.893
2.6 ÷ 10 = 0.26	2.6 ÷ 100 = 0.026	2.6 ÷ 1,000 = 0.0026
0.07 ÷ 10 = 0.007	0.07 ÷ 100 = 0.0007	0.07 ÷ 1,000 = 0.00007

Practice Problems

1.

Text Format	Fraction Format	Decimal Format
Twenty-five and three hundredths	$25\frac{3}{100}$	25.03
Three and sixty-seven hundredths	$3\frac{67}{100}$	3.67
Three tenths	$\frac{3}{10}$	0.3
One hundred twenty-six and nine tenths	$126\frac{9}{10}$	126.9
Nine hundred eighty-seven thousandths	$\frac{987}{1,000}$	0.987
Three hundred twenty-seven and ninety-eight hundredths	$327\frac{98}{100}$	327.98

2.

Decimal	Fraction	Percentage
1.2	$1\frac{2}{10}$	1 and 20 = 120%
3.68	$3\frac{68}{100}$	3 and 68 = 368%
0.25	$\frac{25}{100}$	25%
0.10	$\frac{1}{10}$	10%
0.5	$\frac{5}{10}$	50%
0.075	$\frac{75}{1,000}$	7.5%

3.

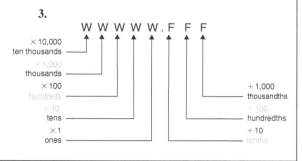

4. 0.4

5. 0.88

6. 0.1

7. 0.384

8. 0.005

9. Estimate: $5 + 5 + 20 + 10 = 40$

Calculation: The numbers can be broken down as: $3 + 7 + 20 + 3 + 10 + 2$

These can be written as smaller equations as follows:

$3 + 7 = 10$

$20 + 3 + 10 + 2 = 20 + 10$ and $3 + 2$, or $30 + 5 = 35$

Adding these results gives the final answer: $10 + 35 = 45$

Comparison: The estimate was 40, and the answer is 45.

10. Estimate: $10 + 20 + 30 + 40 = 100$

Calculation: The numbers can be broken down as: $10 + 1 + 20 + 2 + 30 + 3 + 40 + 2$

These can be written as smaller equations as follows:

$10 + 20 + 30 + 40 = 100$

$1 + 2 + 3 + 2 = 8$

Adding these results gives the final answer: $100 + 8 = 108$

Comparison: The estimate was 100, and the answer is 108.

11. Estimate: $75 - 5 + 10 = 70 + 10 = 80$

Calculation: The numbers can be broken down as: $70 + 6 - 5 + 10 + 2$

These can be written as smaller equations as follows:

$70 + 10 = 80$

$6 - 5 + 2 = 3$

Adding these results gives the final answer: $80 + 3 = 83$

Comparison: The estimate was 80, and the answer is 83.

12. Estimate: $355 - 30 = 325$

Calculation: The numbers can be broken down as: $350 + 6 - 20 - 8$

These can be written as smaller equations as follows:

$350 - 20 = 330$

$6 - 8 = -2$

Adding these results gives the final answer: $330 - 2 = 328$

Comparison: The estimate was 325, and the answer is 328.

13. Estimate: $200 \div 2 = 100$

Calculation: $200 \div 2.2 = 90.9$

Comparison: The estimate was 100, and the answer is 90.9.

14. Estimate: $100 \times 10 = 1,000$

Calculation: The numbers can be broken down as: 90×10 and 90×1

Solving these equations gives:

$90 \times 10 = 900$

$90 \times 1 = 90$

Adding these results gives the final answer: $900 + 90 = 990$

Comparison: The estimate was 1,000, and the answer is 990.

15. Estimate: $25 \times 2 = 50$

Calculation: The numbers can be broken down as: 20×2 and 6×2

Solving these equations gives:

$20 \times 2 = 40$

$6 \times 2 = 12$

Adding these results gives the final answer: $40 + 12 = 52$

Comparison: The estimate was 50, and the answer is 52.

16. Estimate: $3 \times 1 = 3$

Calculation: The numbers can be broken down as: 3×0.2, four times.

Solving these equations gives:

$3 \times 0.2 = 0.6$

$3 \times 0.2 = 0.6$

$3 \times 0.2 = 0.6$

$3 \times 0.2 = 0.6$

Adding these results gives the final answer: $0.6 + 0.6 + 0.6 + 0.6 = 2.4$

Comparison: The estimate was 3, and the answer is 2.4.

17. Estimate: $75 - 25 - 15 - 5 = 50 - 20 = 30$

Calculation: The numbers can be broken down as: $70 + 6 - 20 - 6 - 10 - 3 - 6$

These can be written as smaller equations as follows:

$70 - 20 = 50$

$+ 6 - 6 = 0$

$-10 - 3 - 6 = -19$

Adding these results gives the final answer: $50 + -19$, or $50 - 19$, $= 31$

Comparison: The estimate was 30, and the answer is 31.

18. 18

19. 0.18

20. 2,387.48

21. 0.238748

22. 60

23. 0.006

24. 2,326.7

25. 23.267

26. 23,267

27. 2.3267

28. 232,670

29. 0.23267

30. 1,362.78

31. 13,627.8

32. 136,278

33. 13.6278

34. 1.36278

35. 0.136278

36. 1,860

37. 18,600

38. 186,000

39. 18.6

40. 1.86

41. 0.186

42. 267.8

43. 2,678

44. 26,780

45. 2.678

46. 0.2678

47. 0.02678

48. 3

49. 30

50. 300

51. 0.03

52. 0.003

53. 0.0003

54.

Problem	Foundation Number	× 10	÷ 2
32 × 5	32	320	160
6.5 × 5	6.5	65	32.5
7.36 × 5	7.36	73.6	36.8
0.14 × 5	0.14	1.4	0.7
1.02 × 5	1.02	10.2	5.1

55. $\dfrac{15}{16} = 0.94 = 94\%$

56. $\dfrac{15}{6} = 2.5 = 250\%$

57. C. An estimate of the product of $3.03 \times 4.5 = (3 \times 4) + (3 \times 0.5) = 12 + 1.5 = 13.5$, or 14 mg.

58. $57 + 58 =$ approximately $60 + 60 = 120$.

Subtract to determine the exact number:

$60 - 57 = 3$

$60 - 58 = 2$

$3 + 2 = 5$

$120 - 5 = 115$

The exact answer is 115.

Or, you could add $50 + 50$ and $7 + 8$, which is even simpler!

59. For 9×50: $9 \times 5 = 45$; move the decimal one place to the right for a total of 450 mg.

Chapter 2
Chapter Problems
Addition

1. Estimate: $160 + 210 = 370$

Calculation:

159 is the same as $100 + 50 + 9$

206 is the same as $\underline{200 + \ \ 0 + 6}$

$300 + 50 + 15 = 365$

2. Estimate: $360 + 450 = 810$

Calculation:

361 is the same as $300 + 60 + 1$

457 is the same as $400 + 50 + 7$

$700 + 110 + 8 = 818$

Subtraction

1. Estimate: $260 - 10 = 250$

Calculation: $263 - 10 - 4 =$

$253 - 3 - 1 =$

$250 - 1 = 249$

2. Estimate: $520 - 40 = 480$

Calculation: $515 - 30 - 6 =$

$515 - 15 - 15 - 5 - 1 =$

$500 - 15 - 5 - 1 =$

$500 - 10 - 5 - 5 - 1 =$

$490 - 10 - 1 =$

$480 - 1 = 479$

Adding Decimals

1.
$$\begin{array}{r} 5.80 \\ + \ 30.30 \\ \hline 36.10 \end{array}$$

2.
$$\begin{array}{r} 1{,}869.2345 \\ + \ 70.0000 \\ \hline 1{,}939.2345 \end{array}$$

3.
$$\begin{array}{r} 000.0004 \\ + \ 100.0700 \\ \hline 100.0704 \end{array}$$

Subtracting Decimals

1.
$$\begin{array}{r} 280.40 \\ - \ 005.00 \\ \hline 275.40 \end{array}$$

2.
$$\begin{array}{r} 32.485 \\ - \ 00.010 \\ \hline 32.475 \end{array}$$

3.
$$\begin{array}{r} 218.640 \\ - \ 000.001 \\ \hline 218.639 \end{array}$$

Multiplication

1. Estimate the answer: $40 \times 2 = 80$

Calculate the exact answer:

36×2 can be rearranged as follows: 30×2 and 6×2

30×2 is solved by multiplying 3×2 and adding the zero (multiplying by 10) = 60 and then adding $6 \times 2 = 12$

$60 + 12 = 72$ (The estimated answer was 80.)

2. Estimate the answer: $120 \times 5 = 600$

Calculate the exact answer:

118×5 can be rearranged as follows: 100×5, 10×5, and 8×5

100×5 is solved by multiplying 1×5 and adding two zeros (multiplying by 100) = 500

Then solve the other two pieces: $10 \times 5 = 50$ and $8 \times 5 = 40$

$500 + 50 + 40 = 590$ (The estimated answer was 600.)

3. 1.26

4. 123.56

5. 74.585656

6. 0.0032

7. 468,000

8. 4,680

9. 26

10. 163

Order of Operations

1. $12 \times 11 = 12 \times 10$ and 12×1

$120 + 12 = 132$

Restate the equation:

$80 \div 2 + (132 - 132) =$

$80 \div 2 + (0) =$

$40 + 0 = 40$

2. $14 \times 5 = 10 \times 5$ and 4×5

$50 + 20 = 70$

Restate the equation:

$16 - 8 + 70 \div 2$

Solve the next item:

$70 \div 2 = 35$

Restate the equation:

$16 - 8 + 35 =$

$8 + 35 = 43$

Division

1. Estimate the answer: $200 \div 8$ is less than $200 \div 10 = 20$ and more than $200 \div 4 = 50$.

The calculated answer should be between 20 and 50.

Calculation:

Rearrange the numbers: $200 \div 8$ can be rearranged to $160 \div 8$ and $40 \div 8$.

$160 \div 8 = 20$

$40 \div 8 = 5$

Add the pieces:

$20 + 5 = 25$ mg

The estimated answer was between 20 and 50.

2. Estimate the answer: $153 \div 3$ is more than $150 \div 3 = 50$ and less than $200 \div 3 = 66.67$.

The calculated answer should be between 50 and 66.67.

Calculation:

Rearrange the numbers: $153 \div 3$ can be rearranged to $100 \div 3$, $50 \div 3$, and $3 \div 3$.

$100 \div 3 = 33.3$

$50 \div 3 = 16.67$

$3 \div 3 = 1$

Round 33.3 to the nearest whole number, or 33. Round 16.67 to the nearest whole number, or 17.

Add the pieces:

$$
\begin{array}{r}
33 \\
+ 17 \\
+ 1 \\
\hline
51
\end{array}
$$

The estimated answer was between 50 and 66.67. This checks out.

Multiplying in Manual Mode

1. Foundation number: 54

Multiplier: 83

Estimate: $50 \times 80 = 4{,}000$

Calculation:

$$
\begin{array}{r}
54 \\
\times 83 \\
\hline
162 \\
+ 432\, \\
\hline
4{,}482
\end{array}
$$

Check against the estimate:

Estimate $= 4{,}000$

Answer $= 4{,}482$

2. Foundation number: 26

Multiplier: 77

Estimate: $30 \times 80 = 2{,}400$

Calculation:

$$
\begin{array}{r}
26 \\
\times 77 \\
\hline
182
\end{array}
$$

$$
\begin{array}{r}
26 \\
\times 77 \\
\hline
182 \\
+ 182\, \\
\hline
2{,}002
\end{array}
$$

Check against the estimate:

Estimate $= 2{,}400$

Answer $= 2{,}002$

Multiplying Decimals

1.
$$
\begin{array}{r}
6.3 \\
\times 4 \\
\hline
25.2
\end{array}
$$

2.
$$
\begin{array}{r}
20.28 \\
\times 2 \\
\hline
40.56
\end{array}
$$

3.
$$
\begin{array}{r}
3.87 \\
\times 4.5 \\
\hline
1{,}935
\end{array}
$$

$$
\begin{array}{r}
3.87 \\
\times 4.5 \\
\hline
1935 \\
+ 1548\, \\
\hline
17.415
\end{array}
$$

4. 100.5
$\underline{\times\ 2.5}$
5,025

    100.5
$\underline{\times\ 2.5}$
    5025
$\underline{+\ 2010}$
  251.25

Dividing in Manual Mode

1.   0 9 8 5 8 5
$7\overline{)69\ 0\ 1\ 0\ 0}$

By rounding to the nearest tenth, the answer becomes 985.9.

2.   1 2 8 3
$4\overline{)5\ 1\ 3\ 2}$

This problem works out evenly, but the answer can still be rounded to the nearest tenth, which results in 12.8.

3.   0408.05
$12\overline{)4896.70}$

By rounding to the nearest tenth, the answer becomes 408.1.

Dividing Decimals

1.   123.4
$1\overline{)123.4}$

2.   101.365
$82\overline{)8312.00}$
   $\underline{82}$
   112
    $\underline{82}$
   300
   $\underline{246}$
    540
    $\underline{492}$
    480
    $\underline{410}$
     70

3.   3 3 4 7.5
$8\overline{)26\ 7\ 8\ 0.0}$

Review of Using Estimates

1. Estimate: $5 + 10 + 20 = 35$

2. Estimate: $10 + 10 + 30 = 50$

3. Estimate: $5 + 15 + 20 = 40$

4. Estimate: $50 + 140 + 60 = 250$

5. Estimate: $260 + 300 = 560$

6. Estimate: $150\ \text{lb} \div 2 = 75\ \text{lb}$

Rearrange the numbers: $100 \div 2$ and $60 \div 2$

Calculate: $100 \div 2 = 50$ and $60 \div 2 = 30$

$50 + 30 = 80$

The exact answer is 80 lb.

7. Estimate: 40×5 (Remember the trick of multiplying by 10 and then dividing the answer in half, also called the trick of 5s? $40 \times 10 = 400$; half is 200 for an estimate.)

Rearrange the numbers: $36 \times 7 = 30 \times 7$ and 6×7

Calculate: $30 \times 7 = 210$ and $6 \times 7 = 42$

$210 + 42 = 252$

Practice Problems

1.   36
$\underline{+\ 48}$
  84

2.   28
$\underline{+\ 49}$
  77

3.   66
$\underline{+\ 25}$
  91

4.   45
$\underline{+\ 30}$
  75

5.   126
$\underline{+\ 96}$
 222

6.   88
$\underline{+\ 219}$
 307

7.   165
$\underline{+\ 303}$
 468

8.   49
$\underline{-\ 12}$
  37

9.   3 3
$\underline{-\ 17}$
  16

10.
$$\begin{array}{r} 7\,^{6}\!1 \\ -\ 44 \\ \hline 27 \end{array}$$

11.
$$\begin{array}{r} 3\,^{2}2\,^{1}4 \\ -\ 249 \\ \hline 75 \end{array}$$

12.
$$\begin{array}{r} 10\,^{0}\!^{9}\!1 \\ -\ 74 \\ \hline 27 \end{array}$$

13.
$$\begin{array}{r} 676 \\ -\ 564 \\ \hline 112 \end{array}$$

14.
$$\begin{array}{r} 5\,^{1}2\,^{1}2 \\ -\ 333 \\ \hline 189 \end{array}$$

15.
$$\begin{array}{r} 13 \\ \times\ 7 \\ \hline 91 \end{array}$$

16.
$$\begin{array}{r} 23 \\ \times\ 8 \\ \hline 184 \end{array}$$

17.
$$\begin{array}{r} 45 \\ \times\ 66 \\ \hline 270 \end{array}$$

$$\begin{array}{r} 45 \\ \times\ 66 \\ \hline 270 \\ +\ 2700 \\ \hline 2{,}970 \end{array}$$

18.
$$\begin{array}{r} 50 \\ \times\ 17 \\ \hline 350 \\ +\ 500 \\ \hline 850 \end{array}$$

19.
$$\begin{array}{r} 156 \\ \times\ 60 \\ \hline 9{,}360 \end{array}$$

20.
$$\begin{array}{r} 357 \\ \times\ 230 \\ \hline 0 \\ 10710 \end{array}$$

$$\begin{array}{r} 357 \\ \times\ 230 \\ \hline 0 \\ 10710 \\ +\ 71400 \\ \hline 82{,}110 \end{array}$$

21.
$$\begin{array}{r} 444 \\ \times\ 321 \\ \hline 444 \\ 8880 \\ +\ 133200 \\ \hline 142{,}524 \end{array}$$

22.
$$\begin{array}{r} 2\ 8 \\ 15\overline{)42\ 0} \end{array}$$

23.
$$\begin{array}{r} 5\ 846 \\ 13\overline{)76\ 0\ 0\ 0} \end{array}$$

Round to 5.85.

24.
$$\begin{array}{r} 17\ 142 \\ 7\overline{)12\ 0\ 0\ 0\ 0} \end{array}$$

Round to 17.14.

25.
$$\begin{array}{r} 4\ 295 \\ 44\overline{)189\ 0\ 0\ 0} \end{array}$$

Round to 4.30.

26.
$$\begin{array}{r} 3\ 364 \\ 129\overline{)434\ 0\ 0\ 0} \end{array}$$

Round to 3.36.

27.
$$\begin{array}{r} 10 \\ 30\overline{)300} \end{array}$$

28.
$$\begin{array}{r} 6\ 875 \\ 80\overline{)550\ 0\ 0\ 0} \end{array}$$

Round to 6.86.

29.
$$\begin{array}{r} 8 \\ 125\overline{)1{,}000} \end{array}$$

30.
$$\begin{array}{r} 5.6 \\ +\ 3.8 \\ \hline 9.4 \end{array}$$

31.
$$\begin{array}{r} 6.92 \\ +\ 14.19 \\ \hline 21.11 \end{array}$$

32.
$$\begin{array}{r} 69.48 \\ +\ 597.67 \\ \hline 667.15 \end{array}$$

33.
$$\begin{array}{r} 157.82 \\ +\ 59.46 \\ \hline 217.28 \end{array}$$

34.
$$\begin{array}{r} 548.87 \\ +\ 234.78 \\ \hline 783.65 \end{array}$$

35. 6.4
  − 3.7
  2.7

36. 12.84
  − 9.95
  2.89

37. 356.70
  − 74.56
  282.14

38. 700.06
  − 53.50
  646.56

39. 1,254.730
  −   8.094
  1,246.636

40. 23 − 3 = 20

  4 × 20 = 80

  6 ÷ 2 = 3

  80 + 3 = 83

41. 26 × 2 = 52

  8 ÷ 4 = 2

  52 − 1 = 51

  51 + 5 = 56

  56 + 2 = 58

42. 10 × 2 = 20

  20 × 6 = 120

  120 × 3 = 360

  360 ÷ 2 = 180

  180 + 5 = 185

  185 − 1 = 184

43.

	Estimate	Break it up	Calculate the answer	Check against your estimate
274 + 324	**275 + 325 = 600**	**270 + 4 + 300 + 20 + 4**	**270 + 20 = 290** **4 + 4 = 8** **+ 300** **= 598**	**Estimate = 600** **Answer = 598**
278 − 46	280 − 45 = 235	270 + 8 − 40 − 6	270 − 40 = 230 8 − 6 = 2 = 232	Estimate = 235 Answer = 232
81 × 4	80 × 5 = 400	80 × 4 + 1 × 4	80 × 4 = 320 + 1 × 4 = 4 = 324	Estimate = 400 Answer = 324

44. If one service has 7 ambulances, another service has 9, and the remaining 3 services each have 4, the calculation is: 7 + 9 + (3 × 4) = 16 + 12 = 28 ambulances.

45. A full staff of 35 employees, minus the 4 people who quit, minus the 2 who were fired leaves 29 employees: 35 − 4 − 2 = 29. If you add the 3 new employees to this, you have 29 + 3 = 32 employees. The difference between your full staff and the current number of employees is 3: 35 − 32 = 3. Your service still needs to hire 3 people.

46. Since the bags come in set numbers per box, you need to multiply the number of bags in a box times the number of cases ordered. The calculation is therefore:

(14 × 12) + (13 × 24) = 168 + 312 = 480. There are a total of 480 bags of fluid in the cases your supervisor ordered.

47. There are 365 days in a year. If there were 5,000 calls in 1 year, there was an average of 13.7 calls per day: 5,000 ÷ 365 = 13.7. If you worked 122 days and had an average of 13.7 calls per day, you responded to about 1,671 calls: 122 × 13.7 = 1,671.

48. A patient who takes 4.75 mg of a medication 6 times per day takes 28.5 mg/d: 4.75 × 6 = 28.5. Because there are 7 days in a week, the patient takes 199.5 mg/wk: 28.5 × 7 = 199.5.

49. $33.89 + 24.20 + 29 + 16.65 = 103.74$ gallons

50. Subtract the number of points missed to determine the number of points you earned: $300 - 7.5 - 23.75 - 19.3 = 249.45$ points earned. Your score was therefore $249.45 \div 300 = 0.8315$, which written as a percentage is 83%.

51.
```
  12.3
×   2
  24.6
```

52.
```
  53.14
×    5
 265.70
```

53.
```
    8.2
 × 4.1
    82
 + 328
  33.62
```

54.
```
   25.11
 × 4.63
   7533

   25.11
 × 4.63
   7533
  15066

   25.11
 ×   4.63
   7533
  15066
 + 10044
 116.2593
```

55.
```
   63.9
2)127.8
```

56.
```
   262.147
34)8913.000
   68
   211
   204
    73
    68
    50
    34
   160
   136
   240
   238
     2
```

57.
```
  2 41 3 5  5
4)9 65 4 2  0
```

58.
```
     17512.22
50)875611.000
   50
   375
   350
   256
   250
    61
    50
   111
   100
   110
   100
   100
   100
     0
```

Chapter Problems

Multiplying and Dividing by the Number 1

1. $\dfrac{12}{24} \div \dfrac{3}{3} = \dfrac{4}{8}$

2. $\dfrac{4}{8} \div \dfrac{2}{2} = \dfrac{2}{4}$

3. $\dfrac{2}{4} \div \dfrac{2}{2} = \dfrac{1}{2}$

4. $\dfrac{4}{8} \div \dfrac{4}{4} = \dfrac{1}{2} = 0.5$

5. $\dfrac{2}{4} \div \dfrac{2}{2} = \dfrac{1}{2} = 0.5$

6. $\dfrac{1}{2} = 0.5$

Reducing Fractions With Ease

1. $\dfrac{10}{100} \div \dfrac{10}{10} = \dfrac{1}{10}$

2. $\dfrac{18}{32} \div \dfrac{2}{2} = \dfrac{9}{16}$

3. $\dfrac{90}{255} \div \dfrac{15}{15} = \dfrac{6}{17}$

Examples of Reducing Fractions

1. $\dfrac{6}{168} \div \dfrac{6}{6} = \dfrac{1}{28}$

$$28\overline{)1\ 00\ 0} \quad 0.03\ 5$$

Round to 0.04. Converted to a percentage, this would be 4%.

2. $\dfrac{56}{42} \div \dfrac{7}{7} = \dfrac{8}{6}$

$$6\overline{)8\ 0} \quad 1\ 3$$

3. $\dfrac{24}{1,600} \div \dfrac{8}{8} = \dfrac{3}{200}$

$$200\overline{)3\ 00\ 0} \quad 0.01\ 5$$

Reducing Complicated Fractions: Making Complicated Fractions Simple

1. Cross out the 3s and restate the equation:

$$\frac{28 \times 88}{15 \times 7 \times 44}$$

Restate:

$$\frac{7 \times 4 \times 44 \times 2}{15 \times 7 \times 44}$$

Restate:

$$\frac{4 \times 2}{15} = \frac{8}{15}$$

$$15\overline{)8\ 0\ 0\ 0} \quad 0\ 5\ 3\ 3$$

Round to 0.53. Converted to a percentage, this would be 53%.

2. Cross out the 15s and restate the equation:

$$\frac{5 \times 100}{11 \times 2 \times 25}$$

Restate:

$$\frac{5 \times 25 \times 2 \times 2}{11 \times 2 \times 25}$$

Cross out the 25s and one set of 2s, then restate:

$$\frac{5 \times 2}{11} = \frac{10}{11}$$

Divide:

$$11\overline{)10\ 0\ 00} \quad 0.9\ 09$$

Round to 0.91. Converted to a percentage, this is 91%.

3. Cross out the 21s and reduce the 12 and 6:

$$\frac{12 \times 21 \times 10.5}{6 \times 8 \times 21}$$

Restate:

$$\frac{2 \times 10.5}{8}$$

Rephrase 2×10.5 as:
2×10 and 2×0.5
$2 \times 10 = 20$
$2 \times 0.5 = 1$ (remember 0.5 equals half; half of 2 is 1)
$20 + 1 = 21$

Restate the equation:

$$\frac{21}{8}$$

Divide:

$$8\overline{)21\ 0\ 0\ 0} \quad 2\ 6\ 2\ 5$$

Round to 2.63.

Practice Problems

1. Two examples of how to reduce this fraction follow:

$$\frac{125}{150} \div \frac{5}{5} = \frac{25}{30}$$

$$\frac{125}{150} \div \frac{25}{25} = \frac{5}{6}$$

Note that the first reduction can be further reduced as follows:

$$\frac{25}{30} \div \frac{5}{5} = \frac{5}{6}$$

2. Three examples of how to reduce this fraction follow:

$$\frac{80}{100} \div \frac{2}{2} = \frac{40}{50}$$

$$\frac{80}{100} \div \frac{5}{5} = \frac{16}{20}$$

$$\frac{80}{100} \div \frac{10}{10} = \frac{8}{10}$$

This can be further reduced as follows:

$$\frac{8}{10} \div \frac{2}{2} = \frac{4}{5}$$

3. Two examples of how to reduce this fraction follow:

$$\frac{126}{144} \div \frac{3}{3} = \frac{42}{48}$$

$$\frac{126}{144} \div \frac{2}{2} = \frac{63}{72}$$

These can both be further reduced as follows:

$$\frac{42}{48} \div \frac{6}{6} = \frac{7}{8}$$

$$\frac{63}{72} \div \frac{9}{9} = \frac{7}{8}$$

4. Two examples of how to reduce this fraction follow:

$$\frac{16}{24} \div \frac{2}{2} = \frac{8}{12}$$

$$\frac{16}{24} \div \frac{4}{4} = \frac{4}{6}$$

These can be further reduced as follows:

$$\frac{8}{12} \div \frac{4}{4} = \frac{2}{3}$$

$$\frac{4}{6} \div \frac{2}{2} = \frac{2}{3}$$

5. $\frac{125}{150} \div \frac{5}{5} = \frac{25}{30} \div \frac{5}{5} = \frac{5}{6} = 0.83$

6. $\frac{80}{100} \div \frac{10}{10} = \frac{8}{10} = 0.8$

7. $\frac{126}{144} \div \frac{3}{3} = \frac{42}{48} \div \frac{6}{6} = \frac{7}{8} = 0.875$

8. $\frac{16}{24} \div \frac{4}{4} = \frac{4}{6} \div \frac{2}{2} = \frac{2}{3} = 0.67$

9. $\frac{7}{8}$ cannot be reduced.

$$9) \overline{8}\ \frac{0.8\ 7\ 5}{7\ 0\ 0\ 0}$$

Round to 0.88.

10. $\frac{4}{9}$ cannot be reduced.

$$9)\overline{4\ 0\ 0\ 0}\ {}^{0.4\ 4\ 4}$$

Round to 0.44.

11. $\frac{5}{16}$ cannot be reduced.

$$16)\overline{5\ 0\ 0\ 0}\ {}^{0.3\ 1\ 2}$$

Round to 0.31.

12. $\frac{6}{32} \div \frac{2}{2} = \frac{3}{16}$

$$32)\overline{6\ 0\ 0\ 0}\ {}^{0.1\ 8\ 7}$$

Round to 0.19.

13. $\frac{25}{32}$ cannot be reduced.

$$32)\overline{25\ 0\ 0\ 0}\ {}^{0.7\ 8\ 1}$$

Round to 0.78.

14. $\frac{41}{64}$ cannot be reduced.

$$64)\overline{41\ 0\ 0\ 0}\ {}^{0.6\ 4\ 0}$$

Round to 0.64.

15. $\frac{34}{55}$ cannot be reduced.

$$55)\overline{34\ 0\ 0\ 0}\ {}^{0.6\ 1\ 8}$$

Round to 0.62.

16. $\frac{76}{32} \div \frac{4}{4} = \frac{19}{8}$

$$8)\overline{19.0\ 0\ 0}\ {}^{2.3\ 7\ 5}$$

Round to 2.38.

17. $\frac{28}{5}$ cannot be reduced.

$$5)\overline{28.0}\ {}^{5.6}$$

18. $\dfrac{88}{24} \div \dfrac{8}{8} = \dfrac{11}{3}$

$$3\overline{)11.000} \quad 3.666$$

Round to 3.67.

19. $\dfrac{40}{60} \div \dfrac{20}{20} = \dfrac{2}{3}$

$$3\overline{)2.000} \quad 0.666$$

Round to 0.67.

20. $\dfrac{84}{8} \div \dfrac{4}{4} = \dfrac{21}{2}$

$$2\overline{)21.00} \quad 10.50$$

21. $\dfrac{67}{68}$ cannot be reduced.

$$68\overline{)67.0\,0\,0} \quad 0.9\ 8\ 5$$

Round to 0.99.

22. $\dfrac{63}{62}$ cannot be reduced.

$$62\overline{)63.00\,0} \quad 1.01\ 6$$

Round to 1.02.

23. $\dfrac{104}{58} \div \dfrac{2}{2} = \dfrac{52}{29}$

$$29\overline{)52.0\,0\,0} \quad 1.7\ 9\ 3$$

Round to 1.79.

24. $\dfrac{70}{32} \div \dfrac{2}{2} = \dfrac{35}{16}$

$$16\overline{)35.0\,0\,0} \quad 2.1\ 8\ 7$$

Round to 2.19.

25. $\dfrac{5}{55} \div \dfrac{5}{5} = \dfrac{1}{11}$

$$11\overline{)1.00\,0} \quad 0.09\ 0$$

Round to 0.09.

26. $\dfrac{144}{164} \div \dfrac{2}{2} = \dfrac{72}{82}$

$\dfrac{72}{82} \div \dfrac{2}{2} = \dfrac{36}{41}$

27. $\dfrac{80}{100} \div \dfrac{2}{2} = \dfrac{40}{50}$

$\dfrac{40}{50} \div \dfrac{2}{2} = \dfrac{20}{25}$

$\dfrac{20}{25} \div \dfrac{5}{5} = \dfrac{4}{5}$

28. $\dfrac{18}{27} \div \dfrac{9}{9} = \dfrac{2}{3}$

29. $\dfrac{62}{100} \div \dfrac{2}{2} = \dfrac{31}{50}$

30. $\dfrac{33}{99} \div \dfrac{33}{33} = \dfrac{1}{3}$

31. $\dfrac{25}{100} \div \dfrac{25}{25} = \dfrac{1}{4}$

32. $\dfrac{6}{18} \div \dfrac{6}{6} = \dfrac{1}{3}$

33. $\dfrac{4}{6} \div \dfrac{2}{2} = \dfrac{2}{3}$

$\dfrac{2}{4} \div \dfrac{2}{2} = \dfrac{1}{2}$

34. $\dfrac{18}{24} \div \dfrac{6}{6} = \dfrac{3}{4}$

$\dfrac{6}{9} \div \dfrac{3}{3} = \dfrac{2}{3}$

35. $\dfrac{5 \times 2 \times 2 \times 4 \times 2}{2 \times 2 \times 5} =$

$\dfrac{5 \times 2 \times 2 \times 4 \times 2}{2 \times 2 \times 5} = 4 \times 2$

36. $\dfrac{3 \times 7 \times 4 \times 2}{2 \times 7 \times 4 \times 3} =$

$\dfrac{3 \times 7 \times 4 \times 2}{2 \times 7 \times 4 \times 3} = 1$

37. $\dfrac{2 \times 3 \times 3 \times 3 \times 8 \times 4}{8 \times 3 \times 2}$

$\dfrac{2 \times 3 \times 3 \times 3 \times 8 \times 4}{8 \times 3 \times 2} = 3 \times 3 \times 4$

38. $\dfrac{3 \times 5 \times 4 \times 2 \times 2 \times 3 \times 5}{5 \times 2 \times 3} =$

$\dfrac{3 \times 5 \times 4 \times 2 \times 2 \times 3 \times 5}{5 \times 2 \times 3}$

$= 4 \times 2 \times 3 \times 5$

39. $\dfrac{3 \times 4 \times 5 \times 5 \times 6 \times 5 \times 7}{5 \times 4 \times 6 \times 7}$

$\dfrac{3 \times 4 \times 5 \times 5 \times 6 \times 5 \times 7}{5 \times 4 \times 6 \times 7} = 3 \times 5 \times 5$

40. $\dfrac{5 \times 2 \times 4 \times 5 \times 6 \times 5}{2 \times 4 \times 5} =$

$\dfrac{5 \times 2 \times 4 \times 5 \times 6 \times 5}{2 \times 4 \times 5} = 5 \times 6 \times 5$

41. $\dfrac{11 \times 5 \times 11 \times 2 \times 3 \times 3}{2 \times 11 \times 3} =$

$\dfrac{11 \times 5 \times 11 \times 2 \times 3 \times 3}{2 \times 11 \times 3} = 5 \times 11 \times 3$

42. $\dfrac{3 \times 11 \times 2 \times 4.5 \times 5 \times 2 \times 7}{4.5 \times 2 \times 3 \times 2 \times 7} =$

$\dfrac{3 \times 11 \times 2 \times 4.5 \times 5 \times 2 \times 7}{4.5 \times 2 \times 3 \times 2 \times 7} = 11 \times 5$

43. $\dfrac{7 \times 2 \times 8 \times 7 \times 10 \times 8}{7 \times 7 \times 8} =$

$\dfrac{7 \times 2 \times 8 \times 7 \times 10 \times 8}{7 \times 7 \times 8} = 2 \times 10 \times 8$

44. $\dfrac{23 \times 13 \times 2 \times 29}{29 \times 2 \times 13 \times 23 \times 2} =$

$\dfrac{23 \times 13 \times 2 \times 29}{29 \times 2 \times 13 \times 23 \times 2} = \dfrac{1}{2}$

45. $\dfrac{4 \times 11 \times 7 \times 8 \times 9 \times 9}{4 \times 7 \times 9 \times 11} =$

$\dfrac{4 \times 11 \times 7 \times 8 \times 9 \times 9}{4 \times 7 \times 9 \times 11} = 8 \times 9$

46. $\dfrac{9 \times 4 \times 12 \times 6 \times 10 \times 6 \times 5 \times 3}{9 \times 12 \times 10 \times 5} =$

$\dfrac{9 \times 4 \times 12 \times 6 \times 10 \times 6 \times 5 \times 3}{9 \times 12 \times 10 \times 5}$

$= 4 \times 6 \times 6 \times 3$

47. $\dfrac{400 \times 2 \times 50 \times 3}{400 \times 50} =$

$\dfrac{400 \times 2 \times 50 \times 3}{400 \times 50} = 2 \times 3$

48. $\dfrac{10 \times 100 \times 50 \times 10 \times 10 \times 10}{100 \times 50 \times 10} =$

$\dfrac{10 \times 100 \times 50 \times 10 \times 10 \times 10}{100 \times 50 \times 10}$

$= 10 \times 10 \times 10$

49. $\dfrac{9 \times 5 \times 10 \times 5 \times 11 \times 5 \times 15 \times 5}{9 \times 10 \times 11 \times 15} =$

$\dfrac{9 \times 5 \times 10 \times 5 \times 11 \times 5 \times 15 \times 5}{9 \times 10 \times 11 \times 15}$

$= 5 \times 5 \times 5 \times 5$

50. $\dfrac{23.5 \times 2 \times 38 \times 2 \times 10 \times 5}{38 \times 23.5 \times 10} =$

$\dfrac{23.5 \times 2 \times 38 \times 2 \times 10 \times 5}{38 \times 23.5 \times 10} = 2 \times 2 \times 5$

51. $\dfrac{30 \times 2 \times 30 \times 10 \times 6 \times 7}{30 \times 30 \times 6} =$

$\dfrac{30 \times 2 \times 30 \times 10 \times 6 \times 7}{30 \times 30 \times 6} = 2 \times 10 \times 7$

52. $\dfrac{15 \times 5 \times 15}{15 \times 5 \times 15 \times 5 \times 75} =$

$\dfrac{15 \times 5 \times 15}{15 \times 5 \times 15 \times 5 \times 75} = \dfrac{1}{5} \times 75$

53. $\dfrac{10}{12} = 12\overline{)10.0\,0\,0}^{\,0.8\,3\,3}$

Round to 0.83, or 83%.

54. $\dfrac{5}{8} = 8\overline{)5.0\,0\,0}^{\,0.6\,2\,5}$

Round to 0.63, or 63%.

55. $\dfrac{14}{23} = 23\overline{)14.0\,00}^{\,0.6\,08}$

Round to 0.61, or 61%.

56. $\dfrac{745}{1,240} \div \dfrac{5}{5} = \dfrac{149}{248}$

$248\overline{)149.0\,00}^{\,0.6\,00}$

Round to 0.60, or 60%.

57. $\dfrac{199}{243} = 243\overline{)199.0\,0\,0}$ $\quad\dfrac{0\;8\;1\;8}{}$

Round to 0.82, or 82%.

58. $\dfrac{70}{74} \div \dfrac{2}{2} = \dfrac{35}{37}$

$37\overline{)35.0\,0\,0}$ $\dfrac{0\;9\;4\;5}{}$

Round to 0.95, or 95%.

59. $\dfrac{2}{74} = 74\overline{)2.00\,0}$ $\dfrac{0.02\;7}{}$

Round to 0.03, or 3%.

60. $\dfrac{8}{51} = 51\overline{)8.0\,0\,0}$ $\dfrac{0.1\;5\;6}{}$

Round to 0.16, or 16%.

61. $\dfrac{67}{80} = 80\overline{)67.0\,0\,0}$ $\dfrac{0\;8\;3\;7}{}$

Round to 0.84, or 84%.

62. $\dfrac{56}{75} = 75\overline{)56.0\,0\,0}$ $\dfrac{0\;7\;4\;6}{}$

Round to 0.75, or 75%.

63. $\dfrac{56}{(145 + 56 + 83)} =$

$\dfrac{56}{284} \div \dfrac{4}{4} = \dfrac{14}{71}$

$71\overline{)14.0\,0\,0}$ $\dfrac{0.1\;9\;7}{}$

Round to 0.20, or 20%.

64. $\dfrac{11}{18} = 18\overline{)11.0\,0\,0}$ $\dfrac{0.6\;1\;1}{}$

Round to 0.61, or 61%.

65. $\dfrac{12}{(15 + 12)} =$

$\dfrac{12}{27} \div \dfrac{3}{3} = \dfrac{4}{9}$

$9\overline{)4.0\,0\,0}$ $\dfrac{0.4\;4\;4}{}$

Round to 0.44, or 44%.

66. $\dfrac{333}{744} \div \dfrac{3}{3} = \dfrac{111}{248}$

$248\overline{)111.0\,0\,0}$ $\dfrac{0.4\;4\;7}{}$

Round to 0.45, or 45%.

67. $\dfrac{25}{35} \div \dfrac{5}{5} = \dfrac{5}{7}$

$7\overline{)5.0\,0\,0}$ $\dfrac{0.7\;1\;4}{}$

Round to 0.71, or 71%.

68. $\dfrac{13}{31} = 31\overline{)13.0\,0\,0}$ $\dfrac{0.4\;1\;9}{}$

Round to 0.42, or 42%.

69. $\dfrac{4}{6} \div \dfrac{2}{2} = \dfrac{2}{3}$

$3\overline{)2.0\,0\,0}$ $\dfrac{0.6\;6\;6}{}$

Round to 0.67, or 67%.

70. $\dfrac{34 \times 45 \times 66}{17 \times 9 \times 11} =$

$\dfrac{17 \times 2 \times 9 \times 5 \times 11 \times 6}{17 \times 9 \times 11} =$

$\dfrac{17 \times 2 \times 9 \times 5 \times 11 \times 6}{17 \times 9 \times 11} = 2 \times 5 \times 6$

71. $\dfrac{30 \times 40 \times 50}{3 \times 4 \times 5} =$

$\dfrac{10 \times 3 \times 10 \times 4 \times 10 \times 5}{3 \times 4 \times 5} =$

$\dfrac{10 \times 3 \times 10 \times 4 \times 10 \times 5}{3 \times 4 \times 5}$

$= 10 \times 10 \times 10$

72. $\dfrac{20 \times 80}{10 \times 8} =$

$\dfrac{10 \times 2 \times 10 \times 8}{10 \times 8} =$

$\dfrac{10 \times 2 \times 10 \times 8}{10 \times 8} = 2 \times 10$

73. $\dfrac{40 \times 25 \times 90}{8 \times 5 \times 9} =$

$\dfrac{5 \times 8 \times 5 \times 5 \times 10 \times 9}{8 \times 5 \times 9} =$

$\dfrac{5 \times 8 \times 5 \times 5 \times 10 \times 9}{8 \times 5 \times 9} = 5 \times 5 \times 10$

74. $\dfrac{12 \times 36 \times 32}{4 \times 9 \times 8} =$

$\dfrac{3 \times 4 \times 9 \times 4 \times 8 \times 4}{4 \times 9 \times 8} =$

$\dfrac{3 \times 4 \times 9 \times 4 \times 8 \times 4}{4 \times 9 \times 8} = 3 \times 4 \times 4$

75. $\dfrac{100 \times 200 \times 300}{50 \times 40 \times 30} =$

$\dfrac{50 \times 2 \times 40 \times 5 \times 30 \times 10}{50 \times 40 \times 30} =$

$\dfrac{50 \times 2 \times 40 \times 5 \times 30 \times 10}{50 \times 40 \times 30}$

$= 2 \times 5 \times 10$

76. $\dfrac{44 \times 55 \times 66}{11 \times 11 \times 6} =$

$\dfrac{11 \times 4 \times 11 \times 5 \times 11 \times 6}{11 \times 11 \times 6} =$

$\dfrac{11 \times 4 \times 11 \times 5 \times 11 \times 6}{11 \times 11 \times 6}$

$= 4 \times 5 \times 11$

77. $\dfrac{120 \times 40 \times 500}{60 \times 20 \times 100} =$

$\dfrac{60 \times 2 \times 20 \times 2 \times 100 \times 5}{60 \times 20 \times 100} =$

$\dfrac{60 \times 2 \times 20 \times 2 \times 100 \times 5}{60 \times 20 \times 100} = 2 \times 2 \times 5$

78. $\dfrac{36 \times 90 \times 14}{12 \times 10 \times 7} =$

$\dfrac{12 \times 3 \times 10 \times 9 \times 7 \times 2}{12 \times 10 \times 7} =$

$\dfrac{12 \times 3 \times 10 \times 9 \times 7 \times 2}{12 \times 10 \times 7} = 3 \times 9 \times 2$

79. $\dfrac{16.4 \times 6.4 \times 8}{4.1 \times 3.2 \times 4} =$

$\dfrac{4.1 \times 4 \times 3.2 \times 2 \times 4 \times 2}{4.1 \times 3.2 \times 4} =$

$\dfrac{4.1 \times 4 \times 3.2 \times 2 \times 4 \times 2}{4.1 \times 3.2 \times 4} = 2 \times 4 \times 2$

80. $\dfrac{3.5 \times 4.5 \times 5.5}{7 \times 9 \times 11} =$

$\dfrac{3.5 \times 4.5 \times 5.5}{3.5 \times 2 \times 4.5 \times 2 \times 5.5 \times 2} =$

$\dfrac{3.5 \times 4.5 \times 5.5}{3.5 \times 2 \times 4.5 \times 2 \times 5.5 \times 2} = \dfrac{1}{2 \times 2 \times 2}$

81. $\dfrac{21 \times 2 \times 11}{4 \times 84 \times 22} =$

$\dfrac{21 \times 2 \times 11}{4 \times 21 \times 4 \times 11 \times 2} =$

$\dfrac{21 \times 2 \times 11}{4 \times 21 \times 4 \times 11 \times 2} = \dfrac{1}{4 \times 4}$

82. $\dfrac{10 \times 5 \times 10}{5 \times 2 \times 5} =$

$\dfrac{2 \times 5 \times 5 \times 2 \times 5}{5 \times 2 \times 5} =$

$\dfrac{2 \times 5 \times 5 \times 2 \times 5}{5 \times 2 \times 5} = 2 \times 5$

83. $\dfrac{39 \times 14 \times 16 \times 64}{13 \times 16} =$

$\dfrac{13 \times 3 \times 14 \times 16 \times 64}{13 \times 16} =$

$\dfrac{13 \times 3 \times 14 \times 16 \times 64}{13 \times 16} = 3 \times 14 \times 64$

84. $\dfrac{15 \times 16 \times 7 \times 8}{5 \times 4 \times 7 \times 2} =$

$\dfrac{5 \times 3 \times 4 \times 4 \times 7 \times 4 \times 2}{5 \times 4 \times 7 \times 2} =$

$\dfrac{5 \times 3 \times 4 \times 4 \times 7 \times 4 \times 2}{5 \times 4 \times 7 \times 2} = 3 \times 4 \times 4$

85. $\dfrac{51 \times 17 \times 8}{17 \times 4} =$

$\dfrac{51 \times 17 \times 4 \times 2}{17 \times 4} =$

$\dfrac{51 \times 17 \times 4 \times 2}{17 \times 4} = 51 \times 2$

86. $\dfrac{23 \times 13 \times 14}{69 \times 39 \times 5} =$

$\dfrac{23 \times 13 \times 14}{23 \times 3 \times 13 \times 3 \times 5} =$

$\dfrac{23 \times 13 \times 14}{23 \times 3 \times 13 \times 3 \times 5} = \dfrac{14}{3 \times 3 \times 5}$

Chapter 4
Chapter Problems
Reading and Writing Fractions

1. $\dfrac{2}{6} \div \dfrac{2}{2} = \dfrac{1}{3}$

   One third of the ambulances are responding to calls.

2. $\dfrac{4}{20} \div \dfrac{4}{4} = \dfrac{1}{5}$

   One fifth of the medics are needed to staff the units this weekend. This also equals 0.20, or 20%.

   $$20\overline{)4.00}^{\,0.20}$$

3. $\dfrac{1\text{ L LR}}{4\text{ doses LR}}$

   Convert L to mL:

   $$\dfrac{1,000\text{ mL LR}}{4\text{ doses LR}}$$

   Reduce:

   $$\dfrac{1,000}{4} \div \dfrac{4}{4} = \dfrac{250}{1} = 250\text{ mL LR}$$

   Each of the four doses of lactated Ringer's should equal 250 mL.

Multiplying Fractions

1. $\dfrac{4}{1} \times \dfrac{20}{5} = \dfrac{80}{5}$

   This can be reduced:

   $$\dfrac{80}{5} \div \dfrac{5}{5} = 16$$

2. $\dfrac{11}{6} \times \dfrac{8}{2} = \dfrac{88}{12}$

   This can be reduced:

   $$\dfrac{88}{12} \div \dfrac{4}{4} = \dfrac{22}{3}$$

3. $0 \times \dfrac{6}{8} = 0$

   Note that zero times anything is always zero.

Dividing Fractions

1. $\dfrac{3}{12} \times \dfrac{2}{1} = \dfrac{6}{12}$

   This can be further reduced to:

$$\dfrac{6}{12} \div \dfrac{6}{6} = \dfrac{1}{2}$$

This also equals 0.5, or 50%.

2. $\dfrac{7}{8} \times \dfrac{4}{3} = \dfrac{28}{24}$

   This can be further reduced to:

   $$\dfrac{28}{24} \div \dfrac{4}{4} = \dfrac{7}{6}$$

   This also equals:

   $$6\overline{)7.00}^{\,1.16}$$

   This can be rounded to 1.2 (recall rounding from Chapter 1).

3. $\dfrac{76}{128} \times \dfrac{3}{2} = \dfrac{228}{256}$

   (Recall the manual multiplication method to reach these numbers.)

   $$\begin{array}{r} 76 \\ \times\,3 \\ \hline 228 \end{array}$$

   $$\begin{array}{r} 128 \\ \times\,2 \\ \hline 256 \end{array}$$

   This can be further reduced to:

   $$\dfrac{228}{256} \div \dfrac{4}{4} = \dfrac{57}{64}$$

   Note that if the initial fractions had been reduced to their lowest terms at the outset, the multiplication would have been easier:

   $$\dfrac{76}{128} \div \dfrac{4}{4} = \dfrac{19}{32}$$

   The equation would then progress as follows:

   $$\dfrac{19}{32} \times \dfrac{3}{2} = \dfrac{57}{64}$$

Multiplying and Dividing Complicated Fractions

1. $\dfrac{12}{3} \div \dfrac{7}{8} = \dfrac{12}{3} \times \dfrac{8}{7} = \dfrac{96}{21}$

   This can be reduced as follows:

   $$\dfrac{96}{21} \div \dfrac{3}{3} = \dfrac{32}{7}$$

Note that if you reduce $\frac{12}{3}$ at the outset, you will come up with the same answer:

$$\frac{12}{3} \div \frac{3}{3} = \frac{4}{1}$$

$$\frac{4}{1} \div \frac{7}{8} = \frac{4}{1} \times \frac{8}{7} = \frac{32}{7}$$

This can also be written in decimal form as:

$$7\overline{)32.00} \quad 4.57$$

2. $\dfrac{\frac{12}{1} \times \frac{5}{6}}{\frac{4}{5}} = \dfrac{\frac{60}{6}}{\frac{4}{5}} = \frac{60}{6} \div \frac{4}{5} = \frac{60}{6} \times \frac{5}{4} = \frac{300}{24}$

This can be reduced as follows:

$$\frac{300}{24} \div \frac{12}{12} = \frac{25}{2}$$

If you had reduced the initial fractions before doing the math, it would look like this, and the same answer would result:

$$\frac{60}{6} \div \frac{6}{6} = \frac{10}{1}$$

$$\frac{10}{1} \div \frac{4}{5} = \frac{10}{1} \times \frac{5}{4} = \frac{50}{4}$$

$$\frac{50}{4} \div \frac{2}{2} = \frac{25}{2}$$

In decimal form, this is:

$$2\overline{)25.0} \quad 12.5$$

3. $\dfrac{\frac{9}{18} \times \frac{3}{6}}{\frac{3}{6}} = \dfrac{\frac{27}{108}}{\frac{3}{6}} = \frac{27}{108} \div \frac{3}{6} = \frac{27}{108} \times \frac{6}{3}$

$$= \frac{162}{324}$$

Reducing the fractions first would yield the same result:

$$\frac{9}{18} \div \frac{9}{9} = \frac{1}{2}$$

$$\frac{3}{6} \div \frac{3}{3} = \frac{1}{2}$$

$$\dfrac{\frac{1}{2} \times \frac{1}{2}}{\frac{1}{2}} = \dfrac{\frac{1}{4}}{\frac{1}{2}} = \frac{1}{4} \div \frac{1}{2} = \frac{1}{4} \times \frac{2}{1} = \frac{2}{4}$$

$$\frac{2}{4} \div \frac{2}{2} = \frac{1}{2}$$

This is equal to 0.5 or 50%.

Adding and Subtracting Fractions

1. $\dfrac{1}{10} + \dfrac{4}{10} = \dfrac{5}{10}$

This can be reduced as follows:

$$\frac{5}{10} \div \frac{5}{5} = \frac{1}{2}$$

The answer is $\frac{1}{2}$, which can also be stated as 0.5 or 50%.

2. $\dfrac{3}{4} - \dfrac{2}{4} = \dfrac{1}{4}$

$\frac{1}{4}$, or 0.25, or 25%, is the answer.

Practice Problems

1. $\dfrac{16}{20}$

This can be reduced:

$$\frac{16}{20} \div \frac{4}{4} = \frac{4}{5}$$

2. $\dfrac{20 \text{ mg}}{100 \text{ mg}}$

Reduce:

$$\frac{20}{100} \div \frac{20}{20} = \frac{1}{5}$$

3. $\dfrac{5}{50}$

Reduce:

$$\frac{5}{50} \div \frac{5}{5} = \frac{1}{10}$$

4. $\dfrac{7}{10}$

5. $\dfrac{13}{25}$

6. $\dfrac{2}{3} \times \dfrac{1}{2} = \dfrac{2}{6}$

Reduce:

$$\frac{2}{6} \div \frac{2}{2} = \frac{1}{3}$$

7. $\dfrac{7}{6} \times \dfrac{3}{4} = \dfrac{21}{24}$

Reduce:

$\dfrac{21}{24} \div \dfrac{3}{3} = \dfrac{7}{8}$

8. Reduce first fraction:

$\dfrac{32}{34} \div \dfrac{2}{2} = \dfrac{16}{17}$

Restate the original equation and solve:

$\dfrac{16}{17} \times \dfrac{4}{5} = \dfrac{64}{85}$

9. Restate the equation:

$\dfrac{2}{3} \times \dfrac{2}{1} = \dfrac{4}{3}$

Restate the improper fraction:

$\dfrac{4}{3} = \dfrac{3}{3} + \dfrac{1}{3} = 1\dfrac{1}{3}$

10. Restate the equation:

$\dfrac{7}{6} \times \dfrac{4}{3} = \dfrac{28}{18}$

Reduce:

$\dfrac{28}{18} \div \dfrac{2}{2} = \dfrac{14}{9}$

11. Reduce the first fraction:

$\dfrac{32}{34} \div \dfrac{2}{2} = \dfrac{16}{17}$

Restate the original equation:

$\dfrac{16}{17} \times \dfrac{5}{4} = \dfrac{80}{68}$

Reduce:

$\dfrac{80}{68} \div \dfrac{4}{4} = \dfrac{20}{17}$

Restate the improper fraction:

$\dfrac{20}{17} = \dfrac{17}{17} + \dfrac{3}{17} = 1\dfrac{3}{17}$

12. Work the top half of the fraction:

$\dfrac{2}{3} \times \dfrac{1}{2} = \dfrac{2}{6}$

Reduce:

$\dfrac{2}{6} \div \dfrac{2}{2} = \dfrac{1}{3}$

Restate the original equation:

$\dfrac{1}{3} \div \dfrac{4}{5} =$

Solve:

$\dfrac{1}{3} \times \dfrac{5}{4} = \dfrac{5}{12}$

13. Work the top half of the fraction:

$\dfrac{16}{32} \div 2 =$

$\dfrac{16}{32} \times \dfrac{1}{2} = \dfrac{16}{64}$

Reduce:

$\dfrac{16}{64} \div \dfrac{16}{16} = \dfrac{1}{4}$

Restate the original equation:

$\dfrac{1}{4} \div \dfrac{1}{2} =$

Solve:

$\dfrac{1}{4} \times \dfrac{2}{1} = \dfrac{2}{4}$

Reduce:

$\dfrac{2}{4} \div \dfrac{2}{2} = \dfrac{1}{2}$

14. Reduce $\dfrac{12}{16}$ in the top half of the equation:

$\dfrac{12}{16} \div \dfrac{4}{4} = \dfrac{3}{4}$

Insert the reduced fraction into the top half of the equation and solve:

$\dfrac{3}{4} \times \dfrac{3}{4} = \dfrac{9}{16} =$ top half of equation

Work the bottom half of the original equation:

$\dfrac{1}{2} \div \dfrac{1}{4} =$

Restate:

$\dfrac{1}{2} \times \dfrac{4}{1} = \dfrac{4}{2}$

Reduce:

$$\frac{4}{2} \div \frac{2}{2} = 2 = \text{bottom half of equation}$$

Restate the original equation with the new values for the top and bottom:

$$\frac{\frac{9}{16}}{2} =$$

Restate:

$$\frac{9}{16} \div 2 =$$

Restate again and solve:

$$\frac{9}{16} \times \frac{1}{2} = \frac{9}{32}$$

15. First solve the left half of the equation. Reduce $\frac{12}{24}$:

$$\frac{12}{24} \div \frac{12}{12} = \frac{1}{2}$$

Restate the left half of the equation with the reduced fraction:

$$\frac{1}{2} \div \frac{1}{2} =$$

Restate and solve:

$$\frac{1}{2} \times \frac{2}{1} = \frac{2}{2}$$

Reduce:

$$\frac{2}{2} \div \frac{2}{2} = 1 = \text{left side of original equation}$$

Solve the right half of the equation. Reduce both fractions:

$$\frac{18}{9} \div \frac{9}{9} = 2$$

$$\frac{4}{2} \div \frac{2}{2} = 2$$

Restate with the reduced values and solve:

$$\frac{2}{2} = 1 = \text{right side of original equation}$$

Restate the original equation with the new values and solve this now, very easy, equation:

$$1 \times 1 = 1$$

16. $4 \times 7 = 28$

17. 6 is the common denominator. 3 and 6 both can be divided into 6.

18. $8 \times 10 = 80$

Another possibility is 40 because 8 and 10 both divide evenly into 40 ($8 \times 5 = 40$, $10 \times 4 = 40$).

19. $4 \times 3 = 12$

20. $3 \times 2 = 6$

21. $10 \times 4 = 40$

Another possibility is 20 because 10 and 4 both divide evenly into 20 ($10 \times 2 = 20$, $4 \times 5 = 20$).

22. $6 \times 4 = 24$

Another possibility is 12 because 6 and 4 both divide evenly into 12 ($6 \times 2 = 12$, $4 \times 3 = 12$).

23. 25 and 5 both divide evenly into 100 ($25 \times 4 = 100$, $5 \times 20 = 100$).

24. 4 divides evenly into 100, so 100 is the easiest common denominator.

25. 7 divides evenly into 21, so 21 is the easiest common denominator.

26. Convert fractions to have a common denominator:

$$\frac{3}{4} \times \frac{7}{7} = \frac{21}{28}$$

$$\frac{6}{7} \times \frac{4}{4} = \frac{24}{28}$$

Solve:

$$\frac{21}{28} + \frac{24}{28} = \frac{45}{28}$$

Change from an improper fraction:

$$\frac{45}{28} = \frac{28}{28} + \frac{17}{28} = 1\frac{17}{28}$$

27. Convert second fraction to have a common denominator:

$$\frac{2}{3} \times \frac{2}{2} = \frac{4}{6}$$

Solve:

$$\frac{4}{6} + \frac{4}{6} = \frac{8}{6}$$

Reduce and change from an improper fraction:

$$\frac{8}{6} \div \frac{2}{2} = \frac{4}{3}$$

$$\frac{4}{3} = \frac{3}{3} + \frac{1}{3} = 1\frac{1}{3}$$

28. Convert fractions to have a common denominator:

$$\frac{7}{8} \times \frac{5}{5} = \frac{35}{40}$$

$$\frac{9}{10} \times \frac{4}{4} = \frac{36}{40}$$

Solve and change from an improper fraction:

$$\frac{35}{40} + \frac{36}{40} = \frac{71}{40}$$

$$\frac{71}{40} = \frac{40}{40} + \frac{31}{40} = 1\frac{31}{40}$$

29. Convert fractions to have a common denominator:

$$\frac{2}{3} \times \frac{4}{4} = \frac{8}{12}$$

$$\frac{3}{4} \times \frac{3}{3} = \frac{9}{12}$$

Solve, reduce, and change from an improper fraction:

$$\frac{8}{12} + \frac{9}{12} + \frac{9}{12} = \frac{26}{12}$$

$$\frac{26}{12} \div \frac{2}{2} = \frac{13}{6}$$

$$\frac{13}{6} = \frac{6}{6} + \frac{6}{6} + \frac{1}{6} = 2\frac{1}{6}$$

30. Convert fractions to have a common denominator:

$$\frac{2}{3} \times \frac{2}{2} = \frac{4}{6}$$

$$\frac{1}{2} \times \frac{3}{3} = \frac{3}{6}$$

Solve:

$$\frac{4}{6} - \frac{3}{6} = \frac{1}{6}$$

31. Convert fractions to have a common denominator:

$$\frac{9}{10} \times \frac{2}{2} = \frac{18}{20}$$

$$\frac{3}{4} \times \frac{5}{5} = \frac{15}{20}$$

Solve:

$$\frac{18}{20} - \frac{15}{20} = \frac{3}{20}$$

32. Convert fractions to have a common denominator:

$$\frac{3}{6} \times \frac{2}{2} = \frac{6}{12}$$

$$\frac{1}{4} \times \frac{3}{3} = \frac{3}{12}$$

Solve and reduce:

$$\frac{6}{12} - \frac{3}{12} = \frac{3}{12}$$

$$\frac{3}{12} \div \frac{3}{3} = \frac{1}{4}$$

33. Convert fractions to have a common denominator:

$$\frac{2}{25} \times \frac{4}{4} = \frac{8}{100}$$

$$\frac{1}{5} \times \frac{20}{20} = \frac{20}{100}$$

Solve:

$$\frac{66}{100} - \frac{8}{100} + \frac{20}{100} =$$

$$\frac{58}{100} + \frac{20}{100} = \frac{78}{100}$$

Reduce:

$$\frac{78}{100} \div \frac{2}{2} = \frac{39}{50}$$

34. Convert fractions to have a common denominator:

$$\frac{1}{4} \times \frac{25}{25} = \frac{25}{100}$$

Solve and reduce:

$$\frac{50}{100} - \frac{25}{100} = \frac{25}{100}$$

$$\frac{25}{100} \div \frac{25}{25} = \frac{1}{4}$$

35. Convert fractions to have a common denominator:

$$\frac{2}{7} \times \frac{3}{3} = \frac{6}{21}$$

Solve:

$$\frac{7}{21} - \frac{6}{21} = \frac{1}{21}$$

Chapter 5
Chapter 5
Chapter Problems
The "Cross Multiply and Divide Method"

1. First, reduce the fraction:

$$\frac{11}{14} \div \frac{11}{11} = \frac{1}{4}$$

Restate the original proportion:

$$\frac{1}{4} = \frac{?}{100}$$

Cross multiply and divide:

$$\frac{1}{4} \times 100 = 25$$

2. Cross multiply and divide:

$$\frac{23}{115} \times 10 = ?$$

Reduce where possible. In this case, 10 and 115 can be reduced by 5:

$$\frac{23}{115} \times 10 = ?$$

Restate the equation and solve:

$$\frac{23}{23} \times 2 = 2$$

$$\frac{23}{23} \times 2 = 2$$

3. First, reduce the fraction:

$$\frac{3}{12} \div \frac{3}{3} = \frac{1}{4}$$

Restate the equation and solve:

$$\frac{1}{4} \times 62 =$$

$$\frac{1}{4} \times 62 = \frac{31}{2}$$

$$2\overline{)31.0}^{\,15.5}$$

The answer is 15.5.

Using Proportions to Convert Units of Measure

1. Set up the proportion:

$$\frac{?\ mg}{2\ \mu g} = \frac{1\ mg}{1{,}000\ \mu g}$$

Cross multiply:

$$?\ mg = \frac{1\ mg \times 2\ \mu g}{1{,}000\ \mu g}$$

Solve:

$$?\ mg = 0.002\ mg$$

2. 253 lb = ? kg

Set up the proportion:

$$\frac{?\ kg}{253\ lb} = \frac{1\ kg}{2.2\ lb}$$

Cross multiply:

$$?\ kg = \frac{1\ kg \times 253\ lb}{2.2\ lb}$$

Solve:

$$?\ kg = 115\ kg$$

3. 5 mg = ? μg

Set up the proportion:

$$\frac{?\ \mu g}{5\ mg} = \frac{1{,}000\ \mu g}{1\ mg}$$

Cross multiply:

$$?\ \mu g = \frac{1{,}000\ \mu g \times 5\ mg}{1\ mg}$$

Solve:

$$?\ \mu g = 5{,}000\ \mu g$$

Using Proportion Shorthand to Solve Calculations

1. Flip the equation:

$$\frac{12.5\ g\ D_{50}W}{25\ g\ D_{50}W} = \frac{?\ mL}{50\ mL\ D_{50}W\ solution}$$

Solve:

$$(12.5 \times 50) \div 25 = 25\ mL$$

2. $(25 \times 25) \div 12.5 = 50\ mL$

3. Flip the equation:

$$\frac{?\ g}{25\ g\ D_{50}W} = \frac{25\ mL\ D_{50}W\ solution}{50\ mL\ D_{50}W\ solution}$$

Solve:

$(25 \times 25) \div 50 = 12.5$ g

4. $(50 \times 12.5) \div 25 = 25$ g

Converting Temperatures Between Fahrenheit and Centigrade

1. The formula is:

$$\left(\frac{9}{5} \times °C\right) + 32 = °F$$

$$\left(\frac{9}{5} \times 50\right) + 32 =$$

$$\frac{450}{5} + 32 =$$

$$90 + 32 = 122°F$$

2. The formula is:

$$\frac{5}{9} \times \left(°F - 32\right) = °C$$

$$\frac{5}{9} \times \left(20 - 32\right) =$$

$$\frac{5}{9} \times \left(-12\right) = -6.67°C$$

Concentration Percentages

1. Convert the percentage to g/mL:

$$50\% = \frac{50 \text{ g}}{100 \text{ mL}}$$

Set up the proportion:

$$\frac{50 \text{ g}}{? \text{ mL}} = \frac{50 \text{ g}}{100 \text{ mL}}$$

It is obvious, without calculating, that the answer is 100 mL. Note: If the grams ordered equals the percentage already in the solution, you will administer the entire solution.

2. Convert the percentage to g/mL:

$$10\% = \frac{10 \text{ g}}{100 \text{ mL}}$$

Convert the milligrams to grams:

$$\frac{? \text{ g}}{200 \text{ mg}} = \frac{1 \text{g}}{1,000 \text{ mg}}$$

$$? \text{ g} = \frac{1 \text{ g} \times 200 \text{ mg}}{1000 \text{ mg}}$$

$$? \text{ g} = 0.2 \text{ g}$$

Set up the final proportion:

$$\frac{0.2 \text{ g}}{? \text{ mL}} = \frac{10 \text{ g}}{100 \text{ mL}}$$

Flip and solve:

$$\frac{? \text{ mL}}{0.2 \text{ g}} = \frac{100 \text{ mL}}{10 \text{ g}}$$

$$? \text{ mL} = \frac{100 \text{ mL} \times 0.2 \text{ g}}{10 \text{ g}}$$

$$? \text{ mL} = \frac{20}{10} = 2 \text{ mL}$$

Practice Problems

1. $\dfrac{3 \times 100}{4} = ?$

$$\frac{300}{4} = 75$$

2. $50 \times 2 = 1 \times ?$

$$50 \times 2 = ?$$

$$100 = ?$$

3. $? = \dfrac{3 \times 200}{4}$

$$? = \frac{600}{4}$$

$$? = 150$$

4. $32 \times ? = 4 \times 64$

$$? = \frac{4 \times 64}{32}$$

$$? = \frac{256}{32} = 8$$

5.

Convert this number….	…to this unit of measure	Conversion factor
10 g	10,000 mg	1,000 mg = 1 g
4 mL	0.004 L	1,000 mL = 1 L
76 g	0.076 kg	1,000 g = 1 kg
1,726 mg	0.001726 kg	1,000 mg = 1 g and 1,000 g = 1 kg

First row:

Set up the proportion:

$$\frac{? \text{ mg}}{10 \text{ g}} = \frac{1,000 \text{ mg}}{1 \text{ g}}$$

Cross multiply:

$$? \, mg = \frac{1{,}000 \, mg \times 10 \, g}{1 \, g}$$

Solve:

$$? = 10{,}000 \, mg$$

Second row:
Set up the proportion:

$$\frac{? \, L}{4 \, mL} = \frac{1 \, L}{1{,}000 \, mL}$$

Cross multiply:

$$? \, L = \frac{1 \, L \times 4 \, mL}{1{,}000 \, mL}$$

Solve:

$$? = 0.004 \, L$$

Third row:
Set up the proportion:

$$\frac{? \, kg}{76 \, g} = \frac{1 \, kg}{1{,}000 \, g}$$

Cross multiply:

$$? \, kg = \frac{1 \, kg \times 76 \, g}{1{,}000 \, g}$$

Solve:

$$? = 0.076 \, kg$$

Fourth row:
First, figure out the conversion factor by using the two provided:

$$\frac{1{,}000 \, mg}{1 \, g} \times \frac{1{,}000 \, g}{1 \, kg} = \frac{1{,}000{,}000 \, mg}{1 \, kg}$$

Set up the proportion:

$$\frac{? \, kg}{1{,}726 \, mg} = \frac{1 \, kg}{1{,}000{,}000 \, mg}$$

Cross multiply:

$$? \, kg = \frac{1 \, kg \times 1{,}726 \, mg}{1{,}000{,}000 \, mg}$$

Solve:

$$? = 0.001726 \, kg$$

6. 0.75 g

Conversion factor: 1,000 mg = 1 g

$$750 \, mg \times \frac{1 \, g}{1{,}000 \, mg} = 0.75 \, g$$

7. 3,300 mg

Conversion factor: 1 g = 1,000 mg

$$3.3 \, g \times \frac{1{,}000 \, mg}{1 \, g} = 3{,}300 \, mg$$

8. 25,000 µg

Conversion factor: 1 mg = 1,000 µg

$$25 \, mg \times \frac{1{,}000 \, \mu g}{1 \, mg} = 25{,}000 \, \mu g$$

9. 0.5 mg

Conversion factor: 1,000 µg = 1 mg

$$500 \, \mu g \times \frac{1 \, mg}{1{,}000 \, \mu g} = 0.5 \, mg$$

10. 1,000,000 µg

Conversion factor: 1 mg = 1,000 µg

$$1{,}000 \, mg \times \frac{1{,}000 \, \mu g}{1 \, mg} = 1{,}000{,}000 \, \mu g$$

11. 0.033 L

Conversion factor: 1,000 mL = 1 L

$$33 \, mL \times \frac{1 \, L}{1{,}000 \, mL} = 0.033 \, L$$

12. 2,200 mL

Conversion factor: 1 L = 1,000 mL

$$2.2 \, L \times \frac{1{,}000 \, mL}{1 \, L} = 2{,}200 \, mL$$

13. 0.0074 L

Conversion factor: 1,000 mL = 1 L

$$7.4 \, mL \times \frac{1 \, L}{1{,}000 \, mL} = 0.0074 \, L$$

14. 1.25 L

Conversion factor: 1,000 mL = 1 L

$$1{,}250 \, mL \times \frac{1 \, L}{1{,}000 \, mL} = 1.25 \, L$$

15. 50 mL

Conversion factor: 1 L = 1,000 mL

$$0.05 \, L \times \frac{1{,}000 \, mL}{1 \, L} = 50 \, mL$$

16. 250 μg

Conversion factor: 1 mg = 1,000 μg

$$0.25 \text{ mg} \times \frac{1,000 \text{ μg}}{1 \text{ mg}} = 250 \text{ μg}$$

17. 1,250 mg

Conversion factor: 1 g = 1,000 mg

$$1.25 \text{ g} \times \frac{1,000 \text{ mg}}{1 \text{ g}} = 1,250 \text{ mg}$$

18. 800,000 μg

Conversion factor: 1 mg = 1,000 μg

$$800 \text{ mg} \times \frac{1,000 \text{ μg}}{1 \text{ mg}} = 800,000 \text{ μg}$$

19. 0.0016 g

Conversion factor: 1,000,000 μg = 1 g

$$1,600 \text{ μg} \times \frac{1 \text{ g}}{1,000,000 \text{ μg}} = 0.0016 \text{ g}$$

20. 0.1 L

Conversion factor: 1,000 mL = 1 L

$$100 \text{ mL} \times \frac{1 \text{ L}}{1,000 \text{ mL}} = 0.1 \text{ L}$$

21. 5.0 mL

Conversion factor: 1 L = 1,000 mL

$$0.005 \text{ L} \times \frac{1,000 \text{ mL}}{1 \text{ L}} = 5.0 \text{ mL}$$

22. 0.00675 mg

Conversion factor: 1,000 μg = 1 mg

$$6.75 \text{ μg} \times \frac{1 \text{ mg}}{1,000 \text{ μg}} = 0.00675 \text{ mg}$$

23. 0.989 g

Conversion factor: 1,000 mg = 1 g

$$989 \text{ mg} \times \frac{1 \text{ g}}{1,000 \text{ mg}} = 0.989 \text{ g}$$

24. 50,000,000 μg

Conversion factor: 1 g = 1,000,000 μg

$$50 \text{ g} \times \frac{1,000,000 \text{ μg}}{1 \text{ g}} = 50,000,000 \text{ μg}$$

25. 1,001 μg

Conversion factor: 1 mg = 1,000 μg

$$1.001 \text{ mg} \times \frac{1,000 \text{ μg}}{1 \text{ mg}} = 1,001 \text{ μg}$$

26. 3,500 g

Conversion factor: 1 kg = 1,000 g

$$3.5 \text{ kg} \times \frac{1,000 \text{ g}}{1 \text{ kg}} = 3,500 \text{ g}$$

27. 750 g

Conversion factor: 1 kg = 1,000 g

$$0.75 \text{ kg} \times \frac{1,000 \text{ g}}{1 \text{ kg}} = 750 \text{ g}$$

28. 25 g

Conversion factor: 1 kg = 1,000 g

$$0.025 \text{ kg} \times \frac{1,000 \text{ g}}{1 \text{ kg}} = 25 \text{ g}$$

29. 86,000 mg

Conversion factor: 1 g = 1,000 mg

$$86 \text{ g} \times \frac{1,000 \text{ mg}}{1 \text{ g}} = 86,000 \text{ mg}$$

30. 7,000 g

Conversion factor: 1 kg = 1,000 g

$$7 \text{ kg} \times \frac{1,000 \text{ g}}{1 \text{ kg}} = 7,000 \text{ g}$$

31. 500 g

Conversion factor: 1 kg = 1,000 g

$$0.5 \text{ kg} \times \frac{1,000 \text{ g}}{1 \text{ kg}} = 500 \text{ g}$$

32. 79,000 μg

Conversion factor: 1 mg = 1,000 μg

$$79 \text{ mg} \times \frac{1,000 \text{ μg}}{1 \text{ mg}} = 79,000 \text{ μg}$$

33. 0.005 g

Conversion factor: 1,000,000 μg = 1 g

$$5,000 \text{ μg} \times \frac{1 \text{ g}}{1,000,000 \text{ μg}} = 0.005 \text{ g}$$

34. 400,000 µg

Conversion factor: 1 mg = 1,000 µg

$$400 \text{ mg} \times \frac{1,000 \text{ µg}}{1 \text{ mg}} = 400,000 \text{ µg}$$

35. 0.00000001 kg

Conversion factor: 1,000,000,000 µg = 1 kg

$$10 \text{ µg} \times \frac{1 \text{ kg}}{1,000,000,000 \text{ µg}} = 0.00000001 \text{ kg}$$

36. 7.5 kg

Conversion factor: 1,000 mg = 1 kg

$$7,500 \text{ mg} \times \frac{1 \text{ kg}}{1,000 \text{ mg}} = 7.5 \text{ kg}$$

37. 0.6 kg

Conversion factor: 1,000 g = 1 kg

$$600 \text{ g} \times \frac{1 \text{ kg}}{1,000 \text{ g}} = 0.6 \text{ kg}$$

38. 2.0 kg

Conversion factor: 1,000 g = 1 kg

$$2,000 \text{ g} \times \frac{1 \text{ kg}}{1,000 \text{ g}} = 2.0 \text{ kg}$$

39. The formula is:

$$\frac{5}{9} \times \left(°F - 32\right) = °C$$

$$\frac{5}{9} \times \left(105 - 32\right) =$$

$$\frac{5}{9} \times 73 = 40.56$$

40. The formula is:

$$\frac{5}{9} \times \left(°F - 32\right) = °C$$

$$\frac{5}{9} \times \left(100 - 32\right) =$$

$$\frac{5}{9} \times 68 = 37.78$$

41. The formula is:

$$\left(\frac{9}{5} \times °C\right) + 32 = °F$$

$$\left(\frac{9}{5} \times 38\right) + 32 =$$

$$\frac{342}{5} + 32 =$$

$$68.4 + 32 = 100.4$$

42. The formula is:

$$\left(\frac{9}{5} \times °C\right) + 32 = °F$$

$$\left(\frac{9}{5} \times 36.5\right) + 32 =$$

$$\frac{328.5}{5} + 32 =$$

$$65.7 + 32 = 97.7$$

43. The formula is:

$$\frac{5}{9} \times \left(°F - 32\right) = °C$$

$$\frac{5}{9} \times \left(32 - 32\right) =$$

$$\frac{5}{9} \times 0 = 0$$

44. First, convert milligrams to micrograms because this is a dopamine drip.

$$800 \text{ mg} \times \frac{1,000 \text{ µg}}{1 \text{ mg}} = 800,000 \text{ µg}$$

800,000 µg /500 mL = 1,600 µg/mL

45. First, convert grams to milligrams because this is a lidocaine drip.

$$1 \text{ g} \times \frac{1,000 \text{ mg}}{1 \text{ g}} = 1,000 \text{ mg}$$

1,000 mg/250 mL = 4 mg/mL

46. First, convert milligrams to micrograms because this is a dopamine drip.

$$400 \text{ mg} \times \frac{1,000 \text{ µg}}{1 \text{ mg}} = 400,000 \text{ µg}$$

$$\frac{400,000 \text{ µg}}{250 \text{ mL}} = 1,600 \text{ µg/mL}$$

47. First, convert grams to milligrams because this is a lidocaine drip.

$$2 \text{ g} \times \frac{1,000 \text{ mg}}{1 \text{ g}} = 2,000 \text{ mg}$$

$$\frac{2,000 \text{ mg}}{500 \text{ mL}} = 4 \text{ mg/mL}$$

4 mg/mL × 10 mL = 40 mg

48. First, recall that 1:1,000 means there is 1 g per 1,000 mL. Because the question asks for milligrams and the concentration is in grams, convert grams to milligrams. (Table 5-1 showed that 1 g equals 1,000 mg.)

$$\frac{1,000 \text{ mg}}{1,000 \text{ mL}} = \frac{?}{1 \text{ mL}}$$

? = 1.0 mg

49. 50% solution = 50 g in 100 mL, or 25 g in 50 mL

$$\frac{25}{50} = \frac{5}{?}$$

$$25 \times ? = 50 \times 5$$

$$? = \frac{50 \times 5}{25}$$

$$\frac{250}{25} = 10 \text{ mL}$$

50. 50% solution = 50 g in 100 mL, or 5 g in 10 mL

Because there are 5 g in the 10-mL prefilled syringe and the order is to administer 5 g, a calculation is not needed. By administering the whole prefilled syringe, you will administer the required 5 g.

51. First, convert grams to milligrams: 1 g equals 1,000 mg.

$$\frac{1,000 \text{ mg}}{50 \text{ mL}} = \frac{400 \text{ mg}}{? \text{ mL}}$$

Flip the equation:

$$\frac{?}{400 \text{ mg}} = \frac{50 \text{ mL}}{1,000 \text{ mg}}$$

$$? = \frac{50 \times 400}{1,000}$$

? = 20 mL

52. $\dfrac{500 \text{ mg}}{50 \text{ mL}} = \dfrac{175 \text{ mg}}{? \text{ mL}}$

$$\frac{? \text{ mL}}{175 \text{ mg}} = \frac{50 \text{ mL}}{500 \text{ mg}}$$

$$? = \frac{50 \times 175}{500}$$

? = 17.5 mL

53. 50% solution = 50 g in 100 mL, or 25 g in 50 mL

Because you need to administer 25 g and the prefilled syringe contains 25 g/50 mL, you administer the entire prefilled syringe.

54. 10% solution = 10 g in 100 mL, or 5 g in 50 mL

$$\frac{5 \text{ g}}{50 \text{ mL}} = \frac{4 \text{ g}}{? \text{ mL}}$$

$$\frac{? \text{ mL}}{4 \text{ g}} = \frac{50 \text{ mL}}{5 \text{ g}}$$

$$? = \frac{50 \times 4}{5}$$

? = 40 mL

Because the prefilled syringe contains 20 mL, you will need to administer two prefilled syringes.

55. 25% solution = 25 g in 100 mL, half of which would be 12.5 g in 50 mL

$$\frac{12.5 \text{ g}}{50 \text{ mL}} = \frac{2.75 \text{ g}}{? \text{ mL}}$$

$$\frac{? \text{ mL}}{2.75 \text{ g}} = \frac{50 \text{ mL}}{12.5 \text{ g}}$$

$$? = \frac{50 \times 2.75}{12.5}$$

? = 11 mL

56. Convert grams to milligrams because this is a lidocaine drip.

$$2 \text{ g} \times \frac{1,000 \text{ mg}}{1 \text{ g}} = 2,000 \text{ mg}$$

$$\frac{2,000 \text{ mg}}{500 \text{ mL}} = 4 \text{ mg/mL}$$

$$\frac{4 \text{ mg}}{\text{mL}} = \frac{? \text{ mg}}{3 \text{ mL}}$$

$$\frac{4 \text{ mg} \times 3 \text{ mL}}{\text{mL}} = ?$$

? = 12 mg

The concentration is 4 mg/mL. In 3 mL, there would be 3 times that amount, or 12 mg/3 mL.

57. 60% solution = 60 g in 100 mL, or 30 g in 50 mL

$$\frac{30 \text{ g}}{50 \text{ mL}} = \frac{6 \text{ g}}{? \text{ mL}}$$

$$\frac{? \text{ mL}}{6 \text{ g}} = \frac{50 \text{ mL}}{30 \text{ g}}$$

$$? = \frac{50 \times 6}{30}$$

? = 10 mL

58. 80% solution = 80 g in 100 mL, or 40 g in 50 mL

$$\frac{40\ g}{50\ mL} = \frac{8\ g}{?\ mL}$$

$$\frac{?\ mL}{8\ g} = \frac{50\ mL}{40\ g}$$

$$? = \frac{50 \times 8}{40}$$

$$? = 10\ mL$$

Because the prefilled syringe contains 20 mL, you need to administer half of it.

59. Convert the percentage to g/mL:

$$50\% = \frac{50\ g}{100\ mL}$$

Establish the proportion:

$$\frac{10\ g}{?\ mL} = \frac{50\ g}{100\ mL}$$

Flip and cross multiply to solve:

$$\frac{?\ mL}{10\ g} = \frac{100\ mL}{50\ g}$$

$$?\ mL = \frac{100\ mL \times 10\ g}{50\ g}$$

$$?\ mL = \frac{1,000\ mL}{50\ g} = 20\ mL$$

Chapter 6
Chapter Problems
Solving Rate-Based Problems Using the Number 1

1. First, convert grams to milligrams:

$$1\ g \times \frac{1,000\ mg}{g} = 1,000\ mg$$

Next, reduce the DOH by using the number 1:

$$\frac{1,000\ mg}{250\ mL} \div \frac{250}{250} = \frac{4\ mg}{1\ mL}$$

Plug into the formula:

$$\frac{3\ mg/min}{4\ mg/mL} \times \frac{60\ gtt}{mL} = ?\ gtt/min$$

$$\frac{3\ mg}{min} \times \frac{mL}{4\ mg} \times \frac{60\ gtt}{mL} = ?\ gtt/min$$

Reduce the 60 and 4, and solve:

$$\frac{3\ mg}{min} \times \frac{mL}{1\ mg} \times \frac{15\ gtt}{mL} = 45\ gtt/min$$

The answer is 45 gtt/min.

2. First, convert grams to milligrams:

$$2\ g = 2,000\ mg$$

Reduce the dose on hand by using the number 1:

$$\frac{2,000\ mg}{500\ mL} \div \frac{500}{500} = \frac{4\ mg}{1\ mL}$$

Plug into the formula:

$$\frac{3\ mg/min}{4\ mg/mL} \times \frac{60\ gtt}{mL} = ?\ gtt/min$$

$$\frac{3\ mg}{min} \times \frac{mL}{4\ mg} \times \frac{60\ gtt}{mL} = ?\ gtt/min$$

Reduce the 60 and 4, and solve:

$$\frac{3\ mg}{min} \times \frac{mL}{1\ mg} \times \frac{15\ gtt}{mL} = 45\ gtt/min$$

Dimensional Analysis

1. First, reduce the dose on hand using the number 1.

$$\frac{50\ mg}{5\ mL} \div \frac{5}{5} = \frac{10\ mg}{mL}$$

Then, set up the equation:

$$10\ mg \times \frac{mL}{10\ mg} = 1\ mL$$

2. $63\ mg \times \frac{min}{1.75\ mg} = 36\ min$

3. First convert hours to minutes:

$$2\ h \times \frac{60\ min}{1\ h} = 120\ min$$

Set up the equation:

$$\frac{100\ mL}{120\ min} \times \frac{10\ gtt}{mL} = ?\ gtt/min$$

Reduce and solve:

$$\frac{10 \times 10}{12} = \frac{100}{12} = 8.33\ gtt/min$$

Round to the nearest whole number, or 8 gtt/min.

4. First, convert hours to minutes:

$$\frac{100\ mL}{h} \times \frac{1\ h}{60\ min} = \frac{5\ mL}{3\ min}$$

Set up the equation:

$$\frac{5\ mL}{3\ min} \times \frac{10\ gtt}{mL} = 16.67\ gtt/min$$

Round to the nearest whole number, or 17 gtt/min.

5. First, convert hours to minutes.

$$\frac{120 \text{ mL}}{h} \times \frac{1 h}{60 \text{ min}} = \frac{2 \text{ mL}}{\text{min}}$$

Set up the equation:

$$\frac{2 \text{ mL}}{\text{min}} \times \frac{20 \text{ gtt}}{\text{mL}} = \frac{40 \text{ gtt}}{\text{min}}$$

Note that the 1,000-mL bag does not factor into the equation. This is the dose on hand, but because only 120 mL are needed, there is plenty of normal saline.

The Clock Method

1. First, convert grams to milligrams:

$$2 \text{ g} \times \frac{1,000 \text{ mg}}{g} = 2,000 \text{ mg}$$

Calculate the concentration:

$$\frac{2,000 \text{ mg}}{500 \text{ mL}} \div \frac{500}{500} = \frac{4 \text{ mg}}{\text{mL}}$$

Set up the clock as shown in Figure AK6-1 ▾ :

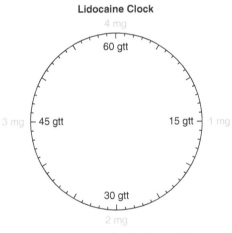

Lidocaine Clock

Figure AK6-1 Lidocaine clock for Practice Problem 1.

According to the clock, you need to administer 60 gtt/min to give 4 mg/min. The answer is 60 gtt/min.

2. Convert milligrams to micrograms:

$$400 \text{ mg} \times \frac{1,000 \text{ µg}}{\text{mg}} = \frac{400,000 \text{ µg}}{\text{mg}}$$

Calculate the concentration:

$$\frac{400,000 \text{ µg}}{250 \text{ mL}} \div \frac{250}{250} = \frac{1,600 \text{ µg}}{\text{mL}}$$

Set up the clock as shown in Figure AK6-2 ▶ :

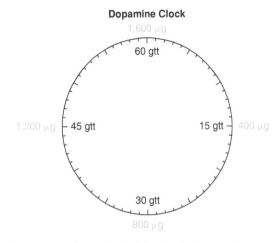

Dopamine Clock

Figure AK6-2 Dopamine clock for Practice Problem 2.

Factor in the patient's weight. First, convert the patient's weight to kilograms:

$$175 \text{ lb} \times \frac{\text{kg}}{2.2 \text{ lb}} = 79.55 \text{ kg}$$

Adjust the DD to accommodate the patient's weight:

$$79.55 \text{ kg} \times \frac{5 \text{ µg}}{\text{kg/min}} = 397.75 \text{ µg/min}$$

Round to 398 µg/min.

Because you need to administer 398 µg/min (almost 400 µg/min), you can see from the clock that you need to administer approximately 15 gtt/min to give the adjusted DD.

Practice Problems

1. $\dfrac{3 \text{ mL}}{150 \text{ µg}} \times 100 \text{ µg} = 2 \text{ mL}$

2. $\dfrac{2 \text{ mL}}{10 \text{ mg}} \times 5 \text{ mg} = 1 \text{ mL}$

3. $\dfrac{2 \text{ mL}}{10 \text{ mg}} \times 8 \text{ mg} = 1.6 \text{ mL}$

4. $\dfrac{10 \text{ mL}}{250 \text{ mg}} \times 100 \text{ mg} = 4 \text{ mL}$

5. $\dfrac{20 \text{ mL}}{40 \text{ mg}} \times 5 \text{ mg} = 2.5 \text{ mL}$

6. First, convert grams to milligrams:

$$1 \text{ g} = 1,000 \text{ mg}$$

$$\frac{10 \text{ mL}}{1,000 \text{ mg}} \times 400 \text{ mg} = 4 \text{ mL}$$

7. $\dfrac{50 \text{ mL}}{100 \text{ mg}} \times 65 \text{ mg} = 32.5 \text{ mL}$

8. $\dfrac{2 \text{ mL}}{4 \text{ mg}} \times 0.2 \text{ mg} = 0.1 \text{ mL}$

9. $\dfrac{10 \text{ mL}}{1 \text{ mg}} \times 0.05 \text{ mg} = 0.5 \text{ mL}$

10. $\dfrac{10 \text{ mL}}{5 \text{ μg}} \times 0.5 \text{ μg} = 1 \text{ mL}$

11. $\dfrac{5 \text{ mL}}{12 \text{ mg}} \times 4 \text{ mg} = 1.67 \text{ mL}$

12. $\dfrac{20 \text{ mL}}{50 \text{ mg}} \times 1.0 \text{ mg} = 0.4 \text{ mL}$

13. First, convert milligrams to micrograms:

$5.0 \text{ mg} \times \dfrac{1,000 \text{ μg}}{\text{mg}} = 5,000 \text{ μg}$

Set up the problem:

$\dfrac{5 \text{ mL}}{5,000 \text{ μg}} \times 250 \text{ μg} = 0.25 \text{ mL}$

14. $\dfrac{1 \text{ min}}{4.5 \text{ mg}} \times 252 \text{ mg} = 56 \text{ min}$

15. First, convert milligrams to micrograms:

$5 \text{ mg} \times \dfrac{1,000 \text{ μg}}{\text{mg}} = 5,000 \text{ μg}$

Set up the problem:

$\dfrac{1 \text{ min}}{100 \text{ μg}} \times 5,000 \text{ μg} = 50 \text{ min}$

16. First, convert milligrams to micrograms.

$0.45 \text{ mg} \times \dfrac{1,000 \text{ μg}}{\text{mg}} = 450 \text{ μg}$

Then set up the problem.

$\dfrac{1 \text{ min}}{10 \text{ μg}} \times 450 \text{ μg} = 45 \text{ min}$

17. First, convert milligrams to micrograms:

$75 \text{ mg} \times \dfrac{1,000 \text{ μg}}{\text{mg}} = 75,000 \text{ μg}$

Set up the problem:

$\dfrac{1 \text{ min}}{1,000 \text{ μg}} \times 75,000 \text{ μg} = 75 \text{ min}$

18. $\dfrac{1 \text{ min}}{1.25 \text{ g}} \times 30 \text{ g} = 24 \text{ min}$

19. $\dfrac{1 \text{ min}}{0.75 \text{ mg}} \times 45 \text{ mg} = 60 \text{ min}$

20. $\dfrac{1 \text{ min}}{0.1 \text{ mg}} \times 10 \text{ mg} = 100 \text{ min}$

21. $\dfrac{1 \text{ min}}{12 \text{ mg}} \times 175 \text{ mg} = 14.58 \text{ min, or } 14.6 \text{ min}$

22. $\dfrac{1 \text{ min}}{0.2 \text{ mg}} \times 60 \text{ mg} = 300 \text{ min}$

23. $\dfrac{1 \text{ min}}{18 \text{ mg}} \times 350 \text{ mg} = 19.44 \text{ min}$

24. First, convert grams to milligrams:

$1.3 \text{ g} \times \dfrac{1,000 \text{ mg}}{\text{g}} = 1,300 \text{ mg}$

Set up the problem:

$\dfrac{1 \text{ min}}{37 \text{ mg}} \times 1,300 \text{ mg} = 35.14 \text{ min}$

25. First, convert grams to milligrams:

$1.67 \text{ g} \times \dfrac{1,000 \text{ mg}}{\text{g}} = 1,670 \text{ mg}$

Set up the problem:

$\dfrac{1 \text{ min}}{11 \text{ mg}} \times 1,670 \text{ mg} = 151.82 \text{ min}$

Round up to the nearest whole number, or 152 min.

26. $50 \text{ mg} \times \dfrac{10 \text{ mL}}{200 \text{ mg}} = 2.5 \text{ mL}$

27. $0.5 \text{ mg} \times \dfrac{10 \text{ mL}}{1.0 \text{ mg}} = 5 \text{ mL}$

28. A 50% solution has 50 g/100 mL of solution. Because you have 50 mL, you have 25 g of medication in the solution. Shown as a proportion, this is:

$\dfrac{50 \text{ g}}{100 \text{ mL}} = \dfrac{? \text{ g}}{50 \text{ mL}}$

$\dfrac{50 \times 50}{100} = 25 \text{ g}$

Another way to find out the DOH is to use the concentration:

$50 \text{ mL} \times \dfrac{0.5 \text{ g}}{\text{mL}} = 25 \text{ g}$

Because the DD is 25 g, and you have determined that you have 25 g in the 50 mL, no further math is needed. You will administer the entire medication vial.

29. $5 \text{ mg} \times \dfrac{10 \text{ mL}}{25 \text{ mg}} = 2 \text{ mL}$

Note that although you were given the time, the time does not factor into the calculation of how much to administer; however, you need to be sure to administer the 2 mL slowly during 5 minutes, as ordered.

30. $1 \text{ g} \times \dfrac{10 \text{ mL}}{4 \text{ g}} = 2.5 \text{ mL}$

31. $1.0 \text{ mg} \times \dfrac{10 \text{ mL}}{2.5 \text{ mg}} = 4 \text{ mL}$

32. $5 \text{ mg} \times \dfrac{2 \text{ mL}}{15 \text{ mg}} = 0.67 \text{ mL}$

Round to the nearest tenth, or 0.7 mL.

33. *Patient 1*

$\dfrac{4 \text{ mg}}{\text{min}} \times 34 \text{ min} = 136 \text{ mg}$

Patient 2

$\dfrac{5 \text{ mg}}{\text{min}} \times 27 \text{ min} = 135 \text{ mg}$

Patient 1 receives more medication.

34. *Patient 1*

First, convert hours to minutes:

$2.6 \text{ h} \times \dfrac{60 \text{ min}}{\text{h}} = 156 \text{ min}$

Set up the problem:

$\dfrac{0.5 \text{ mg}}{\text{min}} \times 156 \text{ min} = 78 \text{ mg}$

Patient 2

$\dfrac{4 \text{ mg}}{\text{min}} \times 20 \text{ min} = 80 \text{ mg}$

Patient 2 receives more medication.

35. *Patient 1*

First, convert hours to minutes:

$3.3 \text{ h} \times \dfrac{60 \text{ min}}{\text{h}} = 198 \text{ min}$

Convert micrograms to milligrams to be able to compare the answer with the answer for Patient 2:

$40 \text{ μg} \times \dfrac{1 \text{ mg}}{1,000 \text{ μg}} = 0.04 \text{ mg}$

Set up the problem:

$\dfrac{0.04 \text{ mg}}{\text{min}} \times 198 \text{ min} = 7.92 \text{ mg}$

Patient 2

$\dfrac{0.2 \text{ mg}}{\text{min}} \times 45 \text{ min} = 9 \text{ mg}$

Patient 2 receives more medication.

36. *Patient 1*

First, convert hours to minutes:

$6.5 \text{ h} \times \dfrac{60 \text{ min}}{\text{h}} = 390 \text{ min}$

Convert micrograms to milligrams to be able to compare the answer with the answer for Patient 2:

$300 \text{ μg} \times \dfrac{1 \text{ mg}}{1,000 \text{ μg}} = 0.3 \text{ mg}$

Then set up the problem.

$\dfrac{0.3 \text{ mg}}{\text{min}} \times 390 \text{ min} = 117 \text{ mg}$

Patient 2

$\dfrac{0.5 \text{ mg}}{\text{min}} \times 187 \text{ min} = 93.5 \text{ mg}$

Patient 1 receives more medication.

37. *Patient 1*

First, convert hours to minutes:

$4.2 \text{ h} \times \dfrac{60 \text{ min}}{\text{h}} = 252 \text{ min}$

Set up the problem:

$\dfrac{7 \text{ mg}}{\text{min}} \times 252 \text{ min} = 1,764 \text{ mg}$

Patient 2

$\dfrac{14 \text{ mg}}{\text{min}} \times 150 \text{ min} = 2,100 \text{ mg}$

Patient 2 receives more medication.

38. First, convert hours to minutes:

$6 \text{ h} \times \dfrac{60 \text{ min}}{\text{h}} = 360 \text{ min}$

Set up the problem:

$\dfrac{300 \text{ mL}}{360 \text{ min}} \times \dfrac{60 \text{ gtt}}{\text{mL}} = 50 \text{ gtt/min}$

39. First, convert hours to minutes:

$5 \text{ h} \times \dfrac{60 \text{ min}}{\text{h}} = 300 \text{ min}$

Set up the problem:

$\dfrac{1,000 \text{ mL}}{300 \text{ min}} \times \dfrac{10 \text{ gtt}}{\text{mL}} = 33.33 \text{ gtt/min}$

Round to the nearest whole number, or 33 gtt/min.

40. First, convert hours to minutes:

$$3\,h \times \frac{60\ min}{h} = 180\ min$$

Then set up the problem.

$$\frac{650\ mL}{180\ min} \times \frac{10\ gtt}{mL} = 36.11\ gtt/min$$

Round to the nearest whole number, or 36 gtt/min.

41. First, convert hours to minutes:

$$18\,h \times \frac{60\ min}{h} = 1{,}080\ min$$

Convert liters to milliliters:

$$2\,L \times \frac{1{,}000\ mL}{L} = 2{,}000\ mL$$

Set up the problem:

$$\frac{2{,}000\ mL}{1{,}080\ min} \times \frac{10\ gtt}{mL} = 18.52\ gtt/min$$

Round to the nearest whole number, or 19 gtt/min.

42. First, convert hours to minutes:

$$2.5\,h \times \frac{60\ min}{h} = 150\ min$$

Convert liters to milliliters:

$$1\,L \times \frac{1{,}000\ mL}{L} = 1{,}000\ mL$$

Set up the problem:

$$\frac{1{,}000\ mL}{150\ min} \times \frac{10\ gtt}{mL} = 66.67\ gtt/min$$

Round to the nearest whole number, or 67 gtt/min.

43. $\dfrac{400\ mL}{90\ min} \times \dfrac{10\ gtt}{mL} = 44.44\ gtt/min$

Round to the nearest whole number, or 44 gtt/min.

44. First, convert hours to minutes:

$$4\,h \times \frac{60\ min}{h} = 240\ min$$

Set up the problem:

$$\frac{1{,}200\ mL}{240\ min} \times \frac{10\ gtt}{mL} = 50\ gtt/min$$

45. First, convert hours to minutes:

$$10\,h \times \frac{60\ min}{h} = 600\ min$$

Set up the problem:

$$\frac{900\ mL}{600\ min} \times \frac{10\ gtt}{mL} = 15\ gtt/min$$

46. $\dfrac{250\ mL}{15\ min} \times \dfrac{10\ gtt}{mL} = 166.67\ gtt/min$

Round to the nearest whole number, or 167 gtt/min.

47. First, convert hours to minutes:

$$3\,h \times \frac{60\ min}{h} = 180\ min$$

Set up the problem:

$$\frac{1{,}000\ mL}{180\ min} \times \frac{10\ gtt}{mL} = 55.56\ gtt/min$$

Round to the nearest whole number, or 56 gtt/min.

48. $\dfrac{250\ mL}{30\ min} \times \dfrac{10\ gtt}{mL} = 83.33\ gtt/min$

Round to the nearest whole number, or 83 gtt/min.

Note that the 500-mL bag does not factor into the calculation. Because the physician ordered 250 mL, the fact that you have a 500-mL bag only tells you that you have enough fluid and will not need a second IV bag. You could drain the fluid you do not use or stop the IV infusion once the correct amount is administered.

49. First, convert grams to milligrams:

$$2\,g \times \frac{1{,}000\ mg}{g} = 2{,}000\ mg$$

Set up the problem:

$$\frac{4\ mg}{min} \times \frac{500\ mL}{2{,}000\ mg} \times \frac{60\ gtt}{mL} = 60\ gtt/min$$

50. $\dfrac{400\ mL}{15\ min} \times \dfrac{10\ gtt}{mL} = 266.67\ gtt/min$

Round to the nearest whole number, or 267 gtt/min.

Note that the 500-mL bag does not factor into your calculation. The fact that you have a 500-mL bag only tells you that you have enough fluid and will not need a second IV bag.

51. $\dfrac{100\ mL}{18\ min} \times \dfrac{10\ gtt}{mL} = 55.56\ gtt/min$

Round to the nearest whole number, or 56 gtt/min.

52. First, convert grams to milligrams:

$$1\,g \times \frac{1{,}000\ mg}{g} = 1{,}000\ mg$$

Set up the problem:

$$\frac{3\ mg}{min} \times \frac{250\ mL}{1{,}000\ mg} \times \frac{60\ gtt}{mL} = 45\ gtt/min$$

53. First, convert grams to milligrams:

$$2\,g \times \frac{1,000\ mg}{g} = 2,000\ mg$$

Calculate the concentration:

$$\frac{2,000\ mg}{500\ mL} \div \frac{500}{500} = \frac{4\ mg}{mL}$$

Set up the clock as shown in Figure AK6-3 ▾ :

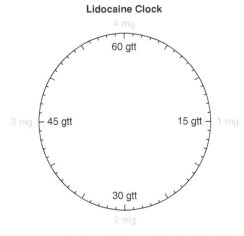

Lidocaine Clock

Figure AK6-3 Lidocaine clock for Practice Problem 53.

According to the clock, you need to administer 30 gtt/min to give 2 mg/min. The answer is 30 gtt/min.

54. First, convert milligrams to micrograms:

$$400\ mg \times \frac{1,000\ \mu g}{mg} = 400,000\ \mu g$$

Calculate the concentration:

$$\frac{400,000\ \mu g}{250\ mL} \div \frac{250}{250} = \frac{1,600\ \mu g}{mL}$$

Set up the clock as shown in Figure AK6-4 ▾ :

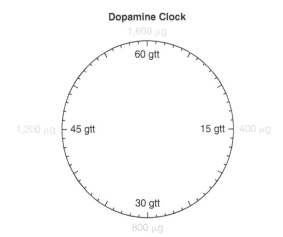

Dopamine Clock

Figure AK6-4 Dopamine clock for Practice Problem 54.

Factor in the patient's weight. First, convert the patient's weight to kilograms:

$$220\ lb \times \frac{kg}{2.2\ lb} = 100\ kg$$

Adjust the DD to accommodate the patient's weight:

$$100\ kg \times \frac{7\ \mu g}{kg/min} = 700\ \mu g/min$$

Because you need to administer 700 µg/min, you can see from the clock that you need to administer between 15 and 30 gtt/min to give the adjusted DD (closer to 30 gtt/min because 700 µg is closer to 800 µg than to 400 µg). Use a proportion to find the exact amount:

$$\frac{30\ gtt}{800\ \mu g} = \frac{gtt}{700\ \mu g}$$

$$\frac{30}{800} \times 700 = 26.25\ gtt$$

Round to 26 gtt/min.

55. First, convert milligrams to micrograms:

$$200\ mg \times \frac{1,000\ \mu g}{mg} = 200,000\ \mu g$$

Calculate the concentration. Because the 10 mL in the vial is less than 10% of 250 mL (which is 25 mL), you do not need to factor the 10 mL into the total volume:

$$\frac{200,000\ \mu g}{250\ mL} \div \frac{250}{250} = \frac{800\ \mu g}{mL}$$

Set up the clock as shown in Figure AK6-5 ▾ :

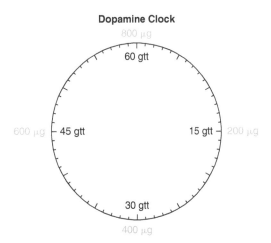

Dopamine Clock

Figure AK6-5 Dopamine clock for Practice Problem 55.

Factor in the patient's weight. The patient's weight is already in kilograms and does not need to be converted.

Adjust the DD to accommodate the patient's weight:

$$80\ \text{kg} \times \frac{5\ \mu\text{g}}{\text{kg/min}} = 400\ \mu\text{g/min}$$

Because you need to administer 400 μg/min, you can see from the clock that you need to administer 30 gtt/min to give the adjusted DD.

Chapter 7
Chapter Problems
Calculating a Weight-Based Dose

1. $185\ \text{lb} \times \dfrac{1\ \text{kg}}{2.2\ \text{lb}} = 84.09\ \text{kg}$

2. $52\ \text{lb} \times \dfrac{1\ \text{kg}}{2.2\ \text{lb}} = 23.64\ \text{kg}$

3. $75\ \text{kg} \times \dfrac{2.2\ \text{lb}}{\text{kg}} = 165\ \text{lb}$

Calculating a Rate for a Weight-Based Medication

1. In this problem, use the method of simplifying the numbers. Start by listing the information:

   DD: 20 μg/kg/min

   DOH: 800 mg in a 500-mL bag of D₅W

   Administration set: 60 gtt/mL

   Patient weight: 201 lb

   Convert pounds to kilograms:

   $201\ \text{lb} \div 2.2\ \text{lb/kg} = 91.36\ \text{kg}$

   Adjust the DD to account for the patient's weight:

   $$\frac{20\ \mu\text{g}}{\text{kg/min}} \times 91.36\ \text{kg} = 1,827.2\ \mu\text{g/min}$$

   Convert and simplify the DOH:

   $$800\ \text{mg} \times \frac{1,000\ \mu\text{g}}{\text{mg}} = 800,000\ \mu\text{g}$$

   $$\frac{800,000\ \mu\text{g}}{500\ \text{mL}} = \frac{?\ \mu\text{g}}{1\ \text{mL}}$$

   $$\frac{800,000\ \mu\text{g}}{500\ \text{mL}} \times 1\ \text{mL} = 1,600\ \mu\text{g in 1 mL of fluid}$$

   Plug into the formula:

   $$\frac{1,827.2\ \mu\text{g/min}}{1,600\ \mu\text{g/mL}} \times \frac{60\ \text{gtt}}{\text{mL}} = ?\ \text{gtt/min}$$

   $$\frac{1,827.2\ \mu\text{g}}{\text{min}} \times \frac{\text{mL}}{1,600\ \mu\text{g}} \times \frac{60\ \text{gtt}}{\text{mL}} = 68.52\ \text{gtt/min}$$

Round to the nearest whole number, or 69 gtt/min.

2. Start by listing the information:

   DD: 12 μg/kg/min

   DOH: 400 mg in a 250-mL bag of D₅W

   Administration set: 60 gtt/mL

   Patient weight: 224 lb

   Convert pounds to kilograms:

   $224\ \text{lb} \div 2.2\ \text{lb/kg} = 101.82\ \text{kg}$

   Adjust the DD to account for the patient's weight:

   $$\frac{12\ \mu\text{g}}{\text{kg/min}} = \frac{?\ \mu\text{g}}{101.82\ \text{kg}}$$

   $$\frac{12\ \mu\text{g}}{\text{kg/min}} \times 101.82\ \text{kg} = 1,221.84\ \mu\text{g/min}$$

   Convert and simplify the DOH:

   $$400\ \text{mg} \times \frac{1,000\ \mu\text{g}}{\text{mg}} = 400,000\ \mu\text{g}$$

   $$\frac{400,000\ \mu\text{g}}{250\ \text{mL}} = \frac{?\ \mu\text{g}}{1\ \text{mL}}$$

   $$\frac{400,000\ \mu\text{g}}{250\ \text{mL}} \times 1\ \text{mL} = 1,600\ \mu\text{g in 1 mL of fluid}$$

   Plug into the formula:

   $$\frac{1,221.84\ \mu\text{g/min}}{1,600\ \mu\text{g/mL}} \times \frac{60\ \text{gtt}}{\text{mL}} = ?\ \text{gtt/min}$$

   $$\frac{1,221.84\ \mu\text{g}}{\text{min}} \times \frac{\text{mL}}{1,600\ \mu\text{g}} \times \frac{60\ \text{gtt}}{\text{mL}} = 45.82\ \text{gtt/min}$$

Round to the nearest whole number, or 46 gtt/min.

3. Although this problem provides a patient scenario rather than just the basic information, do not let it throw you off. It is the same kind of problem as the others. The difference is that it specifically asks for the concentration and the rate, which is not an issue because the concentration is calculated as a standard part of rate calculation.

   Start by listing the information:

   DD: 10 μg/kg/min

   DOH: 800 mg in a 500-mL bag of D₅W

   Administration set: 60 gtt/mL

   Patient weight: 175 lb

   Convert pounds to kilograms:

   $175\ \text{lb} \div 2.2\ \text{lb/kg} = 79.55\ \text{kg}$

   Adjust the DD to account for the patient's weight:

   $$\frac{10\ \mu\text{g}}{\text{kg/min}} = \frac{?\ \mu\text{g}}{79.55\ \text{kg}}$$

$$\frac{10\ \mu g}{kg/min} \times 79.55\ kg\ =\ 795.5\ \mu g/min$$

Simplify the DOH.

$$800\ mg\ \times 1,000\,\frac{\mu g}{mg}\ =\ 800,000\ \mu g$$

$$\frac{800,000\ \mu g}{500\ mL}\ =\ \frac{?\ mg}{1\ mL}$$

$$\frac{800,000\ \mu g}{500\ mL}\ \times 1\ mL\ =\ 1,600\ \mu g\ in\ 1\ mL\ of\ fluid$$

Recall that this problem asked for the concentration. You have just figured it out—1,600 µg/mL.

Plug into the formula:

$$\frac{795.5\ \mu g/min}{1,600\ \mu g/mL}\ \times \frac{60\ gtt}{mL}\ =\ ?\ gtt/min$$

$$\frac{795.5\ \mu g}{min}\ \times \frac{mL}{1,600\ \mu g}\ \times \frac{60\ gtt}{mL}\ =\ 29.83\ gtt/min$$

Round to the nearest whole number, or 30 gtt/min.

Calculating a Pediatric Weight-Based Dose

1. 50 lb ÷ 2.2 lb/kg = 22.72 kg

2. 15 kg × 2.2 lb/kg = 33 lb

3. First, convert 20 pounds to kilograms:

   20 lb ÷ 2.2 lb/kg = 9.09 kg

   Multiply the weight by the dose:

   9.09 kg × 10 mg/kg = 90.9 mg

   Round to 91 mg.

Calculating a Rate for a Pediatric Weight-Based Medication

1. DD: 6 µg/kg/min

   DOH: 200 mg in a 250-mL bag of D_5W

   Administration set: 60 gtt/mL

   Patient weight: 165 lb

   Convert pounds to kilograms:

   $$\frac{165\ lb}{2.2}\ =\ 75\ kg$$

   Adjust the DD to account for the patient's weight:

   $$\frac{6\ \mu g}{kg/min}\ \times 75\ kg\ =\ 450\ \mu g/min$$

Convert and simplify the DOH:

$$200\ mg\ \times \frac{1,000\ \mu g}{mg}\ =\ 200,000\ \mu g$$

$$\frac{200,000\ \mu g}{250\ mL}\ =\ \frac{?\ \mu g}{1\ mL}$$

$$\frac{200,000\ \mu g}{250\ mL}\ \times 1\ mL\ =\ 800\ \mu g\ in\ 1\ mL\ of\ fluid$$

Plug into the formula:

$$\frac{450\ \mu g/min}{800\ \mu g/mL}\ \times \frac{60\ gtt}{mL}\ =\ ?\ gtt/min$$

$$\frac{450\ \mu g}{min}\ \times \frac{mL}{800\ \mu g}\ \times \frac{60\ gtt}{mL}\ =\ 33.75\ gtt/min$$

Round to the nearest whole number, or 34 gtt/min.

2. DD: 5 mg/kg during 40 minutes

   DOH: 500 mg in a 250-mL bag of D_5W

   Administration set: 10 gtt/mL

   Patient weight: 170 lb

   Convert pounds to kilograms:

   $$\frac{170\ lb}{2.2}\ =\ 77.27\ kg$$

   This DD will be easier to work with if the denominator is changed to 1. Do this by dividing the 40 minutes into the 5 mg to find mg/kg/1 min:

   $$\frac{5\ mg}{kg}\ \times \frac{1}{40\ min}\ =\ 0.125\ mg/kg/min$$

   Adjust the DD to account for the patient's weight:

   $$\frac{0.125\ mg}{kg/min}\ \times 77.27\ kg\ =\ 9.66\ mg/min$$

   The DOH does not need to be converted because it and the DD are already in milligrams.

   Simplify the DOH:

   $$\frac{500\ mg}{250\ mL}\ =\ \frac{?\ mg}{1\ mL}$$

   $$\frac{500\ mg}{250\ mL}\ \times 1\ mL\ =\ 2\ mg\ in\ 1\ mL\ of\ fluid$$

   Plug into the formula:

   $$\frac{9.66\ mg/min}{2\ mg/mL}\ \times \frac{10\ gtt}{mL}\ =\ ?\ gtt/min$$

   $$\frac{9.66\ mg}{min}\ \times \frac{mL}{2\ mg}\ \times \frac{10\ gtt}{mL}\ =\ 48.3\ gtt/min$$

   Round to the nearest whole number, or 48 gtt/min.

Rate-Dependent vs Weight-Based Calculations

1. The DD is 1,000 mL/6 h. This is a rate-dependent problem.

   Convert hours to minutes:

   $$6\,h \times \frac{60\ min}{h} = 360\ min$$

   Simplify the DD. First cross out the zeros, then reduce further:

   $$\frac{1,00\cancel{0}\ mL}{36\cancel{0}\ min}$$

   $$\frac{100\ mL}{36\ min} \div \frac{4}{4} = \frac{25}{9}$$

   Set up the equation and solve:

   $$\frac{25\ mL}{9\ min} \times \frac{10\ gtt}{mL} = ?\ gtt/min$$

   $$\frac{25 \times 10\ gtt}{9\ min} = 27.77\ gtt/min$$

   Round to 28 gtt/min.

2. The DD is 5 μg/kg/min. This is a weight-based problem.

   DD: 5 μg/kg/min

   DOH: 400 mg in a 250-mL bag of D_5W

   Administration set: 60 gtt/mL

   Patient weight: 150 lb

   Convert pounds to kilograms:

   $$\frac{150\ lb}{2.2} = 68.18\ kg$$

   Adjust the DD to account for the patient's weight:

   $$\frac{5\ \mu g}{kg/min} \times 68.18\ kg = 340.9\ \mu g/min$$

   Convert and simplify the DOH:

   $$400\ mg \times \frac{1,000\ \mu g}{mg} = 400,000\ \mu g$$

   $$\frac{400,000\ \mu g}{250\ mL} = \frac{?\ \mu g}{1\ mL}$$

   $$\frac{400,000\ \mu g}{250\ mL} \times 1\ mL = 1,600\ \mu g\ in\ 1\ mL\ of\ fluid$$

   Plug into the formula:

   $$\frac{340.9\ \mu g/min}{1,600\ \mu g/mL} \times \frac{60\ gtt}{mL} = ?\ gtt/min$$

   $$\frac{340.9\ \mu g}{min} \times \frac{mL}{1,600\ \mu g} \times \frac{60\ gtt}{mL} = 12.78\ gtt/min$$

Round to the nearest whole number, or 13 gtt/min.

3. The DD is 0.25 mg/kg. This is a weight-based problem.

   Convert pounds to kilograms:

   $$\frac{154\ lb}{2.2} = 70\ kg$$

   Set up the equation and solve:

   $$\frac{0.25\ mg}{kg} \times 70\ kg = 17.5\ mg$$

4. The DD is 500 mL/75 min. This is a rate-dependent problem.

   $$\frac{500\ mL}{75\ min} \times \frac{10\ gtt}{mL} = 66.67\ gtt/min$$

   Round to the nearest whole number, or 67 gtt/min.

Practice Problems

1. Convert pounds to kilograms:

   $$\frac{150\ lb}{2.2} = 68.18\ kg$$

   Calculate the dose to account for the weight:

   $$\frac{1.5\ mg}{kg} \times 68.18\ kg = 102.27\ mg$$

   Set up a proportion:

   $$\frac{10\ mL}{100\ mg} = \frac{?\ mL}{102.27\ mg}$$

   $$\frac{10\ mL \times 102.27\ mg}{100\ mg} = 10.23\ mL$$

   For this medication, you may round this down to 10 mL, and administer the entire prefilled syringe.

2. Convert pounds to kilograms:

   $$\frac{122\ lb}{2.2} = 55.45\ kg$$

   Calculate the dose to account for the weight:

   $$\frac{0.3\ mg}{kg} \times 55.45\ kg = 16.64\ mg$$

   Set up a proportion:

   $$\frac{5\ mL}{50\ mg} = \frac{?\ mL}{16.64\ mg}$$

   $$\frac{5\ mL \times 16.64\ mg}{50\ mg} = 1.66\ mL$$

3. Convert pounds to kilograms:

$$\frac{128 \text{ lb}}{2.2} = 58.18 \text{ kg}$$

Note that mEq stands for milliequivalents, another unit of measure. It does not need to be converted to another unit of measure because the DD and DOH are in milliequivalents.

Calculate the dose to account for the weight:

$$\frac{1.0 \text{ mEq}}{\text{kg}} \times 58.18 \text{ kg} = 58.18 \text{ mEq}$$

Set up a proportion:

$$\frac{50 \text{ mL}}{60 \text{ mEq}} = \frac{? \text{ mL}}{58.18 \text{ mEq}}$$

$$\frac{50 \text{ mL} \times 58.18 \text{ mEq}}{60 \text{ mEq}} = 48.48 \text{ mL}$$

4. Convert pounds to kilograms:

$$\frac{130 \text{ lb}}{2.2} = 59.09 \text{ kg}$$

Calculate the dose to account for the weight:

$$\frac{15 \text{ mg}}{\text{kg}} \times 59.09 \text{ kg} = 886.35 \text{ mg}$$

Set up a proportion:

$$\frac{20 \text{ mL}}{1 \text{ g}} = \frac{? \text{ mL}}{886.35 \text{ mg}}$$

Convert grams to milligrams and solve:

$$\frac{20 \text{ mL} \times 886.35 \text{ mg}}{1,000 \text{ mg}} = 17.73 \text{ mL}$$

5. Convert pounds to kilograms:

$$\frac{185 \text{ lb}}{2.2} = 84.09 \text{ kg}$$

Calculate the dose to account for the weight:

$$\frac{0.25 \text{ mg}}{\text{kg}} \times 84.09 \text{ kg} = 21.02 \text{ mg}$$

Set up a proportion:

$$\frac{10 \text{ mL}}{25 \text{ mg}} = \frac{? \text{ mL}}{21.02 \text{ mg}}$$

$$\frac{10 \text{ mL} \times 21.02 \text{ mg}}{25 \text{ mg}} = 8.41 \text{ mL}$$

6. Convert pounds to kilograms:

$$\frac{142 \text{ lb}}{2.2} = 64.55 \text{ kg}$$

Calculate the dose to account for the weight:

$$\frac{2 \text{ mg}}{\text{kg}} \times 64.55 \text{ kg} = 129.1 \text{ mg}$$

Set up a proportion:

$$\frac{10 \text{ mL}}{150 \text{ mg}} = \frac{? \text{ mL}}{129.1 \text{ mg}}$$

$$\frac{10 \text{ mL} \times 129.1 \text{ mg}}{150 \text{ mg}} = 8.61 \text{ mL}$$

7. Convert pounds to kilograms:

$$\frac{174 \text{ lb}}{2.2} = 79.09 \text{ kg}$$

Calculate the dose to account for the weight:

$$\frac{0.1 \text{ mg}}{\text{kg}} \times 79.09 \text{ kg} = 7.91 \text{ mg}$$

Set up a proportion:

$$\frac{10 \text{ mL}}{10 \text{ mg}} = \frac{? \text{ mL}}{7.91 \text{ mg}}$$

$$\frac{10 \text{ mL} \times 7.91 \text{ mg}}{10 \text{ mg}} = 7.91 \text{ mL}$$

8. Convert pounds to kilograms:

$$\frac{170 \text{ lb}}{2.2} = 77.27 \text{ kg}$$

Calculate the dose to account for the weight:

$$\frac{1.0 \text{ mg}}{\text{kg}} \times 77.27 \text{ kg} = 77.27 \text{ mg}$$

Set up a proportion:

$$\frac{10 \text{ mL}}{100 \text{ mg}} = \frac{? \text{ mL}}{77.27 \text{ mg}}$$

$$\frac{10 \text{ mL} \times 77.27 \text{ mg}}{100 \text{ mg}} = 7.73 \text{ mL}$$

9. Convert pounds to kilograms:

$$\frac{114 \text{ lb}}{2.2} = 51.82 \text{ kg}$$

Calculate the dose to account for the weight:

$$\frac{0.8 \text{ mg}}{\text{kg}} \times 51.82 \text{ kg} = 41.46 \text{ mg}$$

Set up a proportion:

$$\frac{2 \text{ mL}}{100 \text{ mg}} = \frac{? \text{ mL}}{41.46 \text{ mg}}$$

$$\frac{2 \text{ mL} \times 41.46 \text{ mg}}{100 \text{ mg}} = 0.83 \text{ mL}$$

10. Convert pounds to kilograms:

$$\frac{157 \text{ lb}}{2.2} = 71.36 \text{ kg}$$

Calculate the dose to account for the weight:

$$\frac{0.3 \text{ mg}}{\text{kg}} \times 71.36 \text{ kg} = 21.41 \text{ mg}$$

Set up a proportion:

$$\frac{5 \text{ mL}}{50 \text{ mg}} = \frac{? \text{ mL}}{21.41 \text{ mg}}$$

$$\frac{5 \text{ mL} \times 21.41 \text{ mg}}{50 \text{ mg}} = 2.14 \text{ mL}$$

11. Convert pounds to kilograms:

$$\frac{208 \text{ lb}}{2.2} = 94.55 \text{ kg}$$

Calculate the number of milligrams to administer to patient:

$$\frac{1 \text{ mg}}{\text{kg}} \times 94.55 \text{ kg} = 94.55 \text{ mg}$$

Because the prefilled syringe contains 100 mg, set up a proportion to figure out how many milliliters to administer:

$$\frac{10 \text{ mL}}{100 \text{ mg}} = \frac{? \text{ mL}}{94.55 \text{ mg}}$$

$$\frac{10 \text{ mL} \times 94.55 \text{ mg}}{100 \text{ mg}} = 9.46 \text{ mL}$$

12. Convert pounds to kilograms:

$$\frac{133 \text{ lb}}{2.2} = 60.45 \text{ kg}$$

Calculate the number of milligrams to administer:

$$\frac{0.25 \text{ mg}}{\text{kg}} \times 60.45 \text{ kg} = 15.11 \text{ mg}$$

Because the vial contains 20 mg, set up a proportion to figure out how many milliliters to administer:

$$\frac{10 \text{ mL}}{20 \text{ mg}} = \frac{? \text{ mL}}{15.11 \text{ mg}}$$

$$\frac{10 \text{ mL} \times 15.11 \text{ mg}}{20 \text{ mg}} = 7.56 \text{ mL}$$

13. Convert pounds to kilograms:

$$\frac{290 \text{ lb}}{2.2} = 131.82 \text{ kg}$$

Calculate the number of milligrams to be administered:

$$\frac{0.3 \text{ mg}}{\text{kg}} \times 131.82 \text{ kg} = 39.55 \text{ mg}$$

Set up a proportion:

$$\frac{5 \text{ mL}}{50 \text{ mg}} = \frac{? \text{ mL}}{39.55 \text{ mg}}$$

$$\frac{5 \text{ mL} \times 39.55 \text{ mg}}{50 \text{ mg}} = 3.96 \text{ mL}$$

14. Convert pounds to kilograms:

$$\frac{175 \text{ lb}}{2.2} = 79.55 \text{ kg}$$

Calculate the number of milligrams to be administered:

$$\frac{1 \text{ mg}}{\text{kg}} \times 79.55 \text{ kg} = 79.55 \text{ mg}$$

Set up a proportion:

$$\frac{10 \text{ mL}}{100 \text{ mg}} = \frac{? \text{ mL}}{79.55 \text{ mg}}$$

$$\frac{10 \text{ mL} \times 79.55 \text{ mg}}{100 \text{ mg}} = 7.96 \text{ mL}$$

15. Convert pounds to kilograms:

$$\frac{138 \text{ lb}}{2.2} = 62.73 \text{ kg}$$

Calculate the number of milligrams to be administered:

$$\frac{15 \text{ mg}}{\text{kg}} \times 62.73 \text{ kg} = 940.95 \text{ mg}$$

Set up a proportion:

$$\frac{20 \text{ mL}}{1 \text{ g}} = \frac{? \text{ mL}}{940.95 \text{ mg}}$$

Convert grams to milligrams:

$$\frac{20 \text{ mL}}{1,000 \text{ mg}} = \frac{? \text{ mL}}{940.95 \text{ mg}}$$

$$\frac{20 \text{ mL} \times 940.95 \text{ mg}}{1,000 \text{ mg}} = 18.82 \text{ mL}$$

16. Convert pounds to kilograms:

$$\frac{200 \text{ lb}}{2.2} = 90.91 \text{ kg}$$

Calculate the number of milligrams to be administered:

$$\frac{1 \text{ mEq}}{\text{kg}} \times 90.91 \text{ kg} = 90.91 \text{ mEq}$$

Set up a proportion:

$$\frac{50 \text{ mL}}{50 \text{ mEq}} = \frac{? \text{ mL}}{90.91 \text{ mEq}}$$

$$\frac{50 \text{ mL} \times 90.91 \text{ mEq}}{50 \text{ mEq}} = 90.91 \text{ mL}$$

Because the required amount is more than the 50 mEq you have on hand, you will need to administer an entire ampule and an additional 40.91 mL from a second ampule (90.91 mL – 50 mL = 40.91 mL).

17. Convert pounds to kilograms:

$$\frac{184 \text{ lb}}{2.2} = 83.46 \text{ kg}$$

Calculate the number of milligrams to be administered:

$$\frac{0.8 \text{ mg}}{\text{kg}} \times 83.64 \text{ kg} = 66.91 \text{ mg}$$

Set up a proportion:

$$\frac{2 \text{ mL}}{100 \text{ mg}} = \frac{? \text{ mL}}{66.91 \text{ mg}}$$

$$\frac{2 \text{ mL} \times 66.91 \text{ mg}}{100 \text{ mg}} = 1.34 \text{ mL}$$

18. Convert pounds to kilograms:

$$\frac{118 \text{ lb}}{2.2} = 53.64 \text{ kg}$$

Calculate the dose to account for the weight:

$$\frac{1.5 \text{ mg}}{\text{kg}} \times 53.64 \text{ kg} = 80.46 \text{ mg}$$

Set up a proportion:

$$\frac{10 \text{ mL}}{100 \text{ mg}} = \frac{? \text{ mL}}{80.46 \text{ mg}}$$

$$\frac{10 \text{ mL} \times 80.46 \text{ mg}}{100 \text{ mg}} = 8.05 \text{ mL}$$

19. Convert pounds to kilograms:

$$\frac{163 \text{ lb}}{2.2} = 74.09 \text{ kg}$$

Calculate the dose to account for the weight:

$$\frac{0.25 \text{ mg}}{\text{kg}} \times 74.09 \text{ kg} = 18.52 \text{ mg}$$

Set up a proportion:

$$\frac{10 \text{ mL}}{20 \text{ mg}} = \frac{? \text{ mL}}{18.52 \text{ mg}}$$

$$\frac{10 \text{ mL} \times 18.52 \text{ mg}}{20 \text{ mg}} = 9.26 \text{ mL}$$

20. Convert pounds to kilograms:

$$\frac{105 \text{ lb}}{2.2} = 47.73 \text{ kg}$$

Calculate the dose to account for the weight:

$$\frac{15 \text{ mg}}{\text{kg}} \times 47.73 \text{ kg} = 715.95 \text{ mg}$$

Set up a proportion:

$$\frac{20 \text{ mL}}{1 \text{ g}} = \frac{? \text{ mL}}{715.95 \text{ mg}}$$

Convert grams to milligrams and solve:

$$\frac{20 \text{ mL}}{1,000 \text{ mg}} = \frac{? \text{ mL}}{715.95 \text{ mg}}$$

$$\frac{20 \text{ mL} \times 715.95 \text{ mg}}{1,000 \text{ mg}} = 14.32 \text{ mL}$$

21. Convert pounds to kilograms:

$$\frac{200 \text{ lb}}{2.2} = 90.91 \text{ kg}$$

Calculate the dose to account for the weight:

$$\frac{0.3 \text{ mg}}{\text{kg}} \times 90.91 \text{ kg} = 27.27 \text{ mg}$$

Set up a proportion:

$$\frac{5 \text{ mL}}{50 \text{ mg}} = \frac{? \text{ mL}}{27.27 \text{ mg}}$$

$$\frac{5 \text{ mL} \times 27.27 \text{ mg}}{50 \text{ mg}} = 2.73 \text{ mL}$$

22. Convert pounds to kilograms:

$$\frac{144 \text{ lb}}{2.2} = 65.45 \text{ kg}$$

Calculate the dose to account for the weight:

$$\frac{0.8 \text{ mg}}{\text{kg}} \times 65.45 \text{ kg} = 52.36 \text{ mg}$$

Set up a proportion:

$$\frac{2 \text{ mL}}{100 \text{ mg}} = \frac{? \text{ mL}}{52.36 \text{ mg}}$$

$$\frac{2 \text{ mL} \times 52.36 \text{ mg}}{100 \text{ mg}} = 1.05 \text{ mL}$$

23. Convert pounds to kilograms:

$$\frac{100 \text{ lb}}{2.2} = 45.45 \text{ kg}$$

Calculate the dose to account for the weight:

$$\frac{1.0 \text{ mg}}{\text{kg}} \times 45.45 \text{ kg} = 45.45 \text{ mg}$$

Set up a proportion:

$$\frac{10\ \text{mL}}{100\ \text{mg}} = \frac{?\ \text{mL}}{45.45\ \text{mg}}$$

$$\frac{10\ \text{mL} \times 45.45\ \text{mg}}{100\ \text{mg}} = 4.55\ \text{mL}$$

24. Convert pounds to kilograms:

$$\frac{190\ \text{lb}}{2.2} = 86.36\ \text{kg}$$

Calculate the dose to account for the weight:

$$\frac{15\ \text{mg}}{\text{kg}} \times 86.36\ \text{kg} = 1{,}295.4\ \text{mg}$$

Set up a proportion:

$$\frac{20\ \text{mL}}{1\ \text{g}} = \frac{?\ \text{mL}}{1{,}295.4\ \text{mg}}$$

Convert grams to milligrams and solve:

$$\frac{20\ \text{mL} \times 1{,}295.4\ \text{mg}}{1{,}000\ \text{mg}} = 25.91\ \text{mL}$$

Because the vial contains 20 mL and the calculation indicates to administer 25.91 mL, you will need to administer the entire vial and then administer 5.91 mL from a second vial (25.91 mL – 20.0 mL = 5.91 mL).

25. Convert pounds to kilograms:

$$\frac{115\ \text{lb}}{2.2} = 52.27\ \text{kg}$$

Calculate the dose to account for the weight:

$$\frac{1\ \text{mEq}}{\text{kg}} \times 52.27\ \text{kg} = 52.27\ \text{mEq}$$

Set up a proportion:

$$\frac{50\ \text{mL}}{50\ \text{mEq}} = \frac{?\ \text{mL}}{52.27\ \text{mEq}}$$

$$\frac{50\ \text{mL} \times 52.27\ \text{mEq}}{50\ \text{mEq}} = 52.27\ \text{mL}$$

Because the vial contains 50 mL, you will need to administer the entire vial and then administer 2.27 mL from a second vial (52.27 mL – 50 mL = 2.27 mL).

26. Convert pounds to kilograms:

$$\frac{289\ \text{lb}}{2.2} = 131.36\ \text{kg}$$

Calculate the dose to account for the weight:

$$\frac{1.5\ \text{mg}}{\text{kg}} \times 131.36\ \text{kg} = 197.04\ \text{mg}$$

Set up a proportion:

$$\frac{10\ \text{mL}}{100\ \text{mg}} = \frac{?\ \text{mL}}{197.04\ \text{mg}}$$

$$\frac{10\ \text{mL} \times 197.04\ \text{mg}}{100\ \text{mg}} = 19.70\ \text{mL}$$

Because the vial contains 10 mL, you will need to administer the entire vial and then administer 9.7 mL from a second vial (19.70 mL – 10 mL = 9.7 mL).

27. Convert pounds to kilograms:

$$\frac{200\ \text{lb}}{2.2} = 90.91\ \text{kg}$$

Adjust the DD to account for the patient's weight:

$$\frac{1.5\ \text{mg}}{\text{kg}} \times 90.91\ \text{kg} = 136.37\ \text{mg}$$

Simplify the DOH.

$$\frac{150\ \text{mg}}{10\ \text{mL}} = \frac{?\ \text{mL}}{1\ \text{mL}}$$

$$\frac{150\ \text{mg}}{10\ \text{mL}} \times 1\ \text{mL} = 15\ \text{mg in 1 mL of fluid}$$

Set up a proportion (solve using dimensional analysis):

$$136.37\ \text{mg} \times \frac{\text{mL}}{15\ \text{mg}} = 9.09\ \text{mL}$$

Round to 9.1 mL.

28. DD: 20 µg/kg/min

DOH: 800 mg in a 500-mL bag of D_5W

Administration set: 60 gtt/mL

Patient weight: 289 lb

Convert pounds to kilograms:

$$\frac{289\ \text{lb}}{2.2} = 131.36\ \text{kg}$$

Adjust the DD to account for the patient's weight:

$$\frac{20\ \mu\text{g}}{\text{kg/min}} \times 131.36\ \text{kg} = 2{,}627.2\ \mu\text{g/min}$$

Convert and simplify the DOH:

$$800\ \text{mg} \times \frac{1{,}000\ \mu\text{g}}{\text{mg}} = 800{,}000\ \mu\text{g}$$

$$\frac{800{,}000\ \mu\text{g}}{500\ \text{mL}} = \frac{?\ \mu\text{g}}{1\ \text{mL}}$$

$$\frac{800{,}000\ \mu\text{g}}{500\ \text{mL}} \times 1\ \text{mL} = 1{,}600\ \mu\text{g in 1 mL of fluid}$$

Plug into the formula:

$$\frac{\cancel{2,627.2 \ \mu g/min}}{\cancel{1,600 \ \mu g/mL}} \times \frac{60 \ gtt}{mL} = ? \ gtt/min$$

$$\frac{2,627.2 \ \mu g}{min} \times \frac{mL}{1,600 \ \mu g} \times \frac{60 \ gtt}{mL} = 98.52 \ gtt/min$$

Round to the nearest whole number, or 99 gtt/min.

29. DD: 20 μg/kg/min

DOH: 800 mg in a 500-mL bag of D_5W

Administration set: 60 gtt/mL

Patient weight: 169 lb

Convert pounds to kilograms:

$$\frac{169 \ lb}{2.2} = 76.82 \ kg$$

Adjust the DD to account for the patient's weight:

$$\frac{20 \ \mu g}{kg \ /min} \times 76.82 \ \cancel{kg} = 1,536.4 \ \mu g/min$$

Convert and simplify the DOH:

$$800 \ mg \times \frac{1,000 \ \mu g}{mg} = 800,000 \ \mu g$$

$$\frac{800,000 \ \mu g}{500 \ mL} = \frac{? \ \mu g}{1 \ mL}$$

$$\frac{800,000 \ \mu g}{500 \ mL} \times 1 \ mL = 1,600 \ \mu g \ in \ 1 \ mL \ of \ fluid$$

Plug into the formula:

$$\frac{\cancel{1,536.4 \ \mu g/min}}{\cancel{1,600 \ \mu g/mL}} \times \frac{60 \ gtt}{mL} = ? \ gtt/min$$

$$\frac{1,536.4 \ \mu g}{min} \times \frac{mL}{1,600 \ \mu g} \times \frac{60 \ gtt}{mL} = 57.62 \ gtt/min$$

Round to the nearest whole number, or 58 gtt/min.

30. DD: 18 μg/kg/min

DOH: 400 mg in a 250-mL bag of D_5W

Administration set: 60 gtt/mL

Patient weight: 198 lb

Convert pounds to kilograms:

$$\frac{198 \ lb}{2.2} = 90 \ kg$$

Adjust the DD to account for the patient's weight:

$$\frac{18 \ \mu g}{kg \ /min} \times 90 \ \cancel{kg} = 1,620 \ \mu g/min$$

Convert and simplify the DOH:

$$400 \ mg \times \frac{1,000 \ \mu g}{mg} = 400,000 \ \mu g$$

$$\frac{400,000 \ \mu g}{250 \ mL} = \frac{? \ \mu g}{1 \ mL}$$

$$\frac{400,000 \ \mu g}{250 \ mL} \times 1 \ mL = 1,600 \ \mu g \ in \ 1 \ mL \ of \ fluid$$

Plug into the formula:

$$\frac{\cancel{1,620 \ \mu g/min}}{\cancel{1,600 \ \mu g/mL}} \times \frac{60 \ gtt}{mL} = ? \ gtt/min$$

$$\frac{1,620 \ \mu g}{min} \times \frac{mL}{1,600 \ \mu g} \times \frac{60 \ gtt}{mL} = 60.75 \ gtt/min$$

Round to the nearest whole number, or 61 gtt/min.

31. DD: 10 μg/kg/min

DOH: 12.5 mg/mL in a 32-mL prefilled syringe, added to a 250-mL bag of D_5W

Administration set: 60 gtt/mL

Patient weight: 135 lb

At the outset, notice that the prefilled syringe contains 32 mL and the bag contains 250 mL. Remember the rule that the volume in the vial does not need to be factored into the calculation unless it is more than 10% of the bag's volume. In this case, the 32 mL is approximately 13% of the bag's volume:

$$\frac{32 \ mL}{250 \ mL} = 0.128, \ or \ 12.8\%$$

Therefore, be sure to factor the 32 mL into the total volume in your calculations.

Convert pounds to kilograms:

$$\frac{135 \ lb}{2.2} = 61.36 \ kg$$

Adjust the DD to account for the patient's weight:

$$\frac{10 \ \mu g}{kg \ /min} \times 61.36 \ \cancel{kg} = 613.6 \ \mu g/min$$

The DOH is a bit different from the DOH in some of the other problems. First, use dimensional analysis to calculate the total number of milligrams present in the prefilled syringe:

$$\frac{12.5 \ mg}{mL} \times 32 \ \cancel{mL} = 400 \ mg$$

Because you have already added this to the 250-mL bag of D_5W, you have (remember to factor in the 32 mL since this is more than 10% of the bag's volume):

$$\frac{400 \ mg}{250 \ mL \ + \ 32 \ mL}$$

or

$$\frac{400 \text{ mg}}{282 \text{ mL}}$$

Convert milligrams to micrograms and simplify:

$$400 \text{ mg} \times \frac{1{,}000 \text{ µg}}{\text{mg}} = 400{,}000 \text{ µg}$$

$$\frac{400{,}000 \text{ µg}}{282 \text{ mL}} = \frac{? \text{ µg}}{1 \text{ mL}}$$

$$\frac{400{,}000 \text{ µg}}{282 \text{ mL}} \times 1 \text{ mL} = 1{,}418 \text{ µg in 1 mL of fluid}$$

Plug into the formula:

$$\frac{613.6 \text{ µg/min}}{1{,}418 \text{ µg/mL}} \times \frac{60 \text{ gtt}}{\text{mL}} = ? \text{ gtt/min}$$

$$\frac{613.6 \text{ µg}}{\text{min}} \times \frac{\text{mL}}{1{,}418 \text{ µg}} \times \frac{60 \text{ gtt}}{\text{mL}} = 25.96 \text{ gtt/min}$$

Round to the nearest whole number, or 26 gtt/min.

32. DD: 5 µg/kg/min

DOH: 400 mg in a 250-mL bag of D_5W

Administration set: 60 gtt/mL

Patient weight: 80 kg

The patient's weight is already given in kilograms. No conversion is necessary. Adjust the DD to account for the patient's weight:

$$\frac{5 \text{ µg}}{\text{kg/min}} \times 80 \text{ kg} = 400 \text{ µg/min}$$

Convert and simplify the DOH:

$$400 \text{ mg} \times \frac{1{,}000 \text{ µg}}{\text{mg}} = 400{,}000 \text{ µg}$$

$$\frac{400{,}000 \text{ µg}}{250 \text{ mL}} = \frac{? \text{ µg}}{1 \text{ mL}}$$

$$\frac{400{,}000 \text{ µg}}{250 \text{ mL}} \times 1 \text{ mL} = 1{,}600 \text{ µg in 1 mL of fluid}$$

Plug into the formula:

$$\frac{400 \text{ µg/min}}{1{,}600 \text{ µg/mL}} \times \frac{60 \text{ gtt}}{\text{mL}} = ? \text{ gtt/min}$$

$$\frac{400 \text{ µg}}{\text{min}} \times \frac{\text{mL}}{1{,}600 \text{ µg}} \times \frac{60 \text{ gtt}}{\text{mL}} = 15 \text{ gtt/min}$$

33. DD: 15 µg/kg/min

DOH: 800 mg in a 500-mL bag of D_5W

Administration set: 60 gtt/mL

Patient weight: 150 kg

The patient's weight is already in kilograms. Adjust the DD to account for the patient's weight:

$$\frac{15 \text{ µg}}{\text{kg/min}} \times 150 \text{ kg} = 2{,}250 \text{ µg/min}$$

Convert and simplify the DOH:

$$800 \text{ mg} \times \frac{1{,}000 \text{ µg}}{\text{mg}} = 800{,}000 \text{ µg}$$

$$\frac{800{,}000 \text{ µg}}{500 \text{ mL}} = \frac{? \text{ µg}}{1 \text{ mL}}$$

$$\frac{800{,}000 \text{ µg}}{500 \text{ mL}} \times 1 \text{ mL} = 1{,}600 \text{ µg in 1 mL of fluid}$$

Plug into the formula:

$$\frac{2{,}250 \text{ µg/min}}{1{,}600 \text{ µg/mL}} \times \frac{60 \text{ gtt}}{\text{mL}} = ? \text{ gtt/min}$$

$$\frac{2{,}250 \text{ µg}}{\text{min}} \times \frac{\text{mL}}{1{,}600 \text{ µg}} \times \frac{60 \text{ gtt}}{\text{mL}} = 84.38 \text{ gtt/min}$$

Round to the nearest whole number, or 84 gtt/min.

34. DD: 1 mg/min

DOH: 1 g in a 250-mL bag of D_5W

Administration set: 60 gtt/mL

Patient weight: 120 lb

Note that although the patient's weight is given, because the DD does not include weight, the patient's weight is not factored into the calculation. This is a rate-based problem.

Convert and simplify the DOH:

$$1 \text{ g} = 1{,}000 \text{ mg}$$

$$\frac{1{,}000 \text{ mg}}{250 \text{ mL}} = \frac{? \text{ mg}}{1 \text{ mL}}$$

$$\frac{1{,}000 \text{ mg}}{250 \text{ mL}} \times 1 \text{ mL} = 4 \text{ mg in 1 mL of fluid}$$

Plug into the formula:

$$\frac{1 \text{ mg/min}}{4 \text{ mg/mL}} \times \frac{60 \text{ gtt}}{\text{mL}} = ? \text{ gtt/min}$$

$$\frac{1 \text{ mg}}{\text{min}} \times \frac{\text{mL}}{4 \text{ mg}} \times \frac{60 \text{ gtt}}{\text{mL}} = 15 \text{ gtt/min}$$

35. DD: 2 µg/kg/min

DOH: 400 mg in a 250-mL bag of D_5W

Administration set: 60 gtt/mL

Patient weight: 79 kg

The patient's weight is already in kilograms, so there is no need to convert it. Adjust the DD to account for the patient's weight:

$$\frac{2\ \mu g}{kg/min} \times 79\ kg\ =\ 158\ \mu g/min$$

Convert and simplify the DOH:

$$400\ mg\ \times\ \frac{1{,}000\ \mu g}{mg}\ =\ 400{,}000\ \mu g$$

$$\frac{400{,}000\ \mu g}{250\ mL}\ =\ \frac{?\ \mu g}{1\ mL}$$

$$\frac{400{,}000\ \mu g}{250\ mL}\ \times\ 1\ mL\ =\ 1{,}600\ \mu g\ in\ 1\ mL\ of\ fluid$$

Plug into the formula:

$$\frac{158\ \mu g/min}{1{,}600\ \mu g/mL}\ \times\ \frac{60\ gtt}{mL}\ =\ ?\ gtt/min$$

$$\frac{158\ \mu g}{min}\ \times\ \frac{mL}{1{,}600\ \mu g}\ \times\ \frac{60\ gtt}{mL}\ =\ 5.93\ gtt/min$$

Round to the nearest whole number, or 6 gtt/min.

36. DD: 14 µg/kg/min

DOH: 800 mg in a 500-mL bag of D_5W

Administration set: 60 gtt/mL

Patient weight: 129 kg

The weight is already in kilograms. Adjust the DD to account for the patient's weight:

$$\frac{14\ \mu g}{kg/min}\ \times\ 129\ kg\ =\ 1{,}806\ \mu g/min$$

Convert and simplify the DOH:

$$800\ mg\ \times\ \frac{1{,}000\ \mu g}{mg}\ =\ 800{,}000\ \mu g$$

$$\frac{800{,}000\ \mu g}{500\ mL}\ =\ \frac{?\ \mu g}{1\ mL}$$

$$\frac{800{,}000\ \mu g}{500\ mL}\ \times\ 1\ mL\ =\ 1{,}600\ \mu g\ in\ 1\ mL\ of\ fluid$$

Plug into the formula:

$$\frac{1{,}806\ \mu g/min}{1{,}600\ \mu g/mL}\ \times\ \frac{60\ gtt}{mL}\ =\ ?\ gtt/min$$

$$\frac{1{,}806\ \mu g}{min}\ \times\ \frac{mL}{1{,}600\ \mu g}\ \times\ \frac{60\ gtt}{mL}\ =\ 67.73\ gtt/min$$

Round to the nearest whole number, or 68 gtt/min.

37. DD: 10 µg/kg/min

DOH: 400 mg in a 5-mL prefilled syringe

Administration set: 60 gtt/mL

Patient weight: 188 lb

Other: 250-mL bag of fluid

Convert pounds to kilograms:

$$\frac{188\ lb}{2.2}\ =\ 85.45\ kg$$

Adjust the DD to account for the patient's weight:

$$\frac{10\ \mu g}{kg/min}\ \times\ 85.45\ kg\ =\ 854.5\ \mu g/min$$

Convert and simplify the DOH:

$$400\ mg\ \times\ \frac{1{,}000\ \mu g}{mg}\ =\ 400{,}000\ \mu g$$

$$\frac{400{,}000\ \mu g}{250\ mL}\ =\ \frac{?\ \mu g}{1\ mL}$$

$$\frac{400{,}000\ \mu g}{250\ mL}\ \times\ 1\ mL\ =\ 1{,}600\ \mu g\ in\ 1\ mL\ of\ fluid$$

Plug into the formula:

$$\frac{854.4\ \mu g/min}{1{,}600\ \mu g/mL}\ \times\ \frac{60\ gtt}{mL}\ =\ ?\ gtt/min$$

$$\frac{854.5\ \mu g}{min}\ \times\ \frac{mL}{1{,}600\ \mu g}\ \times\ \frac{60\ gtt}{mL}\ =\ 32.04\ gtt/min$$

Round to the nearest whole number, or 32 gtt/min.

38. DD: 12 µg/kg/min

DOH: 800 mg in a 500-mL bag of D_5W

Administration set: 60 gtt/mL

Patient weight: 45 kg

The patient's weight is already in kilograms. Adjust the DD to account for the patient's weight:

$$\frac{12\ \mu g}{kg/min}\ \times\ 45\ kg\ =\ 540\ \mu g/min$$

Convert and simplify the DOH:

$$800\ mg\ \times\ \frac{1{,}000\ \mu g}{mg}\ =\ 800{,}000\ \mu g$$

$$\frac{800{,}000\ \mu g}{500\ mL}\ =\ \frac{?\ \mu g}{1\ mL}$$

$$\frac{800{,}000\ \mu g}{500\ mL}\ \times\ 1\ mL\ =\ 1{,}600\ \mu g\ in\ 1\ mL\ of\ fluid$$

Plug into the formula:

$$\frac{540\ \mu g/min}{1{,}600\ \mu g/mL} \times \frac{60\ gtt}{mL} = ?\ gtt/min$$

$$\frac{540\ \mu g}{min} \times \frac{mL}{1{,}600\ \mu g} \times \frac{60\ gtt}{mL} = 20.25\ gtt/min$$

Round to the nearest whole number, or 20 gtt/min.

39. DD: 15 μg/kg/min

DOH: 800 mg in a 5-mL prefilled syringe

Administration set: 60 gtt/mL

Patient weight: 238 lb

Other: 500-mL bag of D_5W

Convert pounds to kilograms:

$$\frac{238\ lb}{2.2} = 108.18\ kg$$

Adjust the DD to account for the patient's weight:

$$\frac{15\ \mu g}{kg/min} \times 108.18\ kg = 1{,}622.7\ \mu g/min$$

The 800 mg will be added to the 500-mL bag. Convert and simplify the DOH:

$$800\ mg \times \frac{1{,}000\ \mu g}{mg} = 800{,}000\ \mu g$$

$$\frac{800{,}000\ \mu g}{500\ mL} = \frac{?\ \mu g}{1\ mL}$$

$$\frac{800{,}000\ \mu g}{500\ mL} \times 1\ mL = 1{,}600\ \mu g\ in\ 1\ mL\ of\ fluid$$

Plug into the formula:

$$\frac{1{,}622.7\ \mu g/min}{1{,}600\ \mu g/mL} \times \frac{60\ gtt}{mL} = ?\ gtt/min$$

$$\frac{1{,}622.7\ \mu g}{min} \times \frac{mL}{1{,}600\ \mu g} \times \frac{60\ gtt}{mL} = 60.85\ gtt/min$$

Round to the nearest whole number, or 61 gtt/min.

40. DD: 20 μg/kg/min

DOH: 800 mg in a 500-mL bag of D_5W

Administration set: 60 gtt/mL

Patient weight: 160 lb

Convert pounds to kilograms:

$$\frac{160\ lb}{2.2} = 72.73\ kg$$

Adjust the DD to account for the patient's weight:

$$\frac{20\ \mu g}{kg/min} \times 72.73\ kg = 1{,}454.6\ \mu g/min$$

Convert and simplify the DOH:

$$800\ mg \times \frac{1{,}000\ \mu g}{mg} = 800{,}000\ \mu g$$

$$\frac{800{,}000\ \mu g}{500\ mL} = \frac{?\ \mu g}{1\ mL}$$

$$\frac{800{,}000\ \mu g}{500\ mL} \times 1\ mL = 1{,}600\ \mu g\ in\ 1\ mL\ of\ fluid$$

Plug into the formula:

$$\frac{1{,}454.6\ \mu g/min}{1{,}600\ \mu g/mL} \times \frac{60\ gtt}{mL} = ?\ gtt/min$$

$$\frac{1{,}454.6\ \mu g}{min} \times \frac{mL}{1{,}600\ \mu g} \times \frac{60\ gtt}{mL} = 54.55\ gtt/min$$

Round to the nearest whole number, or 55 gtt/min.

41. For problems 41 through 50, because all DDs are given in μg/kg/min, the concentration will be calculated only once and reused each time.

$$800\ mg \times \frac{1{,}000\ \mu g}{mg} = 800{,}000\ \mu g$$

$$\frac{800{,}000\ \mu g}{500\ mL} = \frac{?\ \mu g}{1\ mL}$$

$$\frac{800{,}000\ \mu g}{500\ mL} \times 1\ mL = 1{,}600\ \mu g\ in\ 1\ mL\ of\ fluid$$

The concentration for this set of problems is 1,600 μg/mL.

Convert pounds to kilograms:

$$\frac{193\ lb}{2.2} = 87.73\ kg$$

Adjust the DD to account for the patient's weight:

$$\frac{10\ \mu g}{kg/min} \times 87.73\ kg = 877.3\ \mu g/min$$

Plug into the formula:

$$\frac{877.3\ \mu g/min}{1{,}600\ \mu g/mL} \times \frac{60\ gtt}{mL} = ?\ gtt/min$$

$$\frac{877.3\ \mu g}{min} \times \frac{mL}{1{,}600\ \mu g} \times \frac{60\ gtt}{mL} = 32.90\ gtt/min$$

Round to the nearest whole number, or 33 gtt/min.

42. Convert pounds to kilograms:

$$\frac{269\ lb}{2.2} = 122.27\ kg$$

Adjust the DD to account for the patient's weight:

$$\frac{3\ \mu g}{kg/min} \times 122.27\ kg\ =\ 366.81\ \mu g/min$$

Plug into the formula:

$$\frac{366.81\ \mu g/min}{1,600\ \mu g/mL} \times \frac{60\ gtt}{mL}\ =\ ?\,gtt/min$$

$$\frac{366.81\ \mu g}{min} \times \frac{mL}{1,600\ \mu g} \times \frac{60\ gtt}{mL}\ =\ 13.76\ gtt/min$$

Round to the nearest whole number, or 14 gtt/min.

43. Convert pounds to kilograms:

$$\frac{243\ lb}{2.2}\ =\ 110.45\ kg$$

Adjust the DD to account for the patient's weight:

$$\frac{7\ \mu g}{kg/min} \times 110.45\ kg\ =\ 773.15\ \mu g/min$$

Plug into the formula:

$$\frac{773.15\ \mu g/min}{1,600\ \mu g/mL} \times \frac{60\ gtt}{mL}\ =\ ?\,gtt/min$$

$$\frac{773.15\ \mu g}{min} \times \frac{mL}{1,600\ \mu g} \times \frac{60\ gtt}{mL}\ =\ 28.99\ gtt/min$$

Round to the nearest whole number, or 29 gtt/min.

44. Convert pounds to kilograms:

$$\frac{153\ lb}{2.2}\ =\ 69.55\ kg$$

Adjust the DD to account for the patient's weight:

$$\frac{5\ \mu g}{kg/min} \times 69.55\ kg\ =\ 347.75\ \mu g/min$$

Plug into the formula:

$$\frac{347.75\ \mu g/min}{1,600\ \mu g/mL} \times \frac{60\ gtt}{mL}\ =\ ?\,gtt/min$$

$$\frac{347.75\ \mu g}{min} \times \frac{mL}{1,600\ \mu g} \times \frac{60\ gtt}{mL}\ =\ 13.04\ gtt/min$$

Round to the nearest whole number, or 13 gtt/min.

45. Convert pounds to kilograms:

$$\frac{177\ lb}{2.2}\ =\ 80.45\ kg$$

Adjust the DD to account for the patient's weight:

$$\frac{14\ \mu g}{kg/min} \times 80.45\ kg\ =\ 1,126.3\ \mu g/min$$

Plug into the formula:

$$\frac{1,126.3\ \mu g/min}{1,600\ \mu g/mL} \times \frac{60\ gtt}{mL}\ =\ ?\,gtt/min$$

$$\frac{1,126.3\ \mu g}{min} \times \frac{mL}{1,600\ \mu g} \times \frac{60\ gtt}{mL}\ =\ 42.24\ gtt/min$$

Round to the nearest whole number, or 42 gtt/min.

46. The patient's weight is already in kilograms. Adjust the DD to account for the patient's weight:

$$\frac{20\ \mu g}{kg/min} \times 71\ kg\ =\ 1,420\ \mu g/min$$

Plug into the formula:

$$\frac{1,420\ \mu g/min}{1,600\ \mu g/mL} \times \frac{60\ gtt}{mL}\ =\ ?\,gtt/min$$

$$\frac{1,420\ \mu g}{min} \times \frac{mL}{1,600\ \mu g} \times \frac{60\ gtt}{mL}\ =\ 53.25\,gtt/min$$

Round to the nearest whole number, or 53 gtt/min.

47. The patient's weight is already in kilograms. Adjust the DD to account for the patient's weight:

$$\frac{15\ \mu g}{kg/min} \times 41\ kg\ =\ 615\ \mu g/min$$

Plug into the formula:

$$\frac{615\ \mu g/min}{1,600\ \mu g/mL} \times \frac{60\ gtt}{mL}\ =\ ?\,gtt/min$$

$$\frac{615\ \mu g}{min} \times \frac{mL}{1,600\ \mu g} \times \frac{60\ gtt}{mL}\ =\ 23.06\ gtt/min$$

Round to the nearest whole number, or 23 gtt/min.

48. The patient's weight is already in kilograms. Adjust the DD to account for the patient's weight:

$$\frac{11\ \mu g}{kg/min} \times 50\ kg\ =\ 550\ \mu g/min$$

Plug into the formula:

$$\frac{550\ \mu g/min}{1,600\ \mu g/mL} \times \frac{60\ gtt}{mL}\ =\ ?\,gtt/min$$

$$\frac{550\ \mu g}{min} \times \frac{mL}{1,600\ \mu g} \times \frac{60\ gtt}{mL}\ =\ 20.63\ gtt/min$$

Round to the nearest whole number, or 21 gtt/min.

49. The patient's weight is already in kilograms. Adjust the DD to account for the patient's weight:

$$\frac{4\ \mu g}{kg/min} \times 111\ kg\ =\ 444\ \mu g/min$$

Plug into the formula:

$$\frac{444 \ \mu g/min}{1,600 \ \mu g/mL} \times \frac{60 \ gtt}{mL} = ? \ gtt/min$$

$$\frac{444 \ \mu g}{min} \times \frac{mL}{1,600 \ \mu g} \times \frac{60 \ gtt}{mL} = 16.65 \ gtt/min$$

Round to the nearest whole number, or 17 gtt/min.

50. The patient's weight is already in kilograms. Adjust the DD to account for the patient's weight:

$$\frac{8 \ \mu g}{kg/min} \times 62 \ kg = 496 \ \mu g/min$$

Plug into the formula:

$$\frac{496 \ \mu g/min}{1,600 \ \mu g/mL} \times \frac{60 \ gtt}{mL} = ? \ gtt/min$$

$$\frac{496 \ \mu g}{min} \times \frac{mL}{1,600 \ \mu g} \times \frac{60 \ gtt}{mL} = 18.6 \ gtt/min$$

Round to the nearest whole number, or 19 gtt/min.

51. For problems 51 through 60, all DDs are given in μg/kg/min. The concentration will be calculated only once and reused each time.

$$400 \ mg \times \frac{1,000 \ \mu g}{mg} = 400,000 \ \mu g$$

$$\frac{400,000 \ \mu g}{250 \ mL} = \frac{? \ \mu g}{1 \ mL}$$

$$\frac{400,000 \ \mu g}{250 \ mL} \times 1 \ mL = 1,600 \ \mu g \ in \ 1 \ mL \ of \ fluid$$

The concentration for this set of problems is 1,600 μg/mL.

Convert pounds to kilograms:

$$\frac{173 \ lb}{2.2} = 78.64 \ kg$$

Adjust the DD to account for the patient's weight:

$$\frac{5 \ \mu g}{kg/min} \times 78.64 \ kg = 393.2 \ \mu g/min$$

Plug into the formula:

$$\frac{393.2 \ \mu g/min}{1,600 \ \mu g/mL} \times \frac{60 \ gtt}{mL} = ? \ gtt/min$$

$$\frac{393.2 \ \mu g}{min} \times \frac{mL}{1,600 \ \mu g} \times \frac{60 \ gtt}{mL} = 14.75 \ gtt/min$$

Round to the nearest whole number, or 15 gtt/min.

52. Convert pounds to kilograms:

$$\frac{113 \ lb}{2.2} = 51.36 \ kg$$

Adjust the DD to account for the patient's weight:

$$\frac{10 \ \mu g}{kg/min} \times 51.36 \ kg = 513.6 \ \mu g/min$$

Plug into the formula:

$$\frac{513.6 \ \mu g/min}{1,600 \ \mu g/mL} \times \frac{60 \ gtt}{mL} = ? \ gtt/min$$

$$\frac{513.6 \ \mu g}{min} \times \frac{mL}{1,600 \ \mu g} \times \frac{60 \ gtt}{mL} = 19.26 \ gtt/min$$

Round to the nearest whole number, or 19 gtt/min.

53. Convert pounds to kilograms:

$$\frac{256 \ lb}{2.2} = 116.36 \ kg$$

Adjust the DD to account for the patient's weight:

$$\frac{6 \ \mu g}{kg/min} \times 116.36 \ kg = 698.16 \ \mu g/min$$

Plug into the formula:

$$\frac{698.16 \ \mu g/min}{1,600 \ \mu g/mL} \times \frac{60 \ gtt}{mL} = ? \ gtt/min$$

$$\frac{698.16 \ \mu g}{min} \times \frac{mL}{1,600 \ \mu g} \times \frac{60 \ gtt}{mL} = 26.18 \ gtt/min$$

Round to the nearest whole number, or 26 gtt/min.

54. Convert pounds to kilograms:

$$\frac{300 \ lb}{2.2} = 136.36 \ kg$$

Adjust the DD to account for the patient's weight:

$$\frac{12 \ \mu g}{kg/min} \times 136.36 \ kg = 1,636.32 \ \mu g/min$$

Plug into the formula:

$$\frac{1,636.32 \ \mu g/min}{1,600 \ \mu g/mL} \times \frac{60 \ gtt}{mL} = ? \ gtt/min$$

$$\frac{1,636.32 \ \mu g}{min} \times \frac{mL}{1,600 \ \mu g} \times \frac{60 \ gtt}{mL} = 61.36 \ gtt/min$$

Round to the nearest whole number, or 61 gtt/min.

55. Convert pounds to kilograms:

$$\frac{225 \ lb}{2.2} = 102.27 \ kg$$

Adjust the DD to account for the patient's weight:

$$\frac{18 \ \mu g}{kg/min} \times 102.27 \ kg = 1,840.86 \ \mu g/min$$

Plug into the formula:

$$\frac{1,840.86\ \mu g/min}{1,600\ \mu g/mL} \times \frac{60\ gtt}{mL} = ?\ gtt/min$$

$$\frac{1,840.86\ \mu g}{min} \times \frac{mL}{1,600\ \mu g} \times \frac{60\ gtt}{mL} = 69.03\ gtt/min$$

Round to the nearest whole number, or 69 gtt/min.

56. The patient's weight is already in kilograms. Adjust the DD to account for the patient's weight:

$$\frac{3\ \mu g}{kg/min} \times 32\ kg = 96\ \mu g/min$$

Plug into the formula:

$$\frac{96\ \mu g/min}{1,600\ \mu g/mL} \times \frac{60\ gtt}{mL} = ?\ gtt/min$$

$$\frac{96\ \mu g}{min} \times \frac{mL}{1,600\ \mu g} \times \frac{60\ gtt}{mL} = 3.6\ gtt/min$$

Round to the nearest whole number, or 4 gtt/min.

57. The patient's weight is already in kilograms. Adjust the DD to account for the patient's weight:

$$\frac{2\ \mu g}{kg/min} \times 124\ kg = 248\ \mu g/min$$

Plug into the formula:

$$\frac{248\ \mu g/min}{1,600\ \mu g/mL} \times \frac{60\ gtt}{mL} = ?\ gtt/min$$

$$\frac{248\ \mu g}{min} \times \frac{mL}{1,600\ \mu g} \times \frac{60\ gtt}{mL} = 9.3\ gtt/min$$

Round to the nearest whole number, or 9 gtt/min.

58. The patient's weight is already in kilograms. Adjust the DD to account for the patient's weight:

$$\frac{17\ \mu g}{kg/min} \times 145\ kg = 2,465\ \mu g/min$$

Plug into the formula:

$$\frac{2,465\ \mu g/min}{1,600\ \mu g/mL} \times \frac{60\ gtt}{mL} = ?\ gtt/min$$

$$\frac{2,465\ \mu g}{min} \times \frac{mL}{1,600\ \mu g} \times \frac{60\ gtt}{mL} = 92.44\ gtt/min$$

Round to the nearest whole number, or 92 gtt/min.

59. The patient's weight is already in kilograms. Adjust the DD to account for the patient's weight:

$$\frac{13\ \mu g}{kg/min} \times 106\ kg = 1,378\ \mu g/min$$

Plug into the formula:

$$\frac{1,378\ \mu g/min}{1,600\ \mu g/mL} \times \frac{60\ gtt}{mL} = ?\ gtt/min$$

$$\frac{1,378\ \mu g}{min} \times \frac{mL}{1,600\ \mu g} \times \frac{60\ gtt}{mL} = 51.68\ gtt/min$$

Round to the nearest whole number, or 52 gtt/min.

60. The patient's weight is already in kilograms. Adjust the DD to account for the patient's weight:

$$\frac{20\ \mu g}{kg/min} \times 65\ kg = 1,300\ \mu g/min$$

Plug into the formula:

$$\frac{1,300\ \mu g/min}{1,600\ \mu g/mL} \times \frac{60\ gtt}{mL} = ?\ gtt/min$$

$$\frac{1,300\ \mu g}{min} \times \frac{mL}{1,600\ \mu g} \times \frac{60\ gtt}{mL} = 48.75\ gtt/min$$

Round to the nearest whole number, or 49 gtt/min.

61. Convert pounds to kilograms:

$$\frac{30\ lb}{2.2} = 13.64\ kg$$

Calculate the dose to account for the weight:

$$\frac{0.01\ mg}{kg} \times 13.64\ kg = 0.14\ mg$$

Set up a proportion:

$$\frac{10\ mL}{1.0\ mg} = \frac{?\ mL}{0.14\ mg}$$

$$\frac{10\ mL \times 0.14\ mg}{1.0\ mg} = 1.4\ mL$$

62. Convert pounds to kilograms:

$$\frac{44\ lb}{2.2} = 20\ kg$$

Calculate the dose to account for the weight:

$$\frac{0.1\ mg}{kg} \times 20\ kg = 2\ mg$$

Set up a proportion:

$$\frac{1\ mL}{6\ mg} = \frac{?\ mL}{2\ mg}$$

$$\frac{1\ mL \times 2\ mg}{6\ mg} = 0.33\ mL$$

63. From the previous problem, you know that the patient's weight is 20 kg.

Calculate the dose to account for the weight:

$$\frac{0.2 \text{ mg}}{\text{kg}} \times 20 \text{ kg} = 4 \text{ mg}$$

Set up a proportion:

$$\frac{1 \text{ mL}}{6 \text{ mg}} = \frac{? \text{ mL}}{4 \text{ mg}}$$

$$\frac{1 \text{ mL} \times 4 \text{ mg}}{6 \text{ mg}} = 0.67 \text{ mL}$$

64. Convert pounds to kilograms:

$$\frac{25 \text{ lb}}{2.2} = 11.36 \text{ kg}$$

Calculate the dose to account for the weight:

$$\frac{0.02 \text{ mg}}{\text{kg}} \times 11.36 \text{ kg} = 0.23 \text{ mg}$$

Set up a proportion:

$$\frac{10 \text{ mL}}{1 \text{ mg}} = \frac{? \text{ mL}}{0.23 \text{ mg}}$$

$$\frac{10 \text{ mL} \times 0.23 \text{ mg}}{1 \text{ mg}} = 2.3 \text{ mL}$$

65. Convert pounds to kilograms:

$$\frac{60 \text{ lb}}{2.2} = 27.27 \text{ kg}$$

Calculate the dose to account for the weight:

$$\frac{0.5 \text{ mg}}{\text{kg}} \times 27.27 \text{ kg} = 13.64 \text{ mg}$$

Set up a proportion:

$$\frac{5 \text{ mL}}{20 \text{ mg}} = \frac{? \text{ mL}}{13.64 \text{ mg}}$$

$$\frac{5 \text{ mL} \times 13.64 \text{ mg}}{20 \text{ mg}} = 3.41 \text{ mL}$$

66. Convert pounds to kilograms:

$$\frac{75 \text{ lb}}{2.2} = 34.09 \text{ kg}$$

Calculate the dose to account for the weight:

$$\frac{1 \text{ mg}}{\text{kg}} \times 34.09 \text{ kg} = 34.09 \text{ mg}$$

Set up a proportion:

$$\frac{1 \text{ mL}}{50 \text{ mg}} = \frac{? \text{ mL}}{34.09 \text{ mg}}$$

$$\frac{1 \text{ mL} \times 34.09 \text{ mg}}{50 \text{ mg}} = 0.68 \text{ mL}$$

67. Convert pounds to kilograms:

$$\frac{80 \text{ lb}}{2.2} = 36.36 \text{ kg}$$

Calculate the dose to account for the weight:

$$\frac{0.1 \text{ mg}}{\text{kg}} \times 36.36 \text{ kg} = 3.64 \text{ mg}$$

Set up a proportion:

$$\frac{1 \text{ mL}}{10 \text{ mg}} = \frac{? \text{ mL}}{3.64 \text{ mg}}$$

$$\frac{1 \text{ mL} \times 3.64 \text{ mg}}{10 \text{ mg}} = 0.36 \text{ mL}$$

68. Convert pounds to kilograms:

$$\frac{41 \text{ lb}}{2.2} = 18.64 \text{ kg}$$

Calculate the dose to account for the weight:

$$\frac{0.1 \text{ mg}}{\text{kg}} \times 18.64 \text{ kg} = 1.86 \text{ mg}$$

Set up a proportion:

$$\frac{2 \text{ mL}}{2 \text{ mg}} = \frac{? \text{ mL}}{1.86 \text{ mg}}$$

$$\frac{2 \text{ mL} \times 1.86 \text{ mg}}{2 \text{ mg}} = 1.86 \text{ mL}$$

69. Convert pounds to kilograms:

$$\frac{150 \text{ lb}}{2.2} = 68.18 \text{ kg}$$

Calculate the dose to account for the weight:

$$\frac{1 \text{ mg}}{\text{kg}} \times 68.18 \text{ kg} = 68.18 \text{ mg}$$

Set up a proportion:

$$\frac{10 \text{ mL}}{100 \text{ mg}} = \frac{? \text{ mL}}{68.18 \text{ mg}}$$

$$\frac{10 \text{ mL} \times 68.18 \text{ mg}}{100 \text{ mg}} = 6.82 \text{ mL}$$

70. Convert pounds to kilograms:

$$\frac{74 \text{ lb}}{2.2} = 33.64 \text{ kg}$$

Calculate the dose to account for the weight:

$$\frac{0.03 \text{ mg}}{\text{kg}} \times 33.64 \text{ kg} = 1.01 \text{ mg}$$

Set up a proportion:

$$\frac{1 \text{ mL}}{1 \text{ mg}} = \frac{? \text{ mL}}{1.01 \text{ mg}}$$

$$\frac{1 \text{ mL} \times 1.01 \text{ mg}}{1 \text{ mg}} = 1.01 \text{ mL}$$

For this medication, you may round this down to 1.0 mL, and administer the 1.0 mg in 1 mL of solution that you have on hand.

71. Convert pounds to kilograms:

$$\frac{179 \text{ lb}}{2.2} = 81.36 \text{ kg}$$

Calculate the dose to account for the weight:

$$\frac{1 \text{ μg}}{\text{kg}} \times 81.36 \text{ kg} = 81.36 \text{ μg}$$

Set up a proportion:

$$\frac{1 \text{ mL}}{100 \text{ μg}} = \frac{? \text{ mL}}{81.36 \text{ μg}}$$

$$\frac{1 \text{ mL} \times 13.64 \text{ μg}}{100 \text{ μg}} = 0.81 \text{ mL}$$

72. Convert pounds to kilograms:

$$\frac{72 \text{ lb}}{2.2} = 32.73 \text{ kg}$$

Calculate the dose to account for the weight:

$$\frac{0.05 \text{ mg}}{\text{kg}} \times 32.73 \text{ kg} = 1.64 \text{ mg}$$

Set up a proportion:

$$\frac{2 \text{ mL}}{2 \text{ mg}} = \frac{? \text{ mL}}{1.64 \text{ mg}}$$

$$\frac{2 \text{ mL} \times 1.64 \text{ mg}}{2 \text{ mg}} = 1.64 \text{ mL}$$

73. Convert pounds to kilograms:

$$\frac{45 \text{ lb}}{2.2} = 20.45 \text{ kg}$$

Calculate the dose to account for the weight:

$$\frac{0.3 \text{ mg}}{\text{kg}} \times 20.45 \text{ kg} = 6.14 \text{ mg}$$

Set up a proportion:

$$\frac{1 \text{ mL}}{10 \text{ mg}} = \frac{? \text{ mL}}{6.14 \text{ mg}}$$

$$\frac{1 \text{ mL} \times 6.14 \text{ mg}}{10 \text{ mg}} = 0.61 \text{ mL}$$

74. Convert pounds to kilograms:

$$\frac{160 \text{ lb}}{2.2} = 72.73 \text{ kg}$$

Calculate the dose to account for the weight:

$$\frac{0.1 \text{ mg}}{\text{kg}} \times 72.73 \text{ kg} = 7.27 \text{ mg}$$

Set up a proportion:

$$\frac{1 \text{ mL}}{10 \text{ mg}} = \frac{? \text{ mL}}{7.27 \text{ mg}}$$

$$\frac{1 \text{ mL} \times 7.27 \text{ mg}}{10 \text{ mg}} = 0.73 \text{ mL}$$

75. Convert pounds to kilograms:

$$\frac{27 \text{ lb}}{2.2} = 12.27 \text{ kg}$$

Calculate the dose to account for the weight:

$$\frac{0.4 \text{ mg}}{\text{kg}} \times 12.27 \text{ kg} = 4.91 \text{ mg}$$

Set up a proportion:

$$\frac{1 \text{ mL}}{5 \text{ mg}} = \frac{? \text{ mL}}{4.91 \text{ mg}}$$

$$\frac{1 \text{ mL} \times 4.91 \text{ mg}}{5 \text{ mg}} = 0.98 \text{ mL}$$

76. Convert pounds to kilograms:

$$\frac{148 \text{ lb}}{2.2} = 67.27 \text{ kg}$$

Calculate the dose to account for the weight:

$$\frac{2 \text{ mg}}{\text{kg}} \times 67.27 \text{ kg} = 134.54 \text{ mg}$$

Set up a proportion:

$$\frac{5 \text{ mL}}{250 \text{ mg}} = \frac{? \text{ mL}}{134.54 \text{ mg}}$$

$$\frac{5 \text{ mL} \times 134.54 \text{ mg}}{250 \text{ mg}} = 2.69 \text{ mL}$$

77. Convert pounds to kilograms:

$$\frac{39 \text{ lb}}{2.2} = 17.73 \text{ kg}$$

Calculate the dose to account for the weight:

$$\frac{7 \text{ mg}}{\text{kg}} \times 17.73 \text{ kg} = 124.11 \text{ mg}$$

Set up a proportion:

$$\frac{10 \text{ mL}}{1 \text{ g}} = \frac{? \text{ mL}}{124.11 \text{ mg}}$$

Convert grams to milligrams and solve:

$$\frac{10 \text{ mL} \times 124.11 \text{ mg}}{1,000 \text{ mg}} = 1.24 \text{ mL}$$

78. Convert pounds to kilograms:

$$\frac{40 \text{ lb}}{2.2} = 18.18 \text{ kg}$$

Calculate the dose to account for the weight:

$$\frac{0.5 \text{ mEq}}{\text{kg}} \times 18.18 \text{ kg} = 9.09 \text{ mEq}$$

Set up a proportion:

$$\frac{10 \text{ mL}}{25 \text{ mEq}} = \frac{? \text{ mL}}{9.09 \text{ mEq}}$$

$$\frac{10 \text{ mL} \times 9.09 \text{ mEq}}{25 \text{ mEq}} = 3.64 \text{ mL}$$

Because the order was to administer the dose every 10 minutes, you will administer 3.64 mL every 10 minutes. At the 20-minute mark, you will have given a total of 3.64 mL + 3.64 mL, or 7.28 mL.

79. DD: 2 µg/kg/min

DOH: 400 mg in a 250-mL bag of D_5W

Administration set: 60 gtt/mL

Patient weight: 135 lb

Convert pounds to kilograms:

$$\frac{135 \text{ lb}}{2.2} = 61.36 \text{ kg}$$

Adjust the DD to account for the patient's weight:

$$\frac{2 \text{ µg}}{\text{kg/min}} \times 61.36 \text{ kg} = 122.72 \text{ µg/min}$$

Convert and simplify the DOH:

$$400 \text{ mg} \times \frac{1,000 \text{ µg}}{\text{mg}} = 400,000 \text{ µg}$$

$$\frac{400,000 \text{ µg}}{250 \text{ mL}} = \frac{? \text{ µg}}{1 \text{ mL}}$$

$$\frac{400,000 \text{ µg}}{250 \text{ mL}} \times 1 \text{ mL} = 1,600 \text{ µg in 1 mL of fluid}$$

Plug into the formula:

$$\frac{122.72 \text{ µg/min}}{1,600 \text{ µg/mL}} \times \frac{60 \text{ gtt}}{\text{mL}} = ? \text{ gtt/min}$$

$$\frac{122.72 \text{ µg}}{\text{min}} \times \frac{\text{mL}}{1,600 \text{ µg}} \times \frac{60 \text{ gtt}}{\text{mL}} = 4.60 \text{ gtt/min}$$

Round to the nearest whole number, or 5 gtt/min.

80. DD: 2 µg/kg/min

DOH: 800 mg in a 500-mL bag of D_5W

Administration set: 60 gtt/mL

Patient weight: 105 lb

Convert pounds to kilograms:

$$\frac{105 \text{ lb}}{2.2} = 47.73 \text{ kg}$$

Adjust the DD to account for the patient's weight:

$$\frac{2 \text{ µg}}{\text{kg/min}} \times 47.73 \text{ kg} = 95.46 \text{ µg/min}$$

Convert and simplify the DOH:

$$800 \text{ mg} \times \frac{1,000 \text{ µg}}{\text{mg}} = 800,000 \text{ µg}$$

$$\frac{800,000 \text{ µg}}{500 \text{ mL}} = \frac{? \text{ µg}}{1 \text{ mL}}$$

$$\frac{800,000 \text{ µg}}{500 \text{ mL}} \times 1 \text{ mL} = 1,600 \text{ µg in 1 mL of fluid}$$

Plug into the formula:

$$\frac{95.46 \text{ µg/min}}{1,600 \text{ µg/mL}} \times \frac{60 \text{ gtt}}{\text{mL}} = ? \text{ gtt/min}$$

$$\frac{95.46 \text{ µg}}{\text{min}} \times \frac{\text{mL}}{1,600 \text{ µg}} \times \frac{60 \text{ gtt}}{\text{mL}} = 3.58 \text{ gtt/min}$$

Round to the nearest whole number, or 4 gtt/min.

Chapter 8
Chapter Problems
Chapter 1: The Language of Math: Fractions, Percentages, and Decimals

1. Decimal fraction: $22 \div 8 = 2.75$
Percentage: $2.75 \times 100 = 275\%$

2. Decimal fraction: $14 \div 32 = 0.44 \ (0.4375)$
Percentage: $0.44 \times 100 = 44\%$

3. Decimal fraction: $35 \div 54 = 0.65$
Percentage: $0.65 \times 100 = 65\%$

4. Estimate: $90 + 100 = 190$

Calculation: The numbers can be broken down as: $40 + 40 + 5 + 50 + 40 + 5$

These numbers can be written as smaller equations as follows:

$40 + 40 = 80$

$5 + 5 = 10$

$50 + 40 = 90$

Adding these results gives the final answer: $80 + 10 + 90 = 180$

Comparison: The estimate was 190, and the answer is 180.

5. Estimate: $50 + 30 + 140 = 220$

Calculation: The numbers can be broken down as: $50 + 4 + 20 + 6 + 20 + 30 + 50 + 30 + 8$

These numbers can be written as smaller equations as follows:

$50 + 20 = 70$

$4 + 6 = 10$

$20 + 30 = 50$

$30 + 8 = 38$

and 50

Adding these results gives the final answer: $70 + 10 + 50 + 50 + 38 = 218$

Comparison: The estimate was 220, and the answer is 218.

6. 3

7. 0.03

8. 120

9. 0.012

10. 45,600

11. 0.0456

12. $3 \times 5 \times 7 \times 2$

13. $22 \times 4 \times 6 \times 2$

14. $125 \div 5 \div 5$

15. $38 \div 2 \div 8$

16. $\dfrac{12}{13}$ = 0.923, or 92%

17. $\dfrac{1}{8} \times 12 = \dfrac{12}{8}$ = 1.5 vials, or 150%

18. B. An estimate of the product of $3.03 \times 2.5 = (3 \times 2) + (3 \times 0.5) = 6 + 1.5 = 7.5$, or 8.

19. $16 + 29$ = approximately $15 + 30 = 45$.

Calculation: The numbers can be broken down as: $10 + 6 + 20 + 9$.

These can be written as smaller equations as follows:

$10 + 20 = 30$

$6 + 9 = 15$

Adding these results gives the final answer: $30 + 15 = 45$

Comparison: The estimate was 45, and the answer is 45.

20. $3 \times 20 = 3 \times 2 = 6$; moving the decimal one place to the right (multiplying by 10) = 60

21.
$$\begin{array}{r} 89 \\ +\ 43 \\ \hline 132 \end{array}$$

22.
$$\begin{array}{r} 37 \\ +\ 79 \\ \hline 116 \end{array}$$

23.
$$\begin{array}{r} 159 \\ +\ 73 \\ \hline 232 \end{array}$$

24.
$$\begin{array}{r} 58 \\ +\ 39 \\ \hline 97 \end{array}$$

25.
$$\begin{array}{r} 160 \\ -\ 15 \\ \hline 145 \end{array}$$

26.
$$\begin{array}{r} 311 \\ -\ 33 \\ \hline 278 \end{array}$$

27.
$$\begin{array}{r} 17 \\ \times\ 6 \\ \hline 102 \end{array}$$

28.
$$\begin{array}{r} 47 \\ \times\ 69 \\ \hline 423 \end{array}$$

$$\begin{array}{r} 47 \\ \times\ 69 \\ \hline 423 \\ +\ 2820 \\ \hline 3,243 \end{array}$$

29.
$$\begin{array}{r} 150 \\ \times\ 61 \\ \hline 150 \\ +\ 9000 \\ \hline 9,150 \end{array}$$

30.
$$\begin{array}{r} 328 \\ \times\ 256 \\ \hline 1968 \end{array}$$

$$\begin{array}{r} 328 \\ \times\ 256 \\ \hline 1968 \\ 16400 \end{array}$$

$$\begin{array}{r} 328 \\ \times\ 256 \\ \hline 1968 \\ 16400 \\ +\ 65600 \\ \hline 83,968 \end{array}$$

31. $\dfrac{7.6}{5 \overline{)38.\,0}}$

32. $\dfrac{2.074}{54 \overline{)112.\,00\,0}}$

33. $\dfrac{21.\,5}{8 \overline{)17\,2.\,0}}$

34. $\dfrac{7.75}{32 \overline{)248.\,0\,0}}$

35. $\dfrac{50.5}{4 \overline{)202.\,0}}$

36. $\dfrac{316.0}{13 \overline{)41\,0\,8.0}}$

37. $\begin{array}{r} 8.3 \\ + 4.9 \\ \hline 13.2 \end{array}$

38. $\begin{array}{r} 434.69 \\ + 57.934 \\ \hline 492.624 \end{array}$

39. $\begin{array}{r} 1.1 \\ + 9.7 \\ \hline 10.8 \end{array}$

40. $\begin{array}{r} 974.2 \\ + 13.5 \\ \hline 987.7 \end{array}$

41. $\begin{array}{r} 692.550 \\ - 222.225 \\ \hline 470.325 \end{array}$

42. $\begin{array}{r} 343.51 \\ - 294.93 \\ \hline 48.58 \end{array}$

43. $\begin{array}{r} 5.3 \\ - 2.8 \\ \hline 2.5 \end{array}$

44. $\begin{array}{r} 3102.400 \\ - 4.043 \\ \hline 3,098.357 \end{array}$

45. $2 \times 15 + 6 =$

$30 + 6 = 36$

46. $100 - 4 + 10 + 7 =$

$96 + 17 = 113$

47. $30 \times 7 - 1 + 8 =$

$210 - 1 + 8 =$

$209 + 8 = 217$

48.

	Estimate	Break it up	Calculate the answer	Check against your estimate
$108 - 31$	$110 - 30 = 80$	$100 + 8 - 30 - 1$	$100 - 30 = 70$ $8 - 1 = 7$ $70 + 7 = 77$	Estimate = 80 Answer = 77
77×5	$80 \times 5 = 400$	70×5 $+ 7 \times 5$	$\begin{array}{r} 350 \\ + 35 \\ \hline 385 \end{array}$	Estimate = 400 Answer = 385

49. In one day: $6.75 \times 5 = 33.75$ mg
In one week: $33.75 \times 7 = 236.25$ mg

50. Because the bags come in set numbers per case, multiply the number of bags in a case times the number of cases ordered:

$(10 \times 8) + (12 \times 15) = 80 + 180 = 260$ bags of fluid ordered

51. Because there are 365 days in a year, with 4,200 calls in one year, there was an average of 11.51 calls per day ($4,200 \div 365$). In 261 work days with an average of 11.51 calls per day, you responded to about 3,004 calls (261×11.51).

52. Subtract the number of points missed to determine the number of points you earned: $250 - 11 - 15.5 - 8.2 = 215.3$ points earned. Your score is calculated as follows: $215.3 \div 250 = 0.8612$, which, written as a percentage rounded to a whole number, is 86%.

Chapter 3: Using the Number 1 With Fractions

53. Two examples of how to reduce this fraction follow:

$$\frac{420}{12} \div \frac{2}{2} = \frac{210}{6}$$

$$\frac{420}{12} \div \frac{12}{12} = \frac{35}{1}$$

Note that the first reduction can be further reduced as follows:

$$\frac{210}{6} \div \frac{6}{6} = \frac{35}{1}$$

54. Two examples of how to reduce this fraction follow:

$$\frac{300}{15} \div \frac{5}{5} = \frac{60}{3}$$

$$\frac{300}{15} \div \frac{3}{3} = \frac{100}{5}$$

Note that these fractions can be further reduced as follows, resulting in the same answer:

$$\frac{60}{3} \div \frac{3}{3} = \frac{20}{1}$$

$$\frac{100}{5} \div \frac{5}{5} = \frac{20}{1}$$

55. 0.25

56. 0.125

57. 0.125

58. 2.75

59. 4.4

60. 5.64

61. 0.76

62. 1.40

63. 0.33

64. 1.57

65. 0.25

66. 0.89

67. 0.4

68. 0.33

69. $\frac{150}{120} \div \frac{2}{2} = \frac{75}{60} \div \frac{2}{2} = \frac{37.5}{30}$

70. $\frac{212}{20} \div \frac{2}{2} = \frac{106}{10} \div \frac{2}{2} = \frac{53}{5}$

71. $\frac{550}{25} \div \frac{5}{5} = \frac{110}{5} \div \frac{5}{5} = \frac{22}{1}$

72. $\frac{3 \times 5 \times 7 \times 4 \times 4}{7 \times 2 \times 4 \times 3} = \frac{5 \times 4}{2} = \frac{20}{2} = 10$

73. $\frac{400 \times 3 \times 50 \times 5}{400 \times 50} = 3 \times 5 = 15$

74. $\frac{2}{8} \div \frac{2}{2} = \frac{1}{4}$

$$\frac{8}{10} \div \frac{2}{2} = \frac{4}{5}$$

75. $\frac{14}{28} \div \frac{14}{14} = \frac{1}{2}$

$$\frac{15}{20} \div \frac{5}{5} = \frac{3}{4}$$

76. $1{,}989 \div 3{,}540 = 0.56$, or 56%

77. $18{,}930 \div 27{,}843 = 0.68$, or 68%

78. $33 \div 46 = 0.717$, or 72%

79. $28 \div 45 = 0.62$, or 62%

80. $\frac{48 \times 55 \times 6}{12 \times 11 \times 36} = \frac{12 \times 4 \times 11 \times 5 \times 6}{12 \times 11 \times 6 \times 6}$

$$= \frac{4 \times 5}{6} = \frac{20}{6}$$

81. $\frac{10 \times 4 \times 50}{30 \times 20 \times 100} = \frac{10 \times 4 \times 50}{10 \times 3 \times 4 \times 5 \times 50 \times 2}$

$$= \frac{1}{3 \times 5 \times 2} = \frac{1}{30}$$

82. $\frac{36 \times 9 \times 14}{3 \times 81 \times 7} = \frac{3 \times 12 \times 9 \times 7 \times 2}{3 \times 9 \times 9 \times 7}$

$$= \frac{12 \times 2}{9} = \frac{24}{9}$$

83. $\frac{11.4 \times 26.4 \times 28}{5.7 \times 3.2 \times 7} = \frac{5.7 \times 2 \times 3.2 \times 8.25 \times 7 \times 4}{5.7 \times 3.2 \times 7}$

$$= \frac{2 \times 8.25 \times 4}{1} = \frac{66}{1}$$

84. $\frac{12.3 \times 45.6 \times 78.9}{36.9 \times 91.2 \times 236.7} = \frac{12.3 \times 45.6 \times 78.9}{12.3 \times 3 \times 45.6 \times 2 \times 78.9 \times 3}$

$$= \frac{1}{3 \times 2 \times 3} = \frac{1}{18}$$

Chapter 4: Fun With Fractions

85. $\frac{26}{40}$

Reduce:

$$\frac{26}{40} \div \frac{2}{2} = \frac{13}{20}$$

86. $\frac{15}{25}$

Reduce:

$$\frac{15}{25} \div \frac{5}{5} = \frac{3}{5}$$

87. $\frac{11}{45}$

This fraction cannot be reduced.

88. Neither fraction can be reduced. Solve:

$$\frac{5}{3} \times \frac{7}{2} = \frac{35}{6}$$

89. Reduce the first fraction:

$$\frac{18}{10} \div \frac{2}{2} = \frac{9}{5}$$

Reduce the second fraction:

$$\frac{2}{22} \div \frac{2}{2} = \frac{1}{11}$$

Restate the original equation and solve:

$$\frac{9}{5} \times \frac{1}{11} = \frac{9}{55}$$

90. Reduce the first fraction:

$$\frac{18}{12} \div \frac{6}{6} = \frac{3}{2}$$

Reduce the second fraction:

$$\frac{22}{10} \div \frac{2}{2} = \frac{11}{5}$$

Restate the original equation:

$$\frac{3}{2} \div \frac{11}{5} =$$

Flip and solve:

$$\frac{3}{2} \times \frac{5}{11} = \frac{15}{22}$$

This fraction cannot be reduced.

91. Neither fraction can be reduced.

Restate the equation and solve:

$$\frac{55}{12} \times \frac{2}{7} = \frac{110}{84}$$

Reduce the fraction, then restate the improper fraction:

$$\frac{110}{84} \div \frac{2}{2} = \frac{55}{42}$$

$$\frac{55}{42} = \frac{42}{42} + \frac{13}{42} = 1\frac{13}{42}$$

92. Work the top half of the fraction:

$$\frac{5}{6} \times \frac{4}{8} = \frac{20}{48}$$

Reduce:

$$\frac{20}{48} \div \frac{4}{4} = \frac{5}{12}$$

Restate the original equation:

$$\frac{5}{12} \div \frac{3}{2} =$$

Solve:

$$\frac{5}{12} \times \frac{2}{3} = \frac{10}{36}$$

Reduce:

$$\frac{10}{36} \times \frac{2}{2} = \frac{5}{18}$$

93. Work the top half of the fraction:

$$\frac{1}{2} \times \frac{8}{14} = \frac{8}{28}$$

Reduce:

$$\frac{8}{28} \div \frac{4}{4} = \frac{2}{7}$$

Restate the original equation:

$$\frac{2}{7} \div \frac{1}{3} =$$

Solve:

$$\frac{2}{7} \times \frac{3}{1} = \frac{6}{7}$$

94. 10 is the common denominator.

95. 26 is the common denominator (2×13).

96. Convert fractions and find the common denominator:

$$\frac{1}{6} \times \frac{2}{2} = \frac{2}{12}$$

$$\frac{5}{4} \times \frac{3}{3} = \frac{15}{12}$$

Solve:

$$\frac{2}{12} + \frac{15}{12} = \frac{17}{12}$$

Change from an improper fraction:

$$\frac{17}{12} = \frac{12}{12} + \frac{5}{12} = 1\frac{5}{12}$$

97. Convert fractions and find the common denominator:

$$\frac{3}{8} \times \frac{11}{11} = \frac{33}{88}$$

$$\frac{10}{22} \times \frac{4}{4} = \frac{40}{88}$$

Solve:

$$\frac{33}{88} + \frac{40}{88} = \frac{73}{88}$$

Chapter 5: Ratios and Proportions: Finding the Missing Piece

98. $\dfrac{15 \times 20}{11} = \,?$

$$\frac{300}{11} = 27.27$$

99. $\dfrac{2 \times 18}{34} = \,?$

$$\frac{36}{34} = 1.06$$

100.

Convert this number	to this unit of measure	Conversion factor
100 g	100,000 mg	1,000 mg = 1 g
8 mL	0.008 L	1,000 mL = 1 L
55 g	0.055 kg	1,000 g = 1 kg
924 mg	0.000924 kg	1,000 mg = 1 g and 1,000 g = 1 kg

Calculations:

First row:
Set up the proportion:

$$\frac{?\,\text{mg}}{100\,\text{g}} = \frac{1,000\,\text{mg}}{1\,\text{g}}$$

Cross multiply:

$$?\,\text{mg} = \frac{1,000\,\text{mg} \times 100\,\text{g}}{1\,\text{g}}$$

Solve:

$$? = 100,000\,\text{mg}$$

Second row:
Set up the proportion:

$$\frac{?\,\text{L}}{8\,\text{mL}} = \frac{1\,\text{L}}{1,000\,\text{mL}}$$

Cross multiply:

$$?\,\text{L} = \frac{1\,\text{L} \times 8\,\text{mL}}{1,000\,\text{mL}}$$

Solve:

$$? = 0.008\,\text{L}$$

Third row:
Set up the proportion:

$$\frac{?\,\text{kg}}{55\,\text{g}} = \frac{1\,\text{kg}}{1,000\,\text{g}}$$

Cross multiply:

$$?\,\text{kg} = \frac{1\,\text{kg} \times 55\,\text{g}}{1,000\,\text{g}}$$

Solve:

$$? = 0.055\,\text{kg}$$

Fourth row:
First, figure out the conversion factor by using the two provided:

$$\frac{1,000\,\text{mg}}{1\,\text{g}} \times \frac{1,000\,\text{g}}{1\,\text{kg}} = \frac{1,000,000\,\text{mg}}{1\,\text{kg}}$$

Set up the proportion:

$$\frac{?\,\text{kg}}{924\,\text{mg}} = \frac{1\,\text{kg}}{1,000,000\,\text{mg}}$$

Cross multiply:

$$?\,\text{kg} = \frac{1\,\text{kg} \times 924\,\text{mg}}{1,000,000\,\text{mg}}$$

Solve:

$$? = 0.000924\,\text{kg}$$

101. Conversion factor: 1 g = 1,000 mg

$$8,420\,\text{mg} \times \frac{1\,\text{g}}{1,000\,\text{mg}} = 8.42\,\text{g}$$

102. Conversion factor: 1 g = 1,000 mg

$$4.1\,\text{g} \times \frac{1,000\,\text{mg}}{1\,\text{g}} = 4,100\,\text{mg}$$

103. Conversion factor: 1 mg = 1,000 μg

$$46\,\text{mg} \times \frac{1,000\,\mu\text{g}}{1\,\text{mg}} = 46,000\,\mu\text{g}$$

104. Conversion factor: 1 mg = 1,000 μg

$$50\,\mu\text{g} \times \frac{1\,\text{mg}}{1,000\,\mu\text{g}} = 0.05\,\text{mg}$$

105. Conversion factor: 1 mg = 1,000 μg

$$10,000\,\text{mg} \times \frac{1,000\,\mu\text{g}}{1\,\text{mg}} = 10,000,000\,\mu\text{g}$$

106. The formula is:

$$\left(\frac{9}{5} \times {}^\circ\text{C}\right) + 32 = {}^\circ\text{F}$$

$$\left(\frac{9}{5} \times 33.5\right) + 32 =$$

$$\frac{301.5}{5} + 32 =$$

$$60.3 + 32 = 92.3°F$$

107. The formula is:

$$\frac{5}{9} \times \left(°F - 32\right) = °C$$

$$\frac{5}{9} \times \left(85 - 32\right) =$$

$$\frac{5}{9} \times 53 = 29.4°C$$

108. First, convert milligrams to micrograms:

$$200 \text{ mg} \times \frac{1,000 \text{ μg}}{1 \text{ mg}} = 200,000 \text{ μg}$$

$$\frac{200,000 \text{ μg}}{250 \text{ mL}} = 800 \text{ μg/mL}$$

109. First, convert grams to milligrams:

$$0.5 \text{ g} \times \frac{1,000 \text{ mg}}{1 \text{ g}} = 500 \text{ mg}$$

$$\frac{500 \text{ mg}}{250 \text{ mL}} = 2 \text{ mg/mL}$$

110. First, convert grams to milligrams:
$$1 \text{ g} = 1,000 \text{ mg}$$

$$\frac{100 \text{ mL}}{1,000 \text{ mg}} = \frac{? \text{ mL}}{350 \text{ mg}}$$

$$\frac{100 \text{ mL} \times 350 \text{ mg}}{1,000 \text{ mg}} = 35 \text{ mL}$$

111. $$\frac{10 \text{ mL}}{500 \text{ mg}} = \frac{? \text{ mL}}{175 \text{ mg}}$$

$$\frac{10 \text{ mL} \times 175 \text{ mg}}{500 \text{ mg}} = 3.5 \text{ mL}$$

112. First, convert milligrams to micrograms:
$$1 \text{ mg} = 1,000 \text{ μg}$$

$$\frac{5 \text{ mL}}{1,000 \text{ μg}} = \frac{? \text{ mL}}{275 \text{ μg}}$$

$$\frac{5 \text{ mL} \times 275 \text{ μg}}{1,000 \text{ μg}} = 1.38 \text{ mL}$$

113. First, convert milligrams to micrograms:
$$5 \text{ mg} = 5,000 \text{ μg}$$

$$\frac{1 \text{ mL}}{5,000 \text{ μg}} = \frac{? \text{ mL}}{50 \text{ μg}}$$

$$\frac{1 \text{ mL} \times 50 \text{ μg}}{5,000 \text{ μg}} = 0.01 \text{ mL}$$

114. $$\frac{4}{15} = 0.27 \times 1,489 = 402.03$$

115. $$\frac{3}{8} = 0.375 \times 114 = 42.75$$

116. $$\frac{9}{100} = 0.09 \times 51 = 4.59$$

117. $$\frac{13}{45} = 0.29 \times 660 = 191.4$$

118. $$50\% \text{ dextrose} = \frac{50 \text{ g}}{100 \text{ mL}}$$

Set up the proportion:

$$\frac{? \text{ mL}}{5 \text{ g}} = \frac{100 \text{ mL}}{50 \text{ g}}$$

Solve:

$$? = \frac{100 \text{ mL} \times 5 \text{ g}}{50 \text{ g}}$$

$$? = 10 \text{ mL}$$

Chapter 6: Rate-Dependent Calculations

119. $$\frac{1 \text{ mL}}{1.0 \text{ mg}} \times 0.2 \text{ mg} = 0.2 \text{ mL}$$

120. $$\frac{5 \text{ mL}}{50 \text{ mg}} \times 15 \text{ mg} = 1.5 \text{ mL}$$

121. $$\frac{3 \text{ mL}}{150 \text{ μg}} \times 125 \text{ μg} = 2.5 \text{ mL}$$

122. $$\frac{2 \text{ mL}}{10 \text{ mg}} \times 6 \text{ mg} = 1.2 \text{ mL}$$

123. $$\frac{2 \text{ mL}}{20 \text{ mg}} \times 14 \text{ mg} = 1.4 \text{ mL}$$

124. $$\frac{10 \text{ mL}}{250 \text{ mg}} \times 140 \text{ mg} = 5.6 \text{ mL}$$

125. $$\frac{20 \text{ mL}}{30 \text{ mg}} \times 5 \text{ mg} = 3.33 \text{ mL}$$

126. First, convert grams to milligrams:
$$1 \text{ g} = 1,000 \text{ mg}$$

$$\frac{10 \text{ mL}}{1,000 \text{ mg}} \times 700 \text{ mg} = 7 \text{ mL}$$

127. $$\frac{5 \text{ mL}}{100 \text{ mg}} \times 50 \text{ mg} = 2.5 \text{ mL}$$

128. $$\frac{10 \text{ mL}}{20 \text{ mg}} \times 5 \text{ mg} = 2.5 \text{ mL}$$

129. $\dfrac{1 \text{ min}}{8 \text{ mg}} \times 600 \text{ mg} = 75 \text{ min}$

130. $\dfrac{1 \text{ min}}{3.2 \text{ mg}} \times 412 \text{ mg} = 128.75 \text{ min}$

Round to the nearest whole number, or 129 minutes.

131. First, convert micrograms to milligrams:

$20,000 \text{ µg} \times \dfrac{1 \text{ mg}}{1,000 \text{ µg}} = 20 \text{ mg}$

Then set up the problem:

$\dfrac{1 \text{ min}}{12 \text{ mg}} \times 20 \text{ mg} = 1.67 \text{ min}$

Round to the nearest whole number, or 2 minutes.

132. $\dfrac{1 \text{ min}}{0.75 \text{ mg}} \times 160 \text{ mg} = 213.33 \text{ min}$

Round to the nearest whole number, or 213 minutes.

133. $\dfrac{1 \text{ h}}{1.5 \text{ mg}} \times 80 \text{ mg} = 53.33 \text{ h}$

Round to the nearest whole number, or 53 hours.

134. The units are already in milligrams; there is no need to convert units.

The concentration is given; there is no need to calculate it.

Set up the clock as shown in Figure AK8-1 ▾ .

According to the clock, you need to administer 30 gtt/min to give 2 mg/min. The answer is 30 gtt min.

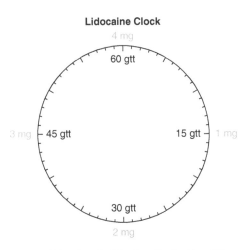

Lidocaine Clock

Figure AK8-1 Lidocaine clock for Practice Problem 134.

135. First, convert grams to milligrams:

$1 \text{ g} \times \dfrac{1,000 \text{ mg}}{\text{g}} = 1,000 \text{ mg}$

Calculate the concentration:

$\dfrac{1,000 \text{ mg}}{250 \text{ mL}} \div \dfrac{250}{250} = 4 \text{ mg/mL}$

Set up the clock as shown in Figure AK8-2 ▾ .

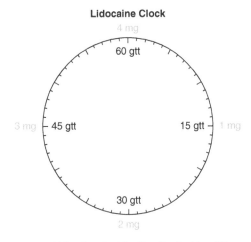

Lidocaine Clock

Figure AK8-2 Lidocaine clock for Practice Problem 135.

According to the clock, you need to administer 45 gtt/min to give 3 mg/min. The answer is 45 gtt/min.

136. Convert milligrams to micrograms:

$400 \text{ mg} \times \dfrac{1,000 \text{ µg}}{\text{mg}} = 400,000 \text{ µg}$

Calculate the concentration:

$\dfrac{400,000 \text{ µg}}{250 \text{ mL}} \div \dfrac{250}{250} = 1,600 \text{ µg/mL}$

Set up the clock as shown in Figure AK8-3 ▶ .

Factor in the patient's weight. First, convert the patient's weight to kilograms:

$145 \text{ lb} \times \dfrac{\text{kg}}{2.2 \text{ lb}} = 65.91 \text{ kg}$

Adjust the desired dose to accommodate the patient's weight:

$65.91 \text{ kg} \times \dfrac{8 \text{ µg}}{\text{kg/min}} = 527.28 \text{ µg/min}$

Round to 527 µg/min.

You need to administer 527 µg/min and can see from the clock that between 15 and 30 gtt/min are needed to give the adjusted desired dose—probably

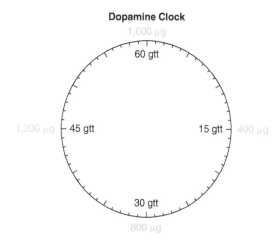

Figure AK8-3 Dopamine clock for Practice Problem 136.

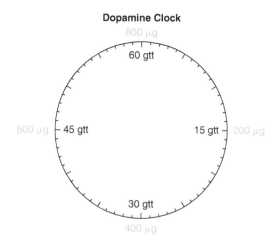

Figure AK8-4 Dopamine clock for Practice Problem 137.

almost halfway between those, or about 23 gtt/min. You can determine the exact amount with a proportion:

$$\frac{15\ \text{gtt}}{400\ \mu\text{g}} = \frac{?\ \text{gtt}}{527\ \mu\text{g}}$$

$$\frac{15\ \text{gtt} \times 527\ \mu\text{g}}{400\ \mu\text{g}} = 19.76\ \text{gtt}$$

Round to 20 gtt/min.

137. Convert milligrams to micrograms:

$$400\ \text{mg} \times \frac{1{,}000\ \mu\text{g}}{\text{mg}} = 400{,}000\ \mu\text{g}$$

Calculate the concentration:

$$\frac{400{,}000\ \mu\text{g}}{500\ \text{mL}} \div \frac{500}{500} = 800\ \mu\text{g/mL}$$

Set up the clock as shown in Figure AK8-4 ▶.

Factor in the patient's weight. First, convert the patient's weight to kilograms:

$$188\ \text{lb} \times \frac{\text{kg}}{2.2\ \text{lb}} = 85.45\ \text{kg}$$

Adjust the desired dose to accommodate the patient's weight:

$$85.45\ \text{kg} \times \frac{2\ \mu\text{g}}{\text{kg/min}} = 170.9\ \mu\text{g/min}$$

Round to 171 μg/min.

You need to administer 171 μg/min and can see from the clock that you need to administer less than 15 gtt/min, probably about 10 gtt/min. You can find out the exact amount with a proportion:

$$\frac{15\ \text{gtt}}{200\ \mu\text{g}} = \frac{?\ \text{gtt}}{171\ \mu\text{g}}$$

$$\frac{15\ \text{gtt} \times 171\ \mu\text{g}}{200\ \mu\text{g}} = 12.83\ \text{gtt}$$

Round to 13 gtt/min.

138. Convert milligrams to micrograms. Note that you have two ampules of 200 mg each, for a total of 400 mg:

$$400\ \text{mg} \times \frac{1{,}000\ \mu\text{g}}{\text{mg}} = 400{,}000\ \mu\text{g}$$

Calculate the concentration:

$$\frac{400{,}000\ \mu\text{g}}{250\ \text{mL}} \div \frac{250}{250} = 1{,}600\ \mu\text{g/mL}$$

Set up the clock as shown in Figure AK8-5 ▼.

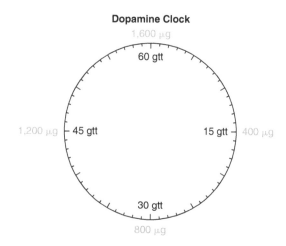

Figure AK8-5 Dopamine clock for Practice Problem 138.

Factor in the patient's weight. First, convert the patient's weight to kilograms:

$$200\ \text{lb}\ \times \frac{\text{kg}}{2.2\ \text{lb}}\ = 90.91\ \text{kg}$$

Adjust the desired dose to accommodate the patient's weight:

$$90.91\ \text{kg}\ \times \frac{5\ \mu\text{g}}{\text{kg/min}}\ = 454.55\ \mu\text{g/min}$$

Round to 455 µg/min.

You need to administer 455 µg/min and can see from the clock that you need to administer a little more than 15 gtt/min. You can find out the exact amount with a proportion:

$$\frac{15\ \text{gtt}}{400\ \mu\text{g}}\ = \frac{?\ \text{gtt}}{455\ \mu\text{g}}$$

$$\frac{15\ \text{gtt}\ \times 455\ \mu\text{g}}{400\ \mu\text{g}}\ = 17.06\ \text{gtt}$$

Round to 17 gtt/min.

139. First, convert hours to minutes:

$$5\ \text{h}\ \times \frac{60\ \text{min}}{\text{h}}\ = 300\ \text{min}$$

Then set up the problem:

$$\frac{750\ \text{mL}}{300\ \text{min}}\ \times \frac{60\ \text{gtt}}{\text{mL}}\ = 150\ \text{gtt/min}$$

140. First, convert hours to minutes:

$$25\ \text{h}\ \times \frac{60\ \text{min}}{\text{h}}\ = 1{,}500\ \text{min}$$

Then set up the problem:

$$\frac{1{,}800\ \text{mL}}{1{,}500\ \text{min}}\ \times \frac{60\ \text{gtt}}{\text{mL}}\ = 72\ \text{gtt/min}$$

141. First, convert hours to minutes:

$$3.5\ \text{h}\ \times \frac{60\ \text{min}}{\text{h}}\ = 210\ \text{min}$$

Then set up the problem:

$$\frac{100\ \text{mL}}{210\ \text{min}}\ \times \frac{60\ \text{gtt}}{\text{mL}}\ = 28.57\ \text{gtt/min}$$

Round to the nearest whole number, or 29 gtt/min.

142. First, convert hours to minutes:

$$3.5\ \text{h}\ \times \frac{60\ \text{min}}{\text{h}}\ = 210\ \text{min}$$

Then set up the problem:

$$\frac{1{,}200\ \text{mL}}{210\ \text{min}}\ \times \frac{60\ \text{gtt}}{\text{mL}}\ = 342.86\ \text{gtt/min}$$

Round to the nearest whole number, or 343 gtt/min.

143. First, convert hours to minutes:

$$4.2\ \text{h}\ \times \frac{60\ \text{min}}{\text{h}}\ = 252\ \text{min}$$

Then set up the problem:

$$\frac{500\ \text{mL}}{252\ \text{min}}\ \times \frac{60\ \text{gtt}}{\text{mL}}\ = 119.05\ \text{gtt/min}$$

Round to the nearest whole number, or 119 gtt/min.

144. $\dfrac{200\ \text{mL}}{30\ \text{min}}\ \times \dfrac{10\ \text{gtt}}{\text{mL}}\ = 66.67\ \text{gtt/min}$

Round to the nearest whole number, or 67 gtt/min.

145. $\dfrac{100\ \text{mL}}{15\ \text{min}}\ \times \dfrac{10\ \text{gtt}}{\text{mL}}\ = 66.67\ \text{gtt/min}$

Round to the nearest whole number, or 67 gtt/min.

Note that the patient's weight does not factor in because the desired dose does not include weight.

Also note that the 500-mL bag does not factor into the calculation. The fact that you have a 500-mL bag only tells you that you have enough medication and will not need a second bag.

146. $\dfrac{400\ \text{mL}}{75\ \text{min}}\ \times \dfrac{10\ \text{gtt}}{\text{mL}}\ = 53.33\ \text{gtt/min}$

Round to the nearest whole number, or 53 gtt/min.

147. Convert hours to minutes:

$$10\ \text{h}\ \times \frac{60\ \text{min}}{1\ \text{h}}\ = 600\ \text{min}$$

Set up the proportion and solve:

$$\frac{1{,}000\ \text{mL}}{600\ \text{min}}\ \times \frac{10\ \text{gtt}}{\text{mL}}\ = 16.67\ \text{gtt/min}$$

Round to the nearest whole number, or 17 gtt/min.

148. Convert hours to minutes:

$$3.3\ \text{h}\ \times \frac{60\ \text{min}}{1\ \text{h}}\ = 198\ \text{min}$$

Set up the proportion and solve:

$$\frac{500\ \text{mL}}{198\ \text{min}}\ \times \frac{10\ \text{gtt}}{\text{mL}}\ = 25.25\ \text{gtt/min}$$

Round to the nearest whole number, or 25 gtt/min.

149. Convert hours to minutes:

$$4.6\,\text{h} \times \frac{60\,\text{min}}{1\,\text{h}} = 276\,\text{min}$$

Set up the proportion and solve:

$$\frac{1{,}250\,\text{mL}}{276\,\text{min}} \times \frac{10\,\text{gtt}}{\text{mL}} = 45.29\,\text{gtt/min}$$

Round to the nearest whole number, or 45 gtt/min.

Chapter 7: Weight-Based Calculations

150. Convert pounds to kilograms:

$$\frac{228\,\text{lb}}{2.2} = 103.64\,\text{kg}$$

Calculate the dose to account for the weight:

$$\frac{1.0\,\text{mg}}{\text{kg}} \times 103.64\,\text{kg} = 103.64\,\text{mg}$$

Set up a proportion:

$$\frac{10\,\text{mL}}{100\,\text{mg}} = \frac{?\,\text{mL}}{103.64\,\text{mg}}$$

$$\frac{10\,\text{mL} \times 103.64\,\text{mg}}{100\,\text{mg}} = 10.36\,\text{mL}$$

Because the prefilled syringe contains 10 mL, you will need to administer all of that, plus 0.36 mL from a second syringe (10.36 mL – 10 mL = 0.36 mL).

151. Convert pounds to kilograms:

$$\frac{153\,\text{lb}}{2.2} = 69.55\,\text{kg}$$

Calculate the dose to account for the weight:

$$\frac{0.25\,\text{mg}}{\text{kg}} \times 69.55\,\text{kg} = 17.39\,\text{mg}$$

Set up a proportion:

$$\frac{10\,\text{mL}}{20\,\text{mg}} = \frac{?\,\text{mL}}{17.39\,\text{mg}}$$

$$\frac{10\,\text{mL} \times 17.39\,\text{mg}}{20\,\text{mg}} = 8.70\,\text{mL}$$

152. Convert pounds to kilograms:

$$\frac{200\,\text{lb}}{2.2} = 90.91\,\text{kg}$$

Calculate the dose to account for the weight:

$$\frac{0.3\,\text{mg}}{\text{kg}} \times 90.91\,\text{kg} = 27.27\,\text{mg}$$

Set up a proportion:

$$\frac{5\,\text{mL}}{50\,\text{mg}} = \frac{?\,\text{mL}}{27.27\,\text{mg}}$$

$$\frac{5\,\text{mL} \times 27.27\,\text{mg}}{50\,\text{mg}} = 2.73\,\text{mL}$$

153. Convert pounds to kilograms:

$$\frac{160\,\text{lb}}{2.2} = 72.73\,\text{kg}$$

Calculate the dose to account for the weight:

$$\frac{0.8\,\text{mg}}{\text{kg}} \times 72.73\,\text{kg} = 58.18\,\text{mg}$$

Set up a proportion:

$$\frac{2\,\text{mL}}{100\,\text{mg}} = \frac{?\,\text{mL}}{58.18\,\text{mg}}$$

$$\frac{2\,\text{mL} \times 58.18\,\text{mg}}{100\,\text{mg}} = 1.16\,\text{mL}$$

154. DD: 15 µg/kg/min

DOH: 800 mg in a 500-mL bag of D_5W

Administration set: 60 gtt/mL

Patient weight: 159 lb

Convert pounds to kilograms:

$$\frac{159\,\text{lb}}{2.2} = 72.27\,\text{kg}$$

Adjust the DD to account for the patient's weight:

$$\frac{15\,\mu\text{g}}{\text{kg/min}} = \frac{?\,\mu\text{g}}{72.27\,\text{kg}}$$

$$\frac{15\,\mu\text{g}}{\text{kg/min}} \times 72.27\,\text{kg} = 1{,}084.05\,\mu\text{g/min}$$

Convert and simplify the DOH:

$$800\,\text{mg} \times \frac{1{,}000\,\mu\text{g}}{\text{mg}} = 800{,}000\,\mu\text{g}$$

$$\frac{800{,}000\,\mu\text{g}}{500\,\text{mL}} = \frac{?\,\mu\text{g}}{1\,\text{mL}}$$

$$\frac{800{,}000\,\mu\text{g}}{500\,\text{mL}} \times 1\,\text{mL} = 1{,}600\,\mu\text{g in 1 mL of fluid}$$

Plug into the formula:

$$\frac{1{,}084.05\,\mu\text{g/min}}{1{,}600\,\mu\text{g/mL}} \times \frac{60\,\text{gtt}}{\text{mL}} = ?\,\text{gtt/min}$$

$$\frac{1{,}084.05\,\mu\text{g}}{\text{min}} \times \frac{\text{mL}}{1{,}600\,\mu\text{g}} \times \frac{60\,\text{gtt}}{\text{mL}} = 40.65\,\text{gtt/min}$$

Round to the nearest whole number, or 41 gtt/min.

155. DD: 20 μg/kg/min

DOH: 400 mg in a 5-mL prefilled syringe and a 250-mL bag of D$_5$W

Administration set: 60 gtt/mL

Patient weight: 176 lb

Convert pounds to kilograms:

$$\frac{176\ \text{lb}}{2.2} = 80\ \text{kg}$$

Adjust the DD to account for the patient's weight:

$$\frac{20\ \mu g}{kg/min} = \frac{?\ \mu g}{80\ \text{kg}}$$

$$\frac{20\ \mu g}{kg/min} \times 80\ \text{kg} = 1{,}600\ \mu g/min$$

Convert and simplify the DOH:

$$400\ \text{mg} \times \frac{1{,}000\ \mu g}{mg} = 400{,}000\ \mu g$$

$$\frac{400{,}000\ \mu g}{250\ \text{mL}} = \frac{?\ \mu g}{1\ \text{mL}}$$

$$\frac{400{,}000\ \mu g}{250\ \text{mL}} \times 1\ \text{mL} = 1{,}600\ \mu g\ \text{in}\ 1\ \text{mL of fluid}$$

Plug into the formula:

$$\frac{1{,}600\ \mu g/min}{1{,}600\ \mu g/mL} \times \frac{60\ \text{gtt}}{mL} = ?\ gtt/min$$

$$\frac{1{,}600\ \mu g}{min} \times \frac{mL}{1{,}600\ \mu g} \times \frac{60\ \text{gtt}}{mL} = 60\ gtt/min$$

156. DD: 14 μg/kg/min

DOH: 800 mg in a 5-mL prefilled syringe, and a 500-mL bag of D$_5$W

Administration set: 60 gtt/mL

Patient weight: 213 lb

Convert pounds to kilograms:

$$\frac{213\ \text{lb}}{2.2} = 96.82\ \text{kg}$$

Adjust the DD to account for the patient's weight:

$$\frac{14\ \mu g}{kg/min} = \frac{?\ \mu g}{96.82\ \text{kg}}$$

$$\frac{14\ \mu g}{kg/min} \times 96.82\ \text{kg} = 1{,}355.48\ \mu g/min$$

Convert and simplify the DOH:

$$800\ \text{mg} \times \frac{1{,}000\ \mu g}{mg} = 800{,}000\ \mu g$$

$$\frac{800{,}000\ \mu g}{500\ \text{mL}} = \frac{?\ \mu g}{1\ \text{mL}}$$

$$\frac{800{,}000\ \mu g}{500\ \text{mL}} \times 1\ \text{mL} = 1{,}600\ \mu g\ \text{in}\ 1\ \text{mL of fluid}$$

Plug into the formula:

$$\frac{1{,}355.48\ \mu g/min}{1{,}600\ \mu g/mL} \times \frac{60\ \text{gtt}}{mL} = ?\ gtt/min$$

$$\frac{1{,}355.48\ \mu g}{min} \times \frac{mL}{1{,}600\ \mu g} \times \frac{60\ \text{gtt}}{mL} = 50.83\ gtt/min$$

Round to the nearest whole number, or 51 gtt/min.

157. For problems 157–162, all of the DDs are given in μg/kg/min; the concentration will be calculated only once and reused each time.

$$800\ \text{mg} \times \frac{1{,}000\ \mu g}{mg} = 800{,}000\ \mu g$$

$$\frac{800{,}000\ \mu g}{500\ \text{mL}} = \frac{?\ \mu g}{1\ \text{mL}}$$

$$\frac{800{,}000\ \mu g}{500\ \text{mL}} \times 1\ \text{mL} = 1{,}600\ \mu g\ \text{in}\ 1\ \text{mL of fluid}$$

The concentration for this set of problems is 1,600 μg/mL. By now you probably know that this is usually the concentration for dopamine.

Convert pounds to kilograms:

$$\frac{194\ \text{lb}}{2.2} = 88.18\ \text{kg}$$

Adjust the DD to account for the patient's weight:

$$\frac{15\ \mu g}{kg/min} = \frac{?\ \mu g}{88.18\ \text{kg}}$$

$$\frac{15\ \mu g}{kg/min} \times 88.18\ \text{kg} = 1{,}322.7\ \mu g/min$$

Plug into the formula:

$$\frac{1{,}322.7\ \mu g/min}{1{,}600\ \mu g/mL} \times \frac{60\ \text{gtt}}{mL} = ?\ gtt/min$$

$$\frac{1{,}322.7\ \mu g}{min} \times \frac{mL}{1{,}600\ \mu g} \times \frac{60\ \text{gtt}}{mL} = 49.60\ gtt/min$$

Round to the nearest whole number, or 50 gtt/min.

158. Convert pounds to kilograms:

$$\frac{229\ \text{lb}}{2.2} = 104.09\ \text{kg}$$

Adjust the DD to account for the patient's weight:

$$\frac{16\ \mu g}{kg/min} = \frac{?\ \mu g}{104.09\ \text{kg}}$$

$$\frac{16\ \mu g}{kg/min} \times 104.09\ kg\ =\ 1{,}665.44\ \mu g/min$$

Plug into the formula:

$$\frac{1{,}665.44\ \mu g/min}{1{,}600\ \mu g/mL} \times \frac{60\ gtt}{mL}\ =\ ?\ gtt/min$$

$$\frac{1{,}665.44\ \mu g}{min} \times \frac{mL}{1{,}600\ \mu g} \times \frac{60\ gtt}{mL}\ =\ 62.45\ gtt/min$$

Round to the nearest whole number, or 62 gtt/min.

159. Convert pounds to kilograms:

$$\frac{143\ lb}{2.2}\ =\ 65\ kg$$

Adjust the DD to account for the patient's weight:

$$\frac{19\ \mu g}{kg/min}\ =\ \frac{?\ \mu g}{65\ kg}$$

$$\frac{19\ \mu g}{kg/min} \times 65\ kg\ =\ 1{,}235\ \mu g/min$$

Plug into the formula:

$$\frac{1{,}235\ \mu g/min}{1{,}600\ \mu g/mL} \times \frac{60\ gtt}{mL}\ =\ ?\ gtt/min$$

$$\frac{1{,}235\ \mu g}{min} \times \frac{mL}{1{,}600\ \mu g} \times \frac{60\ gtt}{mL}\ =\ 46.31\ gtt/min$$

Round to the nearest whole number, or 46 gtt/min.

160. The weight is already in kilograms.

Adjust the DD to account for the patient's weight:

$$\frac{8\ \mu g}{kg/min}\ =\ \frac{?\ \mu g}{79\ kg}$$

$$\frac{8\ \mu g}{kg/min} \times 79\ kg\ =\ 632\ \mu g/min$$

Plug into the formula:

$$\frac{632\ \mu g/min}{1{,}600\ \mu g/mL} \times \frac{60\ gtt}{mL}\ =\ ?\ gtt/min$$

$$\frac{632\ \mu g}{min} \times \frac{mL}{1{,}600\ \mu g} \times \frac{60\ gtt}{mL}\ =\ 23.7\ gtt/min$$

Round to the nearest whole number, or 24 gtt/min.

161. The weight is already in kilograms.

Adjust the DD to account for the patient's weight:

$$\frac{4\ \mu g}{kg/min}\ =\ \frac{?\ \mu g}{24\ kg}$$

$$\frac{4\ \mu g}{kg/min} \times 24\ kg\ =\ 96\ \mu g/min$$

Plug into the formula:

$$\frac{96\ \mu g/min}{1{,}600\ \mu g/mL} \times \frac{60\ gtt}{mL}\ =\ ?\ gtt/min$$

$$\frac{96\ \mu g}{min} \times \frac{mL}{1{,}600\ \mu g} \times \frac{60\ gtt}{mL}\ =\ 3.6\ gtt/min$$

Round to the nearest whole number, or 4 gtt/min.

162. The weight is already in kilograms.

Adjust the DD to account for the patient's weight:

$$\frac{11\ \mu g}{kg/min}\ =\ \frac{?\ \mu g}{55\ kg}$$

$$\frac{11\ \mu g}{kg/min} \times 55\ kg\ =\ 605\ \mu g/min$$

Plug into the formula:

$$\frac{605\ \mu g/min}{1{,}600\ \mu g/mL} \times \frac{60\ gtt}{mL}\ =\ ?\ gtt/min$$

$$\frac{605\ \mu g}{min} \times \frac{mL}{1{,}600\ \mu g} \times \frac{60\ gtt}{mL}\ =\ 22.69\ gtt/min$$

Round to the nearest whole number, or 23 gtt/min.

163. Convert pounds to kilograms:

$$\frac{54\ lb}{2.2}\ =\ 24.55\ kg$$

Calculate the dose to account for the weight:

$$\frac{0.1\ mg}{kg} \times 24.55\ kg\ =\ 2.46\ mg$$

Set up a proportion:

$$\frac{1\ mL}{6\ mg}\ =\ \frac{?\ mL}{2.46\ mg}$$

$$\frac{1\ mL \times 2.46\ mg}{6\ mg}\ =\ 0.41\ mL$$

Round to the nearest tenth, or 0.4 mL.

164. Convert pounds to kilograms:

$$\frac{45\ lb}{2.2}\ =\ 20.45\ kg$$

Calculate the dose to account for the weight:

$$\frac{0.5\ mg}{kg} \times 20.45\ kg\ =\ 10.23\ mg$$

Set up a proportion:

$$\frac{5\ mL}{20\ mg}\ =\ \frac{?\ mL}{10.23\ mg}$$

$$\frac{5\ mL \times 10.23\ mg}{20\ mg}\ =\ 2.56\ mL$$

Round to the nearest tenth, or 2.6 mL.

165. Convert pounds to kilograms:

$$\frac{65 \text{ lb}}{2.2} = 29.55 \text{ kg}$$

Calculate the dose to account for the weight:

$$\frac{1 \text{ mg}}{\text{kg}} \times 29.55 \text{ kg} = 29.55 \text{ mg}$$

Set up a proportion:

$$\frac{1 \text{ mL}}{50 \text{ mg}} = \frac{? \text{ mL}}{29.55 \text{ mg}}$$

$$\frac{1 \text{ mL} \times 29.55 \text{ mg}}{50 \text{ mg}} = 0.59 \text{ mL}$$

Round to the nearest tenth, or 0.6 mL.

166. Convert pounds to kilograms:

$$\frac{60 \text{ lb}}{2.2} = 27.27 \text{ kg}$$

Calculate the dose to account for the weight:

$$\frac{0.1 \text{ mg}}{\text{kg}} \times 27.27 \text{ kg} = 2.73 \text{ mg}$$

Set up a proportion:

$$\frac{1 \text{ mL}}{10 \text{ mg}} = \frac{? \text{ mL}}{2.73 \text{ mg}}$$

$$\frac{1 \text{ mL} \times 2.73 \text{ mg}}{10 \text{ mg}} = 0.27 \text{ mL}$$

Round to the nearest tenth, or 0.3 mL.

167. Convert pounds to kilograms:

$$\frac{54 \text{ lb}}{2.2} = 24.55 \text{ kg}$$

Calculate the dose to account for the weight:

$$\frac{0.03 \text{ mg}}{\text{kg}} \times 24.55 \text{ kg} = 0.74 \text{ mg}$$

Set up a proportion:

$$\frac{1 \text{ mL}}{1 \text{ mg}} = \frac{? \text{ mL}}{0.74 \text{ mg}}$$

$$\frac{1 \text{ mL} \times 0.74 \text{ mg}}{1 \text{ mg}} = 0.74 \text{ mL}$$

Round to the nearest tenth, or 0.7 mL.

168. DD: 2 µg/kg/min

DOH: 400 mg in a 250-mL bag of D_5W

Administration set: 60 gtt/mL

Patient weight: 140 lb

Convert pounds to kilograms:

$$\frac{140 \text{ lb}}{2.2} = 63.64 \text{ kg}$$

Adjust the DD to account for the patient's weight:

$$\frac{2 \text{ µg}}{\text{kg/min}} = \frac{? \text{ µg}}{63.64 \text{ kg}}$$

$$\frac{2 \text{ µg}}{\text{kg/min}} \times 63.64 \text{ kg} = 127.28 \text{ µg/min}$$

Convert and simplify the DOH:

$$400 \text{ mg} \times \frac{1,000 \text{ µg}}{\text{mg}} = 400,000 \text{ µg}$$

$$\frac{400,000 \text{ µg}}{250 \text{ mL}} = \frac{? \text{ µg}}{1 \text{ mL}}$$

$$\frac{400,000 \text{ µg}}{250 \text{ mL}} \times 1 \text{ mL} = 1,600 \text{ µg in 1 mL of fluid}$$

Plug into the formula:

$$\frac{127.28 \text{ µg/min}}{1,600 \text{ µg/mL}} \times \frac{60 \text{ gtt}}{\text{mL}} = ? \text{ gtt/min}$$

$$\frac{127.28 \text{ µg}}{\text{min}} \times \frac{\text{mL}}{1,600 \text{ µg}} \times \frac{60 \text{ gtt}}{\text{mL}} = 4.77 \text{ gtt/min}$$

Round to the nearest whole number, or 5 gtt/min.

169. DD: 5 µg/kg/min

DOH: 800 mg in a 500-mL bag of D_5W

Administration set: 60 gtt/mL

Patient weight: 100 lb

Convert pounds to kilograms:

$$\frac{100 \text{ lb}}{2.2} = 45.45 \text{ kg}$$

Adjust the DD to account for the patient's weight:

$$\frac{5 \text{ µg}}{\text{kg/min}} = \frac{? \text{ µg}}{45.45 \text{ kg}}$$

$$\frac{5 \text{ µg}}{\text{kg/min}} \times 45.45 \text{ kg} = 227.25 \text{ µg/min}$$

Convert and simplify the DOH:

$$800 \text{ mg} \times \frac{1,000 \text{ µg}}{\text{mg}} = 800,000 \text{ µg}$$

$$\frac{800,000 \text{ µg}}{500 \text{ mL}} = \frac{? \text{ µg}}{1 \text{ mL}}$$

$$\frac{800,000 \text{ µg}}{500 \text{ mL}} \times 1 \text{ mL} = 1,600 \text{ µg in 1 mL of fluid}$$

Plug into the formula:

$$\frac{227.25\ \mu g/min}{1,600\ \mu g/mL} \times \frac{60\ gtt}{mL} = ?\ gtt/min$$

$$\frac{227.25\ \mu g}{min} \times \frac{mL}{1,600\ \mu g} \times \frac{60\ gtt}{mL} = 8.52\ gtt/min$$

Round to the nearest whole number, or 9 gtt/min.

170. DD: 6 μg/kg/min

DOH: 400 mg in a 250-mL bag of D_5W

Administration set: 60 gtt/mL

Patient weight: 60 lb

Convert pounds to kilograms:

$$\frac{60\ lb}{2.2} = 27.27\ kg$$

Adjust the DD to account for the patient's weight:

$$\frac{6\ \mu g}{kg/min} = \frac{?\ \mu g}{27.27\ kg}$$

$$\frac{6\ \mu g}{kg/min} \times 27.27\ kg = 163.62\ \mu g/min$$

Convert and simplify the DOH:

$$400\ mg \times \frac{1,000\ \mu g}{mg} = 400,000\ \mu g$$

$$\frac{400,000\ \mu g}{250\ mL} = \frac{?\ \mu g}{1\ mL}$$

$$\frac{400,000\ \mu g}{250\ mL} \times 1\ mL = 1,600\ \mu g\ in\ 1\ mL\ of\ fluid$$

Plug into the formula:

$$\frac{163.62\ \mu g/min}{1,600\ \mu g/mL} \times \frac{60\ gtt}{mL} = ?\ gtt/min$$

$$\frac{163.62\ \mu g}{min} \times \frac{mL}{1,600\ \mu g} \times \frac{60\ gtt}{mL} = 6.14\ gtt/min$$

Round to the nearest whole number, or 6 gtt/min.

171. DD: 10 μg/kg/min

DOH: 400 mg in a 250-mL bag of D_5W

Administration set: 60 gtt/mL

Patient weight: 124 lb

Convert pounds to kilograms:

$$\frac{124\ lb}{2.2} = 56.36\ kg$$

Adjust the DD to account for the patient's weight:

$$\frac{10\ \mu g}{kg/min} = \frac{?\ \mu g}{56.36\ kg}$$

$$\frac{10\ \mu g}{kg/min} \times 56.36\ kg = 563.6\ \mu g/min$$

Convert and simplify the DOH:

$$400\ mg \times \frac{1,000\ \mu g}{mg} = 400,000\ \mu g$$

$$\frac{400,000\ \mu g}{250\ mL} = \frac{?\ \mu g}{1\ mL}$$

$$\frac{400,000\ \mu g}{250\ mL} \times 1\ mL = 1,600\ \mu g\ in\ 1\ mL\ of\ fluid$$

Plug into the formula:

$$\frac{563.6\ \mu g/min}{1,600\ \mu g/mL} \times \frac{60\ gtt}{mL} = ?\ gtt/min$$

$$\frac{563.6\ \mu g}{min} \times \frac{mL}{1,600\ \mu g} \times \frac{60\ gtt}{mL} = 21.14\ gtt/min$$

Round to the nearest whole number, or 21 gtt/min.

172. DD: 12 μg/kg/min

DOH: 400 mg in a 250-mL bag of D_5W

Administration set: 60 gtt/mL

Patient weight: 33 lb

Convert pounds to kilograms:

$$\frac{33\ lb}{2.2} = 15\ kg$$

Adjust the DD to account for the patient's weight:

$$\frac{12\ \mu g}{kg/min} = \frac{?\ \mu g}{15\ kg}$$

$$\frac{12\ \mu g}{kg/min} \times 15\ kg = 180\ \mu g/min$$

Convert and simplify the DOH:

$$400\ mg \times \frac{1,000\ \mu g}{mg} = 400,000\ \mu g$$

$$\frac{400,000\ \mu g}{250\ mL} = \frac{?\ \mu g}{1\ mL}$$

$$\frac{400,000\ \mu g}{250\ mL} \times 1\ mL = 1,600\ \mu g\ in\ 1\ mL\ of\ fluid$$

Plug into the formula:

$$\frac{180\ \mu g/min}{1,600\ \mu g/mL} \times \frac{60\ gtt}{mL} = ?\ gtt/min$$

$$\frac{180\ \mu g}{min} \times \frac{mL}{1,600\ \mu g} \times \frac{60\ gtt}{mL} = 6.75\ gtt/min$$

Round to the nearest whole number, or 7 gtt/min.

administration set The drip chamber and tubing used to move fluid from an IV bag into a patient's vascular system.

ampule A thin-necked, cone-shaped glass vessel; a common way of packaging medications.

apothecary system The oldest system used by pharmacists and chemists, which has been replaced by the metric system in most situations.

clock method A method for calculating drip rates that uses a clock divided into quarters representing the number of drops provided by the administration set and the maximum concentration of the medication to be administered.

colloid solution A solution that contains many high-protein elements used to expand the blood volume because it increases the osmotic pressure within the circulatory system.

common denominator A denominator (bottom part of a fraction) that is the same number in several fractions. For example, $\frac{3}{10}$, $\frac{4}{10}$, and $\frac{5}{10}$ have the common denominator of 10.

concentration A medication's weight per volume.

continuous infusion An infusion that is given for a relatively long period, such as hours or days, at a consistent rate (as opposed to an intermittent infusion); usually used to replace electrolytes or improve fluid balance.

conversion factors The numbers that represent the relationship between two numbers and that can be multiplied or divided to convert from one unit of measure to another.

cross multiply and divide method A method in math in which the numerator (top number) of each side of the fraction is multiplied by the denominator (bottom part) of the opposite side of the fraction.

crystalloid solution A solution that contains electrolytes and nonelectrolytes but not high-protein elements.

decimals Numbers based on the number 10 and that contain a dot (point) between whole numbers (written to the left of the dot) and numbers that are smaller than whole numbers (written to the right of the dot). The numbers to the right of the dot constitute decimal fractions.

denominator The bottom part of a fraction, for example, the 10 in $\frac{1}{10}$.

desired dose (DD) The amount of medication ordered by protocol or a physician.

dimensional analysis A method of calculation in which fractions are set up and like units in the numerators and denominators are cancelled out, resulting in the desired units; for example, mg/min $\times$ mL/mg $\times$ gtt/mL results in gtt/min.

divisor A number that is divided into another number.

dose on hand (DOH) The medication available and how it is packaged.

drip chamber The part of an administration set in which the fluid accumulates so that the tubing remains filled with fluid.

drop factor The number of drops per milliliter, or gtt/mL, that an administration set delivers.

estimate To make an approximation of a number, rather than an actual calculation.

foundation number In multiplication, the first number being multiplied; in division, the number being divided into.

fraction A number expressed using a numerator and a denominator, for example $\frac{1}{10}$.

gtt The unit of measure listed on an administration set, which is short for guttae, meaning drops; when written with milliliters on an administration set, represents the number of drops the set delivers per milliliter.

household system A system of measurement commonly used to measure medications at home, such as teaspoons, fluid ounces, and tablespoons.

improper fraction A fraction in which the numerator is larger than the denominator.

intermittent infusion An infusion that is given for a relatively short period, such as minutes or hours; commonly used to administer low-volume boluses, for example, a small dose repeated every 3 to 5 minutes, such as diazepam to treat a seizure or morphine for pain management. See also continuous infusion and saline lock.

intramuscular A medication route in which medication is administered into muscle (IM).

intravenous A medication route in which medication is administered through a vein (IV).

IV push An IV injection given directly into a vein, through a port in IV tubing, or through an infusion device such as a saline lock; used when a dose is needed quickly.

macrodrip set   A type of administration set that allows 10 to 20 gtt/mL through a large opening between the piercing spike and the drip chamber.

metric system   The system of measurement recognized as the international standard for measurement, which is based on units of 10 and uses decimals.

microdrip set   A type of administration set that allows 60 gtt/mL through the orifice inside the drip chamber.

mixed number   A number written as a whole number and a fraction.

multiple   A number that can be divided by the original number(s) without a remainder. For example; 5, 10, 15, 20, 25, 30, are multiples of 5, and 24 is a multiple of 6 and 4.

multiplier   In multiplication, the second number being multiplied.

numerator   The top part of a fraction, for example, the 1 in $\frac{1}{10}$.

order of operations   The rule in math that indicates that calculations in parentheses must be done first, multiplication and division second, and addition and subtraction last.

parenteral   An alternative way to provide medication to patients without going through the gastrointestinal tract.

percentage   A portion of 100, noted with the "%" sign.

percentage solution   A solution that contains a medication and that is named using a percentage representing the amount of medication in 100 g or 100 mL of solution.

proper fraction   A fraction in which the numerator is smaller than the denominator.

proportion   Two ratios that equal each other in value and are written with an equal sign separating the two ratios.

rate   The number of drops per minute to which the administration set must be set to accomplish the dose ordered.

ratio   An expression in math that states a relationship between two numbers, written as two numbers separated by a colon (1:2).

reduce   To simplify a fraction, accomplished by dividing the same number into the numerator and the denominator.

round   To express a number as a convenient whole number. A rounded number can be used in a mathematical calculation when estimating.

rule of fours   A method for determining the flow rate when the desired dose is rate-based; gtt/mL and concentration are written on a "clock" divided into quarters and compared to facilitate determining how much medication is contained in a certain number of drops.

saline lock   A device used to aid in the process of administering medication quickly into the body; often used to provide an intermittent infusion and to give chemotherapy drugs for cancer treatment.

solute   A component dissolved in a solution, usually expressed as grams, milligrams, or micrograms.

solution   A mixture consisting of a solute and a solvent.

solvent   The liquid component of a solution to which a medication is added, usually expressed as milliliters.

subcutaneous   A medication route in which medication is administered under the skin (SC).

syringe   A device used to inject fluid into or withdraw fluid from the body by way of the vein through an IV catheter. Syringes are also used to administer intramuscular and subcutaneous medications.

total time   The total amount of time during which a medication is to be infused; EMS infusions are usually in minutes.

total volume   The amount of fluid in consideration; includes the amount of fluid in an IV bag and the amount of fluid in a vial of medication that is being added to the bag.

trick of 5s   A method used to make it easier to multiply by 5, in which a number is multiplied by 10 and the answer is then cut in half.

unit of measure   The type of measurement used to note a quantity (volume, weight, length, area, and so forth); units can be in the metric system (for example, mg, g, mL), the British imperial system (for example, pint, quart), or other systems.

volume/volume percentage   A way of naming a solution that states the volume of medication per 100 mL of solution; abbreviated vol/vol.

weight/volume percentage   A way of naming a solution that states the weight of medication per 100 mL of solution; abbreviated wt/vol.

weight/weight percentage   A way of naming a solution that states the weight of medication per 100 g of solution; abbreviated wt/wt.

weight-based calculation   A medication calculation that takes the patient's weight into consideration; for example, if a dose is ordered per kilogram, the dose must be adjusted to correspond to the patient's weight in kilograms.

Index

Note: The letter *f* following a page number denotes a figure. The letter *t* following a page number denotes a table.

Photo Credits

4–1A, 4–1B, 4–2 Courtesy and © Becton, Dickinson and Company; 4–3 © aaaah/ShutterStock, Inc.

Unless otherwise indicated, all photographs and illustrations are under copyright of Jones and Bartlett Publishers.